APPLETON & LANGE'S REVIEW FOR

NATIONAL BOARDS PART I

SECOND EDITION

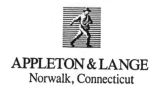

APPLETON & LANGE
Norwalk, Connecticut

0-8385-0119-2

92 93 94 / 10 9 8 7 6 5

Prentice Hall International (UK) Limited, *London*
Prentice Hall of Australia Pty. Limited, *Sydney*
Prentice Hall Canada, Inc., *Toronto*
Prentice Hall Hispanoamericana, S.A., *Mexico*
Prentice Hall India Private Limited, *New Delhi*
Prentice Hall of Japan, Inc., *Tokyo*
Simon & Schuster Asia Pte. Ltd., *Singapore*
Editora Prentice Hall do Brasil Ltda., *Rio de Janeiro*
Prentice Hall, *Englewood Cliffs, New Jersey*

Library of Congress Cataloging-in-Publication Data

Appleton & Lange's review for national boards part I / [edited by]
   Michael Caplan. — 2nd ed.
      p.   cm.
   Rev. ed. of: Appleton's review for national boards part I. c1985.
   Includes bibliographies.
   ISBN 0-8385-0119-2
   1. Medical sciences—Examinations, questions, etc. 2. Medicine—
Examinations, questions, etc. I. Caplan, Michael. II. Appleton's
review for national boards part I. III. Title: Appleton and Lange's
review for national boards part I.
   [DNLM: 1. Medicine—examination questions. W 18 A6494]
R834.5.A664   1989
610′.76—dc20
DNLM/DLC   89-14986
for Library of Congress   CIP

Acquisitions Editor: Jamie Mount Sokol
Production Editor: Charles F. Evans

PRINTED IN THE UNITED STATES OF AMERICA

Table of Contents

Editorial Board

Contributors

Francis J. Chlapowski, PhD
Associate Professor Biochemistry
University of Massachusetts Medical School
Worcester, Massachusetts

Judith Hopfer Deglin, Pharm. D.
Lecturer in Clinical Pharmacy
School of Pharmacy
University of Connecticut
Storrs, Connecticut

Liberato J.A. DiDio, MD, DSc, PhD
Dean of the Graduate School
Chairman and Professor
Department of Anatomy
Medical College of Ohio
Toledo, Ohio

Michael N. Dudley, Pharm. D.
Assistant Professor of Pharmacy
College of Pharmacy
University of Rhode Island
Kingston, Rhode Island

Richard M. Hyde, PhD
Professor
Department of Microbiology and Immunology
College of Medicine
University of Oklahoma
Health Sciences Center
Oklahoma City, Oklahoma

Leonard Kaczmarek, PhD
Assistant Professor of Pharmacology and Physiology
Yale University School of Medicine
New Haven, Connecticut

Melvin Lewis, MB, BS (London), FRCPsych, DCH
Professor of Pediatrics and Psychiatry
Yale University School of Medicine
New Haven, Connecticut

Karen I. Plaisance, Pharm. D.
Assistant Clinical Professor
School of Pharmacy
University of Connecticut
Storrs, Connecticut

David R. Platt, Pharm. D.
Assistant Clinical Professor
School of Pharmacy
University of Connecticut
Storrs, Connecticut

Paul A. Raslavicus, MD
Associate Clinical Professor of Pathology
Tufts University School of Medicine
Boston, Massachusetts

Richard S. Schottenfeld, MD
Assistant Professor of Psychiatry
Yale University School of Medicine
New Haven, Connecticut

Kathleen A. Trotta, MD
Instructor in Pathology
Tufts University School of Medicine
Boston, Massachusetts

Debra Yavner, MD
Instructor in Pathology
Tufts University School of Medicine
Boston, Massachusetts

Richard A. Yeasting, PhD
Associate Professor of Anatomy
Associate Dean for Curriculum
Medical College of Ohio
Toledo, Ohio

Preface

Although there are other review books for the National Medical Boards, *Appleton & Lange's Review for National Boards Part I* has had continued success for several reasons. No other text offers a comprehensive review with cogent explanations and current references coupled with the self-assessment tool of a practice test. Here the reader can assess strengths and weaknesses as well as review cognitive knowledge, and diagnostic and therapeutic skills. Moreover, all of the subjects, question types, and techniques encountered on the official exam are presented in this book offering a current, viable study tool.

This volume is part of a three-book series designed exclusively for candidates for the National Boards Part I, the National Boards Part II, and FLEX. Combined, the three books consist of over 3,400 Board-type questions with detailed explanations, and 13 patient management problems (PMPs).

In order to offer the most complete and accurate review text, we organized a team of authors and editors of various specialties (involved in both academic and clinical settings) from around the country. They were engaged to both research and write questions and PMPs using the parameters set forth by the National Board of Medical Examiners and the Federation of State Medical Boards of the United States. The questions were then reviewed and edited by a specially selected team of experts in the health science question-writing field to ensure content quality and proper format.

Once the guidelines and contents were established, we set to work designing a format for the book that would offer both a style that is easily read, and a sound approach to studying. As a result, the questions are organized by subject and followed by an integrated practice test that presents the material in similar format to that encountered on the exam.

Each of the chapters follows a basic format consisting of two separate lists: the questions, and then the answers and explanations. (At the end of each explanation there is an exact page reference for further study.) The end of each chapter also contains a subspecialty list. This is extremely helpful for assessing areas of strength and weakness and can aid the student in pinpointing areas for concentration during exam preparation. For more general review purposes, we have provided a bibliography list for each of the sections listing all the current reference material applicable to the chapter.

As a result of this process, we believe that you will find the questions, their explanations, and the format of the text to be of the highest caliber and of the greatest assistance to you during your review.

The Editors and the Publisher

Introduction

If you are planning to prepare for National Medical Boards Part I, for the new Foreign Medical Graduate Examination in the Medical Sciences, or for FLEX, then *Appleton & Lange's Review for National Boards Part I* is designed for you. Here, in one package, is a comprehensive review resource with 1200 Board-type basic science multiple-choice questions with referenced, paragraph-length discussions of each answer. In addition, the last 311 questions have been set aside as a practice test for self-assessment purposes.

ORGANIZATION OF THIS BOOK

The book is organized to cover sequentially each of the seven basic science areas specified by the National Board of Medical Examiners (NBME). The seven sections are:

1. **Anatomy** (including gross and microscopic anatomy; neuroanatomy; and development and control mechanisms).
2. **Physiology** (including general and cellular functions; major body system physiology; energy balance; and fluid and electrolyte balance).
3. **Biochemistry** (including energy metabolism; major metabolic pathways of small molecules; major tissue and cellular structures, properties, and functions; biochemical aspects of cellular and molecular biology; and special biochemistry of tissues).
4. **Microbiology** (including microbial structure and composition; cellular metabolism, physiology, and regulation; microbial and molecular genetics; immunology; bacterial pathogens; virology; and medical mycology and parasitology).
5. **Pathology** (including general and systemic pathology; and pathology of syndromes and complex reactions).
6. **Pharmacology** (including general principles; major body system agents; vitamins; chemotherapeutic agents; and poisoning and therapy of intoxication).

7. **Behavioral Sciences** (including behavioral biology; individual, interpersonal, and social behavior; and culture and society).

Appleton & Lange's Review for National Boards Part I is divided into eight chapters, all of which are designed to contribute to your review. Each of the first seven chapters is devoted to one of the basic sciences that will comprise the actual exam. The eighth chapter is a 311-question practice test, which includes questions from all seven basic sciences. Each of the eight chapters is organized in the following order:

1. Questions
2. Answers and explanations
3. Bibliography
4. Subspecialty list

These sections are discussed below in terms of what they contain and how you can use them in the most effective manner.

Questions

Each of the seven basic science chapters contains 127 multiple-choice questions (or "items," in testing parlance). In general, about 50 percent of these are "one best answer–single item" questions, 30 percent are "multiple true-false items," 10 percent are "one best answer–matching sets," and 10 percent are "comparison/matching set" questions. In some cases, a group of two or three questions may be related to a situational theme. In addition, some questions have illustrative material (graphs, x-rays, tables) that require understanding and interpretation on your part. Moreover, questions may be of three levels of difficulty: (1) rote memory question, (2) memory question that requires more understanding of the problem, and (3) a question that requires understanding *and* judgment. In view of the fact that the NBME is moving toward the judgment question and away from the rote memory question, it is the judgment question that we have tried to emphasize throughout this text. Finally, some of the items are stated in the negative. In such instances, we have printed the negative word in capital letters (e.g., "All of the following are correct EXCEPT;" "Which of the following choices is NOT correct;" and "Which of the following is LEAST correct").

One best answer–single item question. This type of question presents a problem or asks a question and is followed by five choices, only **one** of which is entirely correct. The directions preceding this type of question will generally appear as below:

DIRECTIONS (Question 1): Each of the numbered items or incomplete statements in this section is followed by answers or by completions of the statement. Select the <u>ONE</u> lettered answer or completion that is <u>BEST</u> in each case.

An example for this item type follows:

1. An obese 21-yr-old woman complains of increased growth of coarse hair on her lip, chin, chest, and abdomen. She also notes menstrual irregularity with periods of amenorrhea. The most likely cause is

    (A) polycystic ovary disease
    (B) an ovarian tumor
    (C) an adrenal tumor
    (D) Cushing's disease
    (E) familial hirsutism

In this type of question, choices other than the correct answer may be partially correct, but there can only be one *best* answer. In the question above (taken from *Appleton & Lange's Review for National Boards Part II*), the key word is "most." Although ovarian tumors, adrenal tumors, and Cushing's disease are causes of hirsutism (described in the stem of the question), polycystic ovary disease is a much more common cause. Familial hirsutism is not associated with the menstrual irregularities mentioned. Thus, the *most* likely cause of the manifestations described can only be "(A)-polycystic ovary disease."

TABLE 1. STRATEGIES FOR ANSWERING ONE BEST ANSWER–SINGLE ITEM QUESTIONS*

1. Remember that only one choice can be the correct answer.
2. Read the question carefully to be sure that you understand what is being asked.
3. Quickly read each choice for familiarity. (This important step is often not done by test takers.)
4. Go back and consider each choice individually.
5. If a choice is partially correct, tentatively consider it to be incorrect. (This step will help you lessen your choices and increase your odds of choosing the correct choice/answer.)
6. Consider the remaining choices and select the one you think is the answer. At this point, you may want to quickly scan the stem to be sure you understand the question and your answer.
7. Fill in the appropriate circle on the answer sheet. (Even if you do not know the answer, you should at least guess—you are scored on the number of correct answers, so **do not leave any blanks.)**

*Note that steps 2 through 7 should take an average of 50 seconds total. The **actual** examination is timed for an average of 50 seconds per question.

One best answer–matching sets. These questions are essentially matching questions that are always accompanied by the following directions:

DIRECTIONS (Questions 2 through 4): Each group of items in this section consists of lettered headings followed by a set of numbered words or phrases. For each numbered word or phrase, select the <u>ONE</u> lettered heading that is most closely associated with it. <u>Each lettered heading may be selected once, more than once, or not at all.</u>

Any number of questions (usually two to six) may follow the headings:

Questions 2 through 4

For each adverse drug reaction listed below, select the antibiotic with which it is most closely associated.

    (A) tetracycline
    (B) chloramphenicol
    (C) clindamycin
    (D) cefotaxime
    (E) gentamicin

2. Bone marrow suppression

3. Pseudomembranous enterocolitis

4. Acute fatty necrosis of liver

Note that, unlike the single item questions, the choices in the matching sets questions *precede* the actual questions. However, as with the single item questions, only **one** choice can be correct for a given question.

TABLE 2. STRATEGIES FOR ANSWERING ONE BEST ANSWER–MATCHING SETS QUESTIONS

1. Remember that the *lettered choices* are **followed** by the *numbered questions*.
2. As with the single item questions, these questions have only **one** best answer. Therefore apply steps 2 through 7 of the single item strategies.

Comparison/matching set questions. Comparison/matching set questions are, like the one best answer–matching sets questions, essentially matching questions. They are always accompanied by the following general directions and code:

DIRECTIONS (Questions 5 and 6): Each group of items in this section consists of lettered headings followed by a set of numbered words or phrases. For each numbered word or phrase, select

A if the item is associated with (A) only,
B if the item is associated with (B) only,
C if the item is associated with both (A) and (B),
D if the item is associated with neither (A) nor (B).

Any number of questions (usually two to six) may follow the four headings:

Questions 5 and 6

(A) polymyositis
(B) polymyalgia rheumatica
(C) both
(D) neither

5. Pain is a prominent syndrome

6. Associated with internal malignancy in adults

Note that as with the other matching sets questions, the choices precede the actual questions. Once again, only **one** choice can be correct for a given question.

TABLE 3. STRATEGIES FOR ANSWERING COMPARISON/MATCHING SET QUESTIONS

1. Remember that the *lettered choices* are **followed** by the *numbered questions.*
2. As with the one best answer questions, these questions have only **one** best answer.
3. Quickly note what the lettered choices are.
4. Carefully read the question to be sure you understand what is being asked or what its relationship to the lettered choices is.
5. Focus on choices (A) and (B), and use the following sequence to logically determine the correct answer:
    a. If you can determine that (A) is incorrect, your answer must be either B or D.
    b. If you can determine that (B) is incorrect, your answer must be either A or D.
    c. If you can determine that both (A) and (B) are incorrect, your answer must be D.
    d. If you can determine that both (A) and (B) are correct, your answer must be C.*

*Remember, you only have an average of 50 seconds per question.

Multiple true–false items. These questions are considered the most difficult (or tricky), and you should be certain that you understand and follow the code that always accompanies these questions:

DIRECTIONS (Question 7): For each of the items in this section, <u>ONE</u> or <u>MORE</u> of the numbered options is correct. Choose the answer

A if only <u>1, 2 and 3</u> are correct,
B if only <u>1 and 3</u> are correct,
C if only <u>2 and 4</u> are correct,
D if only <u>4</u> is correct,
E if <u>all</u> are correct.

This code is always the same (i.e., "D" would never say "if 3 is correct"), and it is repeated throughout this book at the top of any page on which multiple true–false item questions appear.

SUMMARY OF DIRECTIONS				
A	**B**	**C**	**D**	**E**
1, 2, 3 only	1, 3 only	2, 4 only	4 only	All are correct

A sample question follows:

7. A 12-yr-old boy complains of severe pruritus, especially at night, and is found to have scabies. Effective management includes

(1) treating household pets
(2) treating normal-appearing skin
(3) using griseofulvin
(4) treating asymptomatic family members

You first need to determine which choices are right and wrong, and then which code corresponds to the correct numbers. In the example above, 2 and 4 are both effective management procedures, and therefore (C) is the correct answer to this question.

TABLE 4. STRATEGIES FOR ANSWERING MULTIPLE TRUE–FALSE ITEM QUESTIONS

1. Carefully read and become familiar with the accompanying directions to this tricky question type.
2. Carefully read the stem to be certain that you know what is being asked.
3. Carefully read each of the numbered choices. If you can determine whether any of the choices are true or false, you may find it helpful to place a "+" (true) or a "−" (false) next to the number.
4. Focus on the numbered choices and your true/false notations, and use the following sequence to logically determine the correct answer:
    a. Note that in the answer code choices 1 *and* 3 are *always* both either true or false together. If you are sure that either one is incorrect, your answer must be C or D.
    b. If you are sure that choice 2 *and either* choice 1 *or* 3 are incorrect, your answer must be D.
    c. If you are sure that choices 2 and 4 are incorrect, your answer must be B.*

*Remember, you only have an average of 50 seconds per question. Note that the following two combinations cannot occur: choices 1 and 4 both incorrect; choices 3 and 4 both incorrect.

Answers, Explanations, and References

In each of the sections of this book, the question sections are followed by a section containing the answers, explanations, and references to the questions. This section (1) tells you the answer to each question; (2) gives you an explanation/review of why the answer is correct, background information on the subject matter, and why the other answers are incorrect; and (3) tells you where you can find more in-depth information on the subject matter in other books and/or journals. We encourage you to use this section as a basis for further study and understanding.

If you choose the correct answer to a question, you can then read the explanation (1) for reinforcement and (2) to add to your knowledge about the subject matter (remember that the explanations usually tell not only why the answer is correct, but also why the other choices are incorrect). **If you choose the wrong answer** to a question, you can read the explanation for a learning/ reviewing discussion of the material in the question. Furthermore, you can note the reference cited (e.g., "Joklik et al, pp 103–114"), look up the full source in the bibliography at the end of the section (e.g., "Joklik WK, Willett HP, Amos DB. *Zinsser's Microbiology*. 19th ed. East Norwalk, Conn.: Appleton & Lange; 1988.), and refer to the pages cited for a more in-depth discussion.

Subspecialty Lists

At the end of each section of this book is a subspecialty list for each subject area. These subspecialty lists will help point out your areas of relative weakness and, thus, help you focus your review.

For example, by checking off your incorrect answers on, say, the microbiology list, you may find that a pattern develops in that you are incorrect on most or all of the virology questions. In this case, you could note the references (in the explanation section) for your incorrect answers and read those sources. You might also want to purchase a virology text or review book to do a much more in-depth review. We think that you will find these subspecialty lists very helpful, and we urge you to use them.

Practice Test

The 311-question practice test at the end of the book consists of approximately 45 questions from each of the seven basic sciences. The questions are grouped according to question type (one best answer–single item, one best answer–matching sets, comparison/matching sets, then multiple true–false items), with the subject areas integrated. This format mimics the actual exam and enables you to test your skill at answering questions in all of the basic sciences under simulated examination conditions.

The practice test section is organized in the same format as the seven earlier sections: questions; answers, explanations, and references; bibliography; and subspecialty list (which, here, will also list the major subject heading).

HOW TO USE THIS BOOK

There are two logical ways to get the most value from this book. We will call them Plan A and Plan B.

In Plan A, you go straight to the Practice Test and complete it according to the instructions. Using the subspecialty list, analyze your areas of strength and weakness. This will be a good indicator of your initial knowledge of the subject and will help to identify specific areas for preparation and review. You can now use the first seven chapters of the book to help you improve your relative weak points.

In Plan B, you go through chapters 1 through 7 checking off your answers, and then comparing your choices with the answers and discussions in the book. Once you have completed this process, you can take the Practice Test and see how well prepared you are. If you still have a major weakness, it should be apparent in time for you to take remedial action.

In Plan A, by taking the Practice Test first, you get quick feedback regarding your initial areas of strength and weakness. You may find that you have a good command of the material indicating that perhaps only a cursory review of the first seven chapters is necessary. This, of course, would be good to know early in your exam preparation. On the other hand, you may find that you have many areas of weakness. In this case, you could then focus on these areas in your review—not just with this book, but also with the cited references and with your current textbooks.

It is, however, unlikely that you will not do some studying prior to taking the National Boards (especially since you have this book). Therefore, it may be more realistic to take the Practice Test after you have reviewed the first seven chapters (as in Plan B). This will probably give you a more realistic type of testing situation since very few of us just sit down to a test without studying. In this case, you will have done some reviewing (from superficial to in-depth), and your Practice Test will reflect this studying time. If, after reviewing the first seven chapters and taking the Practice Test, you still have some weaknesses, you can then go back to the first seven chapters and supplement your review with your texts.

SPECIFIC INFORMATION ON THE PART I EXAMINATION

The official source of all information with respect to National Board Examination Part I is the National Board of Medical Examiners (NBME), 3930 Chestnut Street, Philadelphia, PA 19104. Established in 1915, the NBME is a voluntary, nonprofit, independent organization whose sole function is the design, implementation, distribution, and processing of a vast bank of question items, certifying examinations, and evaluative services in the professional medical field.

In order to sit for the Part I examination, a person must be either an officially enrolled medical student or a graduate of an accredited United States or Canadian medical school. It is not necessary to complete any particular year of medical school in order to be a candidate for Part I. Neither is it required to take Part I before Part II.

In applying for Part I, you must use forms supplied by NBME. Remember that registration closes *ten weeks* before the scheduled examination date. Some United States and Canadian medical schools require their students to take Part I even if they are noncandidates. Such students can register as noncandidates at the request of their school. A person who takes Part I as a noncandidate can later change to candidate status and, after payment of a fee, receive certification credit.

Scoring

Because there is no deduction for wrong answers, you should **answer every question.** Your test is scored in the following way:

1. The number of questions answered correctly is totaled. This is called the raw score.
2. The raw score is converted statistically to a "standard" score on a scale of 200 to 800, with the mean set at 500. Each 100 points away from 500 is one standard deviation.
3. Your score is compared statistically with the criteria set by the scores of the second-year medical school candidates for certification in the June administration during the prior four years. This is what is meant by the term, "criterion referenced test."
4. A score of 500 places you around the 50th percentile. A score of 380 is the minimum passing score for Part I; this probably represents about the 12th to 15th percentile. If you answer 50 percent or so of the questions correctly, you will probably receive a passing score.

Remember: You do not have to pass all seven basic science components, although you will receive a standard score in each of them. A score of less than 400 (about the 15th percentile) on any particular area is a real cause for concern as it will certainly drag down your overall score. Likewise, a 600 or better (85th percentile) is an area of great relative strength. (You can use the practice test included in *Appleton & Lange's Review for National Boards Part I* to help determine your areas of strength and weakness well in advance of the actual examination.)

Physical Conditions

The NBME is very concerned that all their exams be administered under uniform conditions in the numerous centers that are used. Except for several No. 2 pencils and an eraser, you are not permitted to bring anything (books, notes, calculators, etc.) into the test room. All examinees receive the same questions at the same session. However, the questions are printed in different sequences in several different booklets, and the booklets are randomly distributed. In addition, examinees are moved to different seats at least once during the test. And, of course, each test is policed by at least one proctor. The object of these maneuvers is to frustrate cheating or even the temptation to cheat.

The number of candidates who fail Part I is larger than you might imagine (especially considering the fact that most of them have already invested two years and thousands of dollars in medical school!). Although you can retake the examination a second time, it is less physically and psychologically taxing to be in the passing group on the first go-around. This is why a review and study plan is so important for your success. We are confident that you will find *Appleton & Lange's Review for National Boards Part I* to be of great assistance during your exam preparation.

Standard Abbreviations

ACTH: adrenocorticotropic hormone
ADH: antidiuretic hormone
ADP: adenosine diphosphate
AFP: α-fetoprotein
AMP: adenosine monophosphate
ATP: adenosine triphosphate
ATPase: adenosine triphosphatase

bid: 2 times a day
BP: blood pressure
BUN: blood urea nitrogen

CT: computed tomography
CBC: complete blood count
CCU: coronary care unit
CNS: central nervous system
CPK: creatine phosphokinase
CSF: cerebrospinal fluid

DNA: deoxyribonucleic acid
DNAse: deoxyribonuclease

ECG: electrocardiogram
EDTA: ethylenediaminetetraacetate
EEG: electroencephalogram
ER: emergency room

FSH: follicle-stimulating hormone

GI: gastrointestinal
GU: genitourinary

HCG: human chorionic gonadotropin
IgA, etc.: immunoglobulin A, etc.
IM: intramuscular(ly)
IQ: intelligence quotient
IU: international unit
IV: intravenous(ly)

KUB: kidney, ureter, and bladder

LDH: lactic dehydrogenase
LH: luteinizing hormone
LSD: lysergic acid diethylamide

mRNA: messenger RNA

PO: oral(ly)
prn: as needed

RBC: red blood cell
RNA: ribonucleic acid
RNAse: ribonuclease
rRNA: ribosomal RNA

SC: subcutaneous(ly)
SGOT: serum glutamic oxaloacetic transaminase
SGPT: serum glutamic pyruvic transaminase

TB: tuberculosis
tRNA: transfer RNA
TSH: thyroid-stimulating hormone
WBC: white blood cell

Anatomy
Questions

DIRECTIONS (Questions 1 through 77): Each of the numbered items or incomplete statements in this section is followed by answers or by completions of the statement. Select the <u>ONE</u> lettered answer or completion that is <u>BEST</u> in each case.

1. Which of the following statements regarding the common bile duct is correct?

    (A) it lies to the left of the hepatic artery

    (B) it descends anterior to the first part of the duodenum

    (C) it crosses the uncinate process of the pancreas

    (D) it joins the main pancreatic duct and they together pass into the second part of the duodenum

    (E) it lies in front of the superior vena cava

2. Which of the following statements correctly applies to the right kidney?

    (A) the second portion of the duodenum lies anterior to its medial border

    (B) its superior extremity reaches the upper border of the 5th thoracic vertebra

    (C) its inferior extremity is closer to the median plane than its superior pole

    (D) it is usually somewhat longer than the left kidney

    (E) it is in contact laterally with the spleen

3. Which of the following structures is associated with the small intestine?

    (A) teniae coli

    (B) mesentery

    (C) sacculations

    (D) epiploic appendages

    (E) haustra coli

4. The common bile duct is located in which of the following ligaments?

    (A) falciform

    (B) hepatogastric

    (C) hepatoduodenal

    (D) hepatocolic

    (E) gastrolienal

5. Which of the following is NOT typically a branch of the axillary artery?

    (A) thyrocervical trunk

    (B) subscapular

    (C) highest intercostal

    (D) lateral thoracic

    (E) posterior humeral circumflex

6. Which of the following structures passes through the scapular notch?

    (A) suprascapular nerve

    (B) subscapular artery

    (C) long thoracic nerve

    (D) suprascapular artery

    (E) subscapular nerve

7. The spermatozoa are stored in which of the following structures?

    (A) seminal vesicles

    (B) testes

    (C) ductus deferens

    (D) spermatic cord

    (E) epididymis

8. The accessory glands of the male genital organs include the

    (A) testes, ductus deferentes, reservoir of spermatozoa, seminal vesicles, ejaculatory ducts, and penis

    (B) testes, seminal vesicles, prostate, and bulbourethral glands

    (C) testes, ductus deferentes, seminal vesicles, and penis

    (D) seminal vesicles, prostate, bulbourethral glands, and urethral glands

    (E) testes, prostate, and bulbourethral glands

9. The middle cerebral artery is a continuation of the

   (A) external carotid artery
   ✓ (B) internal carotid artery
   (C) vertebral artery
   (D) basilar artery
   (E) interior choroid artery

10. The beginning of the thoracic duct is known as the

    (A) intestinal lymph trunk
    (B) broncomediastinal lymph trunk
    (C) jugular lymph trunk
    (D) subclavian lymph trunk
    ✓ (E) cisterna chyli

11. The root of the left lung is ventral to which of the following structures?

    (A) inferior vena cava
    ✓ (B) thoracic aorta
    (C) left phrenic nerve
    (D) pericardiacophrenic vessels
    (E) anterior pulmonary plexuses of nerves

12. Which of the following nerves innervates the gluteus maximus muscle?

    (A) pudendal
    (B) sciatic
    (C) femoral
    (D) inferior gluteal
    (E) obturator

13. The platysma is innervated by

    (A) the mandibular division of cranial nerve V
    (B) the maxillary division of cranial nerve V
    (C) cranial nerve XI (accessory)
    (D) the cervical branch of cranial nerve VII
    (E) cranial nerve XII (hypoglossal)

14. Enclosed in the superior edge of each broad ligament is

    (A) each ovary
    (B) the uterus
    (C) each uterine tube
    (D) the round ligament
    (E) the parametrium

15. The saphenous nerve is the terminal branch of which of the following nerves?

    (A) peroneal
    (B) tibial
    (C) femoral

(D) obturator
(E) pudendal

16. The oculomotor nerve (cranial nerve III) is usually located between

    (A) the anterior inferior cerebellar and internal acoustic arteries
    (B) the posterior communicating and posterior cerebral arteries
    (C) the optic chiasm and mamillary bodies
    (D) the superior cerebellar and posterior cerebral arteries
    (E) none of the above structures

17. All of the following synapse in the thalamus proper EXCEPT

    (A) sensory fibers conveying pain and temperature from the face
    (B) fibers from the dentate nucleus
    (C) sensory fibers conveying proprioception from the body
    (D) sensory fibers conveying pressure and touch from the face and body
    (E) fibers conveying olfactory sensations

18. The neurons of the granular layer of the cerebellar cortex are most directly derived from the

    (A) ventricular zone of the neural tube
    (B) external granular layer neuroblasts
    (C) deep cerebellar nuclei
    (D) inferior olivary nucleus
    (E) basal plate

19. The term sphenomeniscus is sometimes given to which of the following structures?

    (A) piriformis muscle
    (B) sphenomandibular ligament
    (C) terminal end of the maxillary artery
    (D) pterygopalatine fossa
    (E) superior belly of the lateral pterygoid muscle

20. All of the following statements regarding the maxillary artery are true EXCEPT that

    (A) it arises in the parotid gland behind the neck of the mandible as a branch of the external carotid
    (B) the branches of its first (mandibular) portion supply the muscles of mastication and the buccinator
    (C) the nerves that accompany the branches of its third (final) portion are derived from the maxillary nerve

(D) one of its branches, the inferior alveolar artery, supplies the chin and lower teeth

(E) one of its branches, the sphenopalatine artery, supplies the nasal cavity (conchae, meatuses, septum, paranasal sinuses)

21. For descriptive purposes, the body may be viewed as divided into planes described as

(A) frontal, sagittal, posterior, and inferior

(B) cranial, medial, posterior, longitudinal, and dorsal

(C) posterior, lateral, anterior, plantar, and cephalic

(D) sagittal, plantar, frontal, transverse, and ventral

(E) plantar, posterior, lateral, horizontal, and transverse

22. The internal female genitalia comprise the

(A) ovaries, uterine tubes, uterus, and vagina

(B) ovaries, oviducts, uterus, vagina, and clitoris

(C) ovaries, uterine tubes, cervix, and pudendum

(D) ovaries, uterine horns, uterus, cervix, and labia

(E) ovaries, uterine horns, uterus, vagina, and hymen

23. Which of the following statements concerning the female genital system is true?

(A) the round ligament extends from the uterus to the labia minora

(B) the posterior aspect of the vagina can be palpated by means of rectal digital exploration

(C) the uterovesical pouch is located posterior to the uterus

(D) perimetrium is loose connective tissue between layers of parametrium

(E) the mesovarium, or mesometrium, attaches the ovary to the uterus

24. Which of the following statements regarding the structure of the perineum is true?

(A) the superficial perineal space lodges the root of the penis or clitoris and its associated muscles

(B) the superficial perineal space is delineated by the inferior and superior fasciae of the urogenital diaphragm

(C) the male perineal space is occupied by the urinary bladder and seminal vesicles

(D) the female perineal space is occupied by the neck of the uterus

(E) the perineal body is located at the level of each ischial tuberosity

25. Which of the following statements concerning the genital system is correct?

(A) spermatozoa are formed in the testes and are stored in the reservoir of spermatozoa

(B) the seminal vesicle is a single median organ in which the urine and the sperm are mixed together

(C) the prostate contains the terminations of the epididymis and the ejaculatory ducts

(D) the urethra is the canal that conveys urine and ejaculate in both sexes

(E) the ampullae of the ductus deferentes open distally to the utricle of the prostatic urethra

26. Which of the following structures is located in the wall of the left atrium?

(A) terminal crest

(B) opening of the coronary sinus

(C) limbus fossae ovalis

(D) septomarginal trabecula

(E) valvula foraminis ovalis

27. The bare area of the liver is limited above and below by the laminae of the

(A) round (teres) ligament

(B) coronary ligament

(C) right and left triangular ligaments

(D) hepatorenal ligament

(E) gastrophrenic ligament

28. Which of the following statements applies to the accessory pancreatic duct?

(A) it empties into the duodenal cap

(B) it empties at the greater duodenal papilla

(C) it develops within the ventral pancreatic primordium

(D) it drains the tail of the pancreas

(E) none of the above

29. Which of the following statements regarding the digestive system is true?

(A) the gastrolienal ligament extends between the greater curvature of the stomach and the medial margin of the kidney

(B) the gastrophrenic ligament establishes the connection between the stomach and the anterior aspect of the pancreas

(C) the coronary ligament and the right and left triangular ligaments are connections between the small and large intestine

(D) the adult bursa omentalis, or lesser peritoneal sac, is a space behind the stomach

(E) the gastrohepatic ligament is the midportion of the greater omentum

30. The clinical importance of the posterior inferior cerebellar artery is that it in part supplies the

   (A) spinal cord
   (B) medulla oblongata
   (C) cerebellum
   (D) pons
   (E) cerebrum

31. The arterial circle of Willis is formed by the internal carotid arteries and the branches of the

   (A) external carotid artery
   (B) vertebral artery
   (C) basilar artery
   (D) middle meningeal artery
   (E) anterior temporal artery

32. The blood supply of the spinal cord is provided by all of the following arteries EXCEPT

   (A) a single anterior spinal artery derived from the vertebral arteries
   (B) paired posterior spinal arteries derived from vertebral arteries
   (C) anterior and posterior radicular arteries formed by segmental arteries
   (D) medullary arteries that reinforce the segmental supply
   (E) inferior posterior cerebellopontine arteries

33. Which of the following statements regarding the anatomy of the urinary bladder is true?

   (A) the orientation of the smooth muscle layers in the urinary bladder wall is easily discernible
   (B) the mucosa of the bladder is lined with transitional epithelium that does not rest on a lamina propria
   (C) the muscle coat of the urinary bladder consists of bundles of smooth muscle collectively called detrusor urinae muscle
   (D) the transitional epithelium of the bladder is highly keratinized
   (E) the serous coat surrounds the entire bladder, including the prostate gland

34. The muscles of the urogenital diaphragm include the

   (A) superficial transverse perineus muscle and sphincter urethrae muscle
   (B) deep and superficial transverse perineus muscles
   (C) deep transverse perineus and sphincter urethrae muscles
   (D) sphincter urethrae and sphincter ani internus muscles

   (E) sphincter urethrae and sphincter vesicae urinariae muscles

35. The cavernous, or erectile, tissues of the penis include the

   (A) corpora cavernosa penis and prepuce
   (B) corpora spongiosa penis and glans penis
   (C) frenulum of the prepuce, glans penis, and corpus spongiosum penis
   (D) corpora cavernosa penis and corpus spongiosum penis
   (E) corpora spongiosa penis and corpus scrotalis penis

36. Which of the following statements concerning the genital system is true?

   (A) the tunica dartos of the scrotum is directly continuous with the subcutaneous tissue of the abdominal wall
   (B) the ilioinguinal nerve traverses the inguinal canal deep to the inguinal ring, where it gives off the posterior scrotal nerves
   (C) the iliohypogastric nerve, also called the subcostal nerve, is a pelvic nerve
   (D) the inferior epigastric artery is a terminal branch of the internal thoracic artery and descends in the rectus sheath posterior to the rectus abdominis muscle
   (E) the pampiniform plexus is made up of nerves that supply the cervix

37. The horizontal fissure and the inferior part of the oblique fissure form the boundaries of which of the following?

   (A) apex of the left lung
   (B) lingula of the left lung
   (C) middle lobe of the right lung
   (D) superior lobe of the right lung
   (E) inferior lobe of the left lung

38. Failure of the tracheoesophageal septum to form produces

   (A) a tracheoesophageal fistula
   (B) an azygos lobe of the lung
   (C) hypoplasia of the lung
   (D) a laryngeal web
   (E) agenesis of the lung

39. The parathyroid gland is correctly described as

   (A) three pairs of yellowish structures located on the deep surface of the lateral lobes of the thyroid
   (B) two pairs of structures encased in the thymus

(C) three pairs of glands located in the anterior aspect of the thyroid lobes

(D) two pairs of small structures embedded in the capsule of the thyroid on its posterior aspect

(E) directly dependent on the secretion of the pineal gland

40. The superior ophthalmic vein enters the cavernous sinus via the

(A) foramen rotundum
(B) foramen ovale
(C) inferior orbital fissure
(D) superior orbital fissure
(E) optic foramen

41. The lymphatic trunk that collects lymph from the inferior limbs and abdomen and receives tributaries from the left side of the thorax, neck, and head is the

(A) lacteal vessel
(B) thoracic duct
(C) right lymphatic duct
(D) cervical duct
(E) left lymphatic duct

42. The crura of both the clitoris and penis are covered by the musculus

(A) bulbocavernosus
(B) transversus perinei superficialis
(C) transversus perinei profundus
(D) ischiocavernosus
(E) bulbospongiosus

43. Which of the following structures is not included in the female pudendum?

(A) ovaries
(B) mons pubis
(C) clitoris
(D) bulb of the vestibule
(E) greater vestibular glands

44. The morphologic equivalent of the penis is the

(A) vestibule of the vagina
(B) hymen
(C) clitoris
(D) vestibular gland
(E) vulva

45. The broad ligament does not enclose which of the following structures?

(A) uterine tubes
(B) ovarian ligaments

(C) uterine arteries
(D) uterovaginal plexus of nerves
(E) greater vestibular glands

46. The orifices on the colliculus seminalis at either side of the prostatic utricle are associated with the

(A) vestibular canals
(B) urethral lacunae
(C) ductus deferentes
(D) ejaculatory ducts
(E) seminal ducts

47. The bulbourethral glands of the male are embedded in the fibers of which of the following muscles?

(A) sphincter urethrae
(B) ischiocavernosus
(C) superficial transverse perineus
(D) bulbospongiosus
(E) none of the above

48. Which of the following structures are lined by ciliated, pseudostratified epithelium containing goblet cells and have cartilage plates, mucous glands, and smooth muscle?

(A) alveolar ducts
(B) terminal bronchioles
(C) respiratory bronchioles
(D) alveolar sacs
(E) secondary bronchi

49. The extrinsic muscles of the larynx are described as

(A) moving the upper part of the larynx
(B) moving the larynx as a whole
(C) circular and oval
(D) including the stylothyroid
(E) all unpaired and median

50. Which of the following statements correctly applies to the left bronchus?

(A) it is shorter than the right bronchus
(B) it passes under the aortic arch
(C) it is the more direct continuation of the trachea
(D) it is usually larger in diameter than the right bronchus
(E) foreign bodies are more apt to lodge in it

51. The middle lobe of the right lung has two segments, described as

    (A) lateral and medial
    (B) superior and inferior
    (C) lingular and apical
    (D) posterior and anterior
    (E) ventral and dorsal

52. The posterior mediastinum contains all of the following structures EXCEPT the

    (A) thymus
    (B) thoracic duct
    (C) aorta
    (D) esophagus
    (E) splanchnic nerves

53. All of the following statements correctly describe the cupula of the pleura EXCEPT that

    (A) it is at the level of the first rib
    (B) it is strengthened by a thickening of endothoracic fascia to protect it and the lung
    (C) it is strengthened by a thickening of the pulmonary ligament
    (D) the sympathetic trunk, first thoracic nerve, and vessels of the first intercostal space lie behind it
    (E) it is associated with the apex of the lung

54. Which of the following structures usually runs in the free edge of the lesser omentum?

    (A) portal vein
    (B) hepatic artery
    (C) common bile duct
    (D) right gastroepiploic artery
    (E) splenic artery

55. Which of the following arteries does not provide meningeal branches for the dura?

    (A) maxillary
    (B) ophthalmic
    (C) vertebral
    (D) occipital
    (E) superficial temporal

56. Which of the following structures extends in the midline of the cranial cavity from the crista galli to the internal occipital protuberance?

    (A) falx cerebri
    (B) tentorium cerebelli
    (C) falx cerebelli
    (D) diaphragma sellae
    (E) leptomeninges

57. The spinal cord normally comprises 31 segments. The 31st segment is located at what spinal column level?

    (A) T-12
    (B) L-1–2
    (C) L-4–5
    (D) S-4–5
    (E) C-1

58. All of the following nuclei are associated with the ascending auditory pathway EXCEPT the

    (A) inferior colliculus
    (B) superior olivary nucleus
    (C) lateral lemniscus nucleus
    (D) medial geniculate body
    (E) inferior olivary nucleus

59. The gentle stroking of the skin immediately lateral to the umbilicus results in the conveying of this tickling sensation to the spinal cord via spinal nerve

    (A) C-5
    (B) T-1
    (C) T-10
    (D) L-1
    (E) S-1

60. Nerve fibers that convey pain and temperature sensations are part of which major sensory tract?

    (A) fasciculus gracilis
    (B) fasciculus cuneatus
    (C) anterior spinocerebellar tract
    (D) lateral spinothalamic tract
    (E) corticospinal tract

61. Which of the following encapsulated receptors is the largest and most widely distributed?

    (A) tactile corpuscles of Meissner
    (B) end bulbs
    (C) pacinian corpuscles
    (D) Golgi-Mazzoni corpuscles
    (E) neuromuscular spindles

62. All of the following tracts synapse on the final common pathway EXCEPT the

    (A) rubrospinal tract
    (B) corticospinal tract
    (C) vestibulospinal tract
    (D) reticulospinal tract
    (E) spinothalamic tract

63. The cartilages of the larynx are correctly described as

(A) occurring singly and median in location

(B) thyroid, cricoid, epiglottic, arytenoid, corniculate, and cuneiform

(C) ossified before puberty

(D) responsible for the jugular notch

(E) thyroid, parathyroid, cricoid, epiglottic, valleculae, arytenoid, and cuneiform

64. All of the following statements concerning the trigeminal nerve and nuclei are true EXCEPT that

(A) most of the primary afferent cell bodies are in the main sensory nucleus

(B) some primary afferent cell bodies (for proprioception) are located in the mesencephalic nucleus

(C) fibers from the ophthalmic division are most medially placed in the spinal tract

(D) the *major* efferent pathway from the spinal nucleus is the contralateral ventral trigeminothalamic tract

(E) the motor nucleus projects to the mandibular division

65. All of the following structures contain endolymph EXCEPT the

(A) ductus reuniens

(B) saccule

(C) ampulla

(D) vestibular duct (scala vestibuli)

(E) cochlear duct (scala media)

66. Tumors derived from Schwann's cells characteristically arise in the cerebellopontine angle, where they lie in close anatomic relationship to all of the following structures EXCEPT the

(A) superior cerebellar peduncle

(B) middle cerebellar peduncle

(C) inferior cerebellar peduncle

(D) seventh cranial nerve

(E) flocculus of the cerebellum

Questions 67 and 68

The figure below represents a cross-section through the spinal cord.

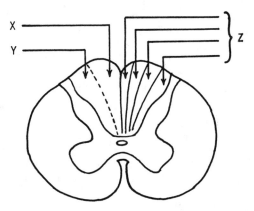

67. Nerve fibers that comprise tract Y in the figure are usually found at which spinal cord levels?

(A) all spinal cord levels

(B) L-5 and above

(C) L-1 and above

(D) T-12 and above

(E) T-6 and above

68. In the figure above, the spatial arrangement of fibers in the half or part of the posterior white funiculus designated by the letter Z, from medial to lateral positions, is

(A) sacral, lumbar, thoracic, and cervical

(B) cervical, thoracic, lumbar, and sacral

(C) lumbar, sacral, cervical, and thoracic

(D) cervical, sacral, thoracic, and lumbar

(E) lumbar, thoracic, cervical, and trigeminal

69. All of the following statements concerning the larynx are correct EXCEPT that

(A) the internal laryngeal nerve supplies the internal muscles of the larynx

(B) the inferior laryngeal nerve supplies the internal muscles of the larynx

(C) the inferior laryngeal nerve is a branch of the vagus nerve

(D) the superior laryngeal nerve is a branch of the vagus nerve

(E) the internal laryngeal nerve is a branch of the superior laryngeal nerve

70. Main efferent pathways from the hypothalamus include all of the following EXCEPT the

(A) mamillothalamic tract

(B) mamillotegmental tract

(C) medial forebrain bundle

(D) stria terminalis

(E) hypothalamohypophyseal tract

71. The conducting system of the adult heart comprises all of the following except for the

(A) sinoatrial (SA) node
(B) atrioventricular (AV) node
(C) atrioventricular (AV) bundle
(D) subendocardial plexuses of conducting myofibers
(E) crista terminalis

72. The infundibulum is an area of the heart associated with the

(A) opening of the pulmonary artery (from the right ventricle)
(B) opening of the aorta (from the left ventricle)
(C) right AV opening
(D) left AV opening
(E) opening of the coronary sinus into the right atrium

73. The nodule and lunula of the heart are features of the

(A) right AV valve
(B) left AV valve
(C) semilunar valves
(D) right atrium
(E) left atrium

74. Which of the following statements concerning the heart and great vessels is true?

(A) the SA node is supplied by the vena cava
(B) the SA node is drained by the left coronary artery in 60 percent of cases
(C) the SA node is supplied by an atrial branch of the right coronary artery in most cases
(D) the SA node and the AV node are drained by the second septal artery of the anterior interventricular artery
(E) the AV node is drained by the left coronary artery, the circumflex artery, and the anterior interventricular artery

75. Which of the following statements concerning the heart and great vessels is true?

(A) the pericardium has a closer relationship with the SA node than with the AV node
(B) the right vagus nerve has more control on the AV node than on the SA node
(C) the epicardium contains subendocardial Purkinje fibers for conduction purposes
(D) the pars membranacea is the upper portion of the interatrial septum in children
(E) the AV node is located in the right aspect of the superior vena cava, at the level of the sulcus terminalis

76. The left coronary artery gives off which of the following branches?

(A) conus artery
(B) nodal artery
(C) posterior interventricular artery
(D) circumflex branch
(E) none of the above

77. Which of the following statements concerning the lymphatics is true?

(A) an aggregate is an isolated but important lymph node
(B) no single body organ is primarily made up of lymphatic tissue
(C) lymph is formed near the surface of the skin
(D) hematogenic organs produce white blood cells (WBCs) only
(E) lymph nodes polarize infection and disease

DIRECTIONS (Questions 78 through 87): Each group of items in this section consists of lettered headings followed by a set of numbered words or phrases. For each numbered word or phrase, select the ONE lettered heading that is most closely associated with it. Each lettered heading may be selected once, more than once, or not at all.

Questions 78 through 81

(A) dorsal scapular artery
(B) inferior thyroid artery
(C) costocervical trunk
(D) transverse cervical artery
(E) suprascapular artery

78. The artery that passes over the superior transverse ligament of the scapula.

79. The artery has an intimate relation to the brachial plexus, passing frequently either above or below the middle trunk.

80. It divides into the highest intercostal and the deep cervical arteries.

81. It turns medialward behind the carotid sheath and passes variably behind, in front of, or between strands of the cervical sympathetic trunk.

Questions 82 through 85

For each muscle listed, choose the branchial arch from which it arises.

(A) branchial arch I
(B) branchial arch II
(C) branchial arch III

(D) branchial arch IV

(E) branchial arch VI

82. Stylohyoid

83. Stylopharyngeus

84. Masseter

85. Buccinator

Questions 86 and 87

For each description below, choose the nerve with which it is associated.

(A) ulnar

(B) radial

(C) median

(D) musculocutaneous

(E) axillary

86. The largest nerve derived from the medial cord of the brachial plexus and carries nerve fibers from the 8th cervical and 1st thoracic nerves.

87. The nerve pierces the coracobrachialis muscles.

DIRECTIONS (Questions 88 through 100): Each group of items in this section consists of lettered headings followed by a set of numbered words or phrases. For each numbered word or phrase, select

A if the item is associated with (A) <u>only</u>,

B if the item is associated with (B) <u>only</u>,

C if the item is associated with <u>both</u> (A) <u>and</u> (B),

D if the item is associated with <u>neither</u> (A) <u>nor</u> (B).

Questions 88 through 92

(A) sinoatrial (SA) node

(B) atrioventricular (AV) node

(C) both

(D) neither

88. Specialized myocardium

89. Located at the cephalic end of the sulcus terminalis

90. Receives its blood supply from the anterior interventricular artery

91. The right vagal and right sympathetic branches ending chiefly in this region

92. The pacemaker of the heart

Questions 93 through 96

(A) obturator nerve

(B) femoral nerve

(C) both

(D) neither

93. It arises from the lumbar nerves 2, 3, and 4

94. It is the principal preaxial nerve of the lumbar plexus

95. It gives rise to the saphenous nerve

96. It innervates the abductors of the thigh

Questions 97 through 100

(A) receives preganglionic fibers from the superior salivatory nucleus

(B) sends postganglionic fibers to the lacrimal glands

(C) both

(D) neither

97. The otic ganglion

98. The pterygopalatine ganglion

99. The submandibular ganglion

100. The ciliary ganglion

DIRECTIONS (Questions 101 through 127): For each of the items in this section, <u>ONE</u> or <u>MORE</u> of the numbered options is correct. Choose the answer

A if only <u>1, 2, and 3</u> are correct,

B if only <u>1 and 3</u> are correct,

C if only <u>2 and 4</u> are correct,

D if only <u>4</u> is correct,

E if <u>all</u> are correct.

101. Preganglionic parasympathetic fibers are located in which of the following nerves?

(1) greater petrosal

(2) chorda tympani

(3) deep petrosal

(4) abducens

SUMMARY OF DIRECTIONS				
A	**B**	**C**	**D**	**E**
1, 2, 3 only	1, 3 only	2, 4 only	4 only	All are correct

102. The development of the pancreas is correctly described by which of the following statements?

    (1) the dorsal pancreatic rudiment develops from the wall of the foregut, and the ventral pancreatic rudiment arises from the hepatic diverticulum
    (2) the ventral pancreatic rudiment duct becomes a portion of the definitive duct
    (3) a portion of the dorsal pancreatic rudiment duct becomes the accessory duct
    (4) the ventral pancreatic rudiment becomes apposed to the embryonic right surface of the dorsal pancreatic rudiment

103. The hair cells of the cristae ampullares are known to

    (1) receive afferent innervation from neurons located in the spiral ganglion
    (2) be stimulated by the movement of endolymph
    (3) usually be activated when the head moves forward
    (4) respond to angular acceleration

104. The medial longitudinal fasciculus is correctly described as

    (1) containing fibers from the vestibular nuclei that synapse in the nuclei of cranial nerves III, IV, and VI
    (2) originating from the same vestibular nuclei as the lateral vestibulospinal tract
    (3) composed of secondary vestibular fibers
    (4) carrying sensory impulses that originate in the auditory pathway

105. The blood supply to the pars distalis is correctly described as

    (1) arising in large part from vessels in the pars nervosa
    (2) arising in large part from a capillary plexus in the hypothalamus
    (3) containing an extremely high concentration of oxytocin
    (4) containing peptides that are secreted by hypothalamic neurons

106. The visual system is correctly described by which of the following statements?

    (1) a light shining onto the retina through the pupil will pass through pigment epithelium before passing through the outer nuclear layer
    (2) "rounding up" of the lens increases its refractive power
    (3) the fovea centralis lies medial to the optic disk
    (4) the ora serrata is the transition area between the nervous and nonnervous retina

107. Olfactory receptors are located in the

    (1) olfactory bulb
    (2) olfactory cortex
    (3) olfactory tract
    (4) nasal mucosa

108. Modalities of general sensation conducted ipsilaterally in the spinal cord include

    (1) vibratory sense
    (2) muscle, joint, and tendon sense
    (3) two-point touch discrimination
    (4) sensations of coolness and warmth

109. The cerebellum receives fibers from the

    (1) pontine nuclei
    (2) vestibular nuclei
    (3) nucleus dorsalis of Clarke
    (4) inferior olivary nucleus

110. Characteristic signs of neocerebellar dysfunction include

    (1) ataxic movements
    (2) dysmetria
    (3) intention tremor
    (4) synergy of movements

111. A bullet wound at spinal cord level C-8 that completely destroys both dorsal funiculi would result in a total deficit of sensory modalities conveyed via the

    (1) fasciculus gracilis
    (2) spinothalamic tracts
    (3) fasciculus cuneatus
    (4) spinocerebellar tracts

112. A spinal cord segment is defined as that portion of the spinal cord that furnishes dorsal and ventral rootlets to a single pair of spinal nerves At the midthoracic level, what modalities are conveyed via that pair of spinal nerves?

 (1) sensory fibers
 (2) autonomic sympathetic fibers
 (3) motor fibers
 (4) autonomic parasympathetic fibers

113. the embryonic dorsal mesentery gives rise to the

 (1) lesser omentum
 (2) greater omentum
 (3) falciform ligament
 (4) mesentery of jejunoileum

114. Structures that are always interposed between the fetal and maternal blood in the human placenta include the

 (1) fetal capillary endothelium
 (2) maternal capillary endothelium
 (3) syncytiotrophoblast
 (4) cytotrophoblast

115. The proctodeum is correctly described as being

 (1) covered by epithelium of endodermal origin
 (2) partially covered by columnar epithelium
 (3) derived from the yolk sac
 (4) created by mesenchymal condensations around the cloacal membrane

116. The adrenal medulla is correctly described as

 (1) developing from embryonic coelomic epithelium
 (2) receiving preganglionic sympathetic fibers
 (3) releasing hormones in response to corticotropin (ACTH) stimulation
 (4) developing after the adrenal cortex begins to develop

117. Axons contained in the hypothalamohypophyseal tract are known to

 (1) terminate on the walls of the hypothalamic-hypophyseal portal vessels
 (2) contain vasopressin (ADH) bound to neurophysin
 (3) originate exclusively from neurons in the septal area
 (4) contain Herring bodies

118. The neurohypophysis is correctly described as

 (1) originating from embryonic neural tissue
 (2) storing peptide hormones produced by neurons located in the hypothalamus
 (3) containing pituicytes
 (4) involved in the milk ejection reflex

119. Human limb development is correctly described by which of the following statements?

 (1) myogenic processes take place in the mesenchyme surrounding limb skeletal blastemas to give rise to the limb musculature
 (2) during early stages of limb development, hindlimbs are more advanced structurally than are forelimb buds
 (3) developing hindlimbs undergo a series of rotational changes during which they rotate medially about 90 degrees
 (4) limb buds initially appear as small elevations from each side of the embryo during the second week of development

120. The midgut intestinal loop is correctly described as

 (1) giving rise to the entire small intestine
 (2) forming the cecum in its proximal limb
 (3) rotating some 270 degrees counterclockwise (viewed from its front) while herniated into the umbilical cord
 (4) undergoing all of its rotation around the axis of the superior mesenteric artery

121. Embryonic development of the pancreas is correctly described by which of the following statements?

 (1) the body and tail of the adult pancreas are derived from the ventral pancreas
 (2) the pancreatic acinar cells are derived from foregut endoderm
 (3) the connective tissue of the septa and duct walls is derived from foregut endoderm
 (4) the portion of the major pancreatic duct that enters the duodenum is derived from the ventral pancreas

SUMMARY OF DIRECTIONS				
A	**B**	**C**	**D**	**E**
1, 2, 3 only	1, 3 only	2, 4 only	4 only	All are correct

122. Which of the following statements may correctly describe skeletal development in embryonic human limbs?

    (1) individuation of the skeletal elements occurs in distal-to-proximal sequence (e.g., metacarpals develop before the radius, and carpals develop before the humerus)

    (2) differentiation of limb bud mesenchymal cells into chondrocytes involves a process known as condensation

    (3) migration of ectodermal cells into the limb bud mesenchyme is commonly thought to contribute to the pool of cells that will become chondrocytes

    (4) ossification sites in the cartilaginous models of the long limb bones are first apparent in the shaft (diaphysis) and later appear in the ends of the model to form the epiphyses

123. The cranial division of the parasympathetic nervous system supplies visceral structures in the

    (1) head
    (2) thorax
    (3) abdomen
    (4) pelvis

124. An articular disk is found in which of the following joints?

    (1) sternoclavicular joint
    (2) temporomandibular joint
    (3) distal radiulnar joint
    (4) knee joint

125. The second branchial arch is correctly described as

    (1) giving rise to the buccinator muscle
    (2) having derivatives that are innervated by mandibular division of the trigeminal nerve
    (3) forming a portion of the temporal bone
    (4) containing Meckel's cartilage

126. Synovial fluid (synovia) is found in

    (1) synovial joints
    (2) intermuscular bursae
    (3) tendon sheaths
    (4) the nucleus pulposus of intervertebral disks

127. The pars distalis is correctly described as

    (1) derived from embryonic oral ectoderm
    (2) containing axons that originate from the hypothalamohypophyseal tract
    (3) containing basophilic cells that produce gonadotropic hormones
    (4) the site of release for vasopressin (ADH) and oxytocin

Answers and Explanations

1. **The answer is D.** The common bile duct lies to the right of the hepatic artery and anterior to the portal vein. It descends behind the first portion of the duodenum and then crosses the posterior surface of the head of the pancreas. It lies in front of the inferior vena cava. The common bile duct and the main pancreatic duct meet one another and, together, pass obliquely through the posteromedial wall of the second part of the duodenum. *(Woodburne, p 462)*

2. **The answer is A.** The second portion of the duodenum lies anterior to the medial border of the right kidney. The superior extremities reach the upper border of the body of the 12th thoracic vertebra; their inferior extremities lie at the level of the 3rd lumbar vertebra and farther from the median plan than are the superior poles. The left kidney is somewhat longer than the right kidney. *(Woodburne, p 448)*

3. **The answer is B.** Three surface features serve to distinguish isolated loops of the small or large intestine. The large intestine has teniae coli, sacculations or haustra coli, and epiploic appendages. The mesentery is the peritoneal reflection from the body wall to the small intestine. *(Woodburne, pp 472–473)*

4. **The answer is C.** The hepatoduodenal ligament transmits the hepatic artery, the portal vein, and the common bile duct. The lesser omentum is a continuous sheet extending from the liver to the stomach that includes both the hepatogastric and hepatoduodenal ligaments. *(Gardner et al, pp 107–108)*

5. **The answer is A.** The axillary artery supplies the adjacent muscles and has the following six branches: (1) the highest, or superior, thoracic, (2) the thoracoacromial, (3) the lateral thoracic, (4) the subscapular, (5) the anterior humeral circumflex, and (6) the posterior humeral circumflex. These branches show great variation in their level of origin and pattern of branching. The thyrocervical trunk is a branch of the first portion of the subclavian artery. *(Gardner et al, pp 107–108)*

6. **The answer is A.** The suprascapular nerve passes through the scapular notch and is separated from the suprascapular artery by the superior transverse scapular ligament. *(Woodburne, pp 88–89)*

7. **The answer is E.** The epididymis is a C-shaped structure applied to the posterior margin of the testis and overlapping the adjacent part of the lateral surface. The spermatozoa are stored in it until they are emitted. *(Gardner et al, p 476)*

8. **The answer is D.** The male accessory genital glands contribute secretions to the seminal fluid and consist of the seminal vesicles, the prostate, the bulbourethral glands, and the urethral glands. The other choices listed in the question are to be rejected because they include at least one structure that is not an accessory gland (e.g., ductus deferentes, testes, penis). *(Gardner et al, pp 47,474–476)*

9. **The answer is B.** The middle cerebral artery is one of the two terminal branches of the internal carotid artery, the other being the anterior cerebral artery. Since the middle cerebral artery is larger than the anterior one, it is considered the continuation of the internal carotid artery. It gives rise to numerous branches on the surface of the insula. *(Gardner et al, p 606)*

10. **The answer is E.** The cisterna chyli, or the beginning of the thoracic duct, receives the right and left lumbar trunks. *(Woodburne, p 493)*

11. **The answer is B.** The root of the left lung is ventral to the thoracic aorta and inferior to its arch. Ventral to both roots are the phrenic nerves, the pericardiacophrenic vessels, and the anterior pulmonary plexuses of nerves. *(Woodburne, p 396)*

12. **The answer is D.** The inferior gluteal nerve, a postaxial branch of the sacral plexus with fibers

from L5 and S1 and S2 is the sole supply of the gluteus maximus. The pudendal nerve innervates muscles of the perineum. The femoral, sciatic, and obturator nerves innervate muscles of the lower limb. *(Woodburne, p 577)*

13. **The answer is D.** The facial nerve is cranial nerve VII, and, as its name indicates, it supplies the facial musculature, which includes also a cervicofacial muscle, the platysma. The latter is supplied by the cervical branch of the facial nerve. None of the other nerves listed in the question supply the m. platysma. *(Gardner et al, p 692)*

14. **The answer is C.** The broad ligament extends from each side of the uterus to the lateral wall of the pelvis. Between its two layers of peritoneum, the broad ligament contains the parametrium, which is composed of connective tissue and smooth muscles. The round ligament is inserted into the uterus near the entrance of the uterine tube. The ovary is attached to the posterior aspect of the broad ligament by means of the mesovarium. The uterine tubes are enclosed in the superior margin of the broad ligament. *(Gardner et al, p 485)*

15. **The answer is C.** The saphenous nerve is the terminal branch of the femoral nerve. Arising from the femoral nerve in the femoral triangle, it enters the adductor canal, where it crosses the femoral vessels anteriorly from their lateral to their medial side. *(Woodburne, p 570)*

16. **The answer is D.** The oculomor nerve (cranial nerve III) arises from the midbrain and passes between the superior cerebellar and posterior cerebral arteries. The other structures listed in the question do not have major relationships with the oculomotor nerve. *(Gardner et al, p 611)*

17. **The answer is E.** The sensory fibers conveying pain, temperature, touch, and proprioception from the head and body synapse in the posterior medial and posterior lateral nucleus of the thalamus, respectively. Some fibers from the dentate nucleus terminate in the ventral lateral and ventral anterior thalamic nuclei. The thalamic nuclei then send projection fibers to appropriate cerebral cortical areas. Olfactory sensations are not relayed via the thalamus en route to the cerebral cortex. *(Heimer, pp 331–335)*

18. **The answer is B.** During development of the cerebellum, the neuroblasts of the ventricular zone migrate to the surface of the neural tube. There the neuroblasts continue to multiply, and soon they move away from the surface to produce the definitive, somewhat centrally located granular layer. The deep cerebellar nuclei are derived from cells found near the ventricular surface of the cerebellum. The cells of the inferior olivary nucleus are derived from alar plate of the myelencephalon. The basal plate of the developing neural tube does not serve in the formation and development of the cerebellum. *(Heimer, pp 15,16)*

19. **The answer is E.** The designation of sphenomeniscus is sometimes given to the uppermost portion of the lateral pterygoid muscle, reflecting its separate origin and special insertion. *(Woodburne, p 252)*

20. **The answer is B.** Branches of the first, or mandibular, part of the maxillary artery include the deep auricular and anterior tympanic arteries, middle meningeal artery, accessory meningeal artery, and the inferior alveolar artery. They generally provide arterial blood to the tympanic membrane, the dura and skull, and the teeth of the mandible. They do not supply the muscles of mastication or the buccinator, which are supplied by the second part of the maxillary artery. *(Gardner et al, 674)*

21. **The answer is C.** The body is considered as a solid geometric figure (like a coffin) viewed in the following six planes: (1) cephalic, cranial, or superior, (2) plantar, podalic, or inferior, (3) lateral (right), (4) lateral (left), (5) anterior or ventral, and (6) posterior or dorsal. The trunk has the same planes, except inferiorly the lowest horizontal or transverse plane, tangential to the tip of the coccyx, is described as caudal. *(Gardner et al, pp 4–5)*

22. **The answer is A.** The female genital organs consist of an internal and an external group. The internal organs are situated within the pelvis and include the ovaries, uterine tubes, uterus, and vagina. The external organs are located below the urogenital diaphragm and below and in front of the pubic arch. They include the mons pubis, labia, clitoris, vestibular bulb, and greater vestibular glands. *(Gardner et al, p 475)*

23. **The answer is B.** In females, digital exploration via the rectum allows palpation of the posterior surface of the vagina and other organs. The round ligament does not reach the labia minora; the uterovesical pouch is anterior to the uterus; the perimetrium is the peritoneal covering of the uterus. The mesovarium is not synonymous with the mesometrium, since it connects the ovary to the broad ligament. *(Gardner et al, pp 483–490)*

24. **The answer is A.** The superficial perineal space is limited superiorly by the inferior fascia of the urogenital diaphragm and inferiorly by the deep perineal fascia, the latter attached to the posterior border of the urogenital diaphragm and on each side to the ischiopubic ramus. The root of the penis or of the clitoris and the corresponding muscles are contained within the superficial perineal space.

This space does not contain the urinary bladder and the seminal vesicles in males or the neck of the uterus in females. The perineal body is located in the median plane between the urogenital diaphragm and the anal canal. (*Gardner et al, pp 502–507*)

25. **The answer is A.** The seminal vesicles are paired organs located posterior to the urinary bladder. They secrete a fluid that contributes to the semen. The prostate does not contain the terminations of the epididymis, which are attached to the testes. The urethra does not convey semen in females. The ductus deferentes are not related to the utricle. Spermatozoa are produced in the testes, or male gonads, and stored in the junction between the tail of the epididymis and the ductus deferens, or reservoir of spermatozoa. (*Gardner et al, p 475*)

26. **The answer is E.** The right atrium has a posteriorly situated, thin-walled sinus venarum and an anterior, more muscular portion. The terminal crest separates the two parts. The posterior, or interatrial, septal wall contains an oval, depressed, thinned-out area, the fossa ovalis. Its prominent oval margin is known as the limbus fossae ovalis. The coronary sinus opens into the right atrium. The valvula foraminis ovalis is located on the interseptal wall of the left atrium. (*Woodburne, p 380*)

27. **The answer is B.** A posterior portion of the diaphragmatic aspect of the liver is devoid of peritoneum, and the hepatic parenchyma covered by its capsule is in direct contact with the epimysium of the diaphragm musculature. This portion is called the bare area, or naked area, of the liver and is similar to that of the posterior aspect of the gastric fundus. The bare area is limited superiorly and inferiorly by the laminae of the coronary ligament. (*Gardner et al, p 406*)

28. **The answer is E.** The accessory pancreatic duct empties at the lesser duodenal papilla, which is located in the second portion of the duodenum. The main pancreatic duct drains the tail, body, neck, and part of the head of the pancreas. (*Woodburne, pp 451–452*)

29. **The answer is D.** The omental bursa, or lesser peritoneal cavity, is a retrogastric space in adults. It communicates with the general peritoneal cavity, or greater sac, through the epiploic foramen. It is sometimes found to be continuous with the cavity of the greater omentum. The coronary, right, and left ligaments serve the liver, not the intestines. The gastrohepatic ligament is the major portion of the lesser omentum. (*Gardner et al, pp 377–380*)

30. **The answer is B.** The posterior inferior cerebellar artery supplies the cerebellum, the choroid plexus of the fourth ventricle, and the medulla oblongata. Its partial supply of the medulla oblongata is of particular clinical importance. This vessel, which is the largest branch of the vertebral artery, forms medial and lateral branches. (*Gardner et al, p 611*)

31. **The answer is C.** The circulus arteriosus cerebri, or arterial circle of Willis, is formed by anastomoses among the four arteries that supply the brain: the two vertebral arteries (branches of the basilar artery) and the two internal carotid arteries. The basilar artery originates the branches (vertebral arteries) that form the circle with the right and left internal carotid arteries. The external carotid, middle meningeal, and anterior temporal arteries are structurally unrelated to the circle of Willis. (*Gardner et al, p 612*)

32. **The answer is E.** The blood supply of the spinal cord is provided by the anterior spinal artery and two posterior spinal arteries, all derived from the vertebral arteries. These three longitudinal arteries are reinforced by radicular arteries and medullary arteries, or feeders, originated from the ascending cervical, deep cervical, vertebral, posterior intercostal, and lateral sacral arteries. There are no inferior posterior cerebellopontine arteries to supply the spinal cord. (*Gardner et al, pp 545–548,611*)

33. **The answer is C.** The muscle coat of the urinary bladder is made up of bundles, the orientation of which is not easy to dissect and follow. The transitional epithelium of the mucous lining of the urinary bladder rests on a lamina propria and is not keratinized. The serous coat incompletely surrounds the urinary bladder. The smooth muscle bundles of the bladder form the detrusor urinae. (*Gardner et al, pp 467–470*)

34. **The answer is C.** The musculature of the pelvis comprises the superior pelvic diaphragm, the urogenital diaphragm, and the inferior perineal muscles. The urogenital diaphragm, found in the anterior or urogenital triangle (trigone), is made up of two muscles: the deep transverse muscle of the perineum and the sphincter (membranous) of the urethra. (*Gardner et al, pp 505–507*)

35. **The answer is D.** The cavernous or erectile tissues of the penis are the two corpora cavernosa, situated on the dorsum and sides of the male organ for copulation. These corpora cavernosa limit a median groove on the urethral surface, where the corpus spongiosum, smaller than the corpus cavernosum, is located. (*Gardner et al, p 509*)

36. **The answer is A.** The tunica dartos is the continuation in the scrotum or testicular pouch of the subcutaneous tissue or tela of the abdominal wall. It is continuous with the superficial perineal fascia and with the superficial fascia of the penis. The ilioinguinal nerve gives off the anterior, not the posterior, scrotal (labial) nerves. The iliohypogastric nerve is an abdominal nerve. The inferior epigastric artery is a branch of the external iliac artery. The pampiniform plexus is made up of veins (in the spermatic cord), not of nerves. (*Gardner et al, pp 479,507–508*)

37. **The answer is C.** The oblique fissure separates a superior lobe from the inferior lobe. A further subdivision of the superior lobe of the right lung is made by the horizontal fissure. The horizontal fissure and the inferior part of the oblique fissure form the boundaries of the middle lobe of the right lobe. (*Woodburne, p 392*)

38. **The answer is A.** If the tracheoesophageal septum is not formed in a given region or is broken after it has formed, a tracheoesophageal fistula will result. A laryngeal web results from a lack of tissue breakdown at the appropriate time. An azygos lobe of the lung is created if pulmonary tissue develops medial to the presumptive azygos vein. Hypoplasia and agenesis of the lung would result from impaired tissue interactions during development. (*Moore, pp 216–224*)

39. **The answer is D.** The parathyroid glands are four minute endocrine glands partially embedded in the medial half of the posterior aspect of each lobe of the thyroid gland. They develop as outgrowths from the third and fourth branchial pouches. The parathyroids secrete a hormone (parathormone) that is necessary for calcium metabolism. Parathyroidectomy may lead to tetany, which is preventable by the administration of calcium salts or parathyroid extracts. There is no relationship between the pineal and parathyroid glands. (*Gardner et al, p 699*)

40. **The answer is D.** The superior and inferior ophthalmic veins drain the orbit. The superior accompanies the ophthalmic artery and, after passing through the superior orbital fissure, terminates in the cavernous sinus. Such topography eliminates the foramen rotundum, foramen ovale, optic foramen, and inferior orbital fissure as venous adjuncts. (*Gardner et al, p 639*)

41. **The answer is B.** The thoracic duct collects lymph from the inferior limbs and abdomen and receives tributaries from the left side of the thorax, neck, and head. The right lymphatic duct is found in the opposite side. The cervical ducts are small and restricted to the neck, and the left lymphatic duct usually is absent. Lacteals are projections of the small intestine that carry chyle that is produced during digestion. (*Gardner et al, p 335*)

42. **The answer is D.** The crura of both the clitoris and penis are covered by the ischiocavernosus muscle. This muscle compresses the crus and retards the return of blood through the veins, thus causing the organ to remain erect. The other muscles listed also are common to the urogenital regions of both males and females. (*Gardner et al, pp 508,511*)

43. **The answer is A.** Both the urethral and vaginal openings come to the surface in the vestibule. Also included in the female pudendum are the mons pubis, the clitoris, an erectile mass known as the bulb of the vestibule, and the greater vestibular glands. The internal female genital organs include the ovaries, the uterine tubes, the uterus, and the vagina. (*Woodburne, pp 511,537*)

44. **The answer is C.** The vestibule of the vagina is the cleft that contains the orifices of the urethra, vagina, and greater vestibular glands and is limited by the labia minora. The hymen is a fold of skin that partially closes the orifice of the vagina. The greater vestibular glands are bilateral, situated behind the vestibular bulb. The vulva, or pudendum, consists of the female external genital organs. The clitoris is made up of erectile tissue and is homologous to the penis. (*Gardner et al, p 511*)

45. **The answer is E.** The broad ligament encloses the uterine tube, the ovarian ligament, part of the round ligament, the uterine artery and venous plexus, the uterovaginal plexus of nerves, and part of the ureter. The greater vestibular glands are located in the pudendum. (*Woodburne, pp 538,540*)

46. **The answer is D.** The male urethra presents posteriorly a median ridge, the urethral crest, which is continuous above with the uvula of the urinary bladder. The crest shows an enlargement termed the colliculus seminalis at the level of the prostatic portion of the urethra. At the apex of the colliculus seminalis opens the prostatic utricle (small uterus), sided by the orifices of the ejaculatory ducts. The vestibular canals are found in females; urethral lacunae are numerous small pits; the ductus deferentes and the seminal ducts do not reach the colliculus seminalis. (*Gardner et al, p 478*)

47. **The answer is A.** The bulbospongiosus muscle in the male overlies the bulb of the penis. The ischiocavernosus muscles cover the crura of the penis. The superficial transverse perineus muscles arise on either side from the anterior and medial portions of the ischial tuberosity. The pea-size bulbourethral glands of the male are embedded in the fibers of the sphincter urethrae muscle. (*Woodburne, pp 513–514*)

48. **The answer is E.** The secondary bronchi are lined with ciliated, pseudostratified epithelium containing goblet cells and have cartilage plates, mucous glands, and smooth muscle. Bronchioles have ciliated columnar epithelium and goblet cells and lack cartilage in their walls. Terminal bronchioles are lined by ciliated cuboidal epithelium and are completely invested by smooth muscle. The respiratory bronchioles exhibit scattered alveoli, functional units. *(Woodburne, pp 394–396)*

49. **The answer is B.** The laryngeal extrinsic muscles are those that move the larynx as a whole. These muscles move more than just the superior part of the larynx. They are classified as elevators and depressors and not as circular and oval. The extrinsic muscles of the larynx are not all unpaired and median, since they are bilaterally represented. There is no muscle called the stylothyroid. *(Gardner et al, pp 765–766)*

50. **The answer is B.** The right bronchus is shorter, straighter, and larger, and, since it is the more direct continuation of the trachea, foreign bodies are more apt to lodge in it. The left bronchus is smaller in diameter but almost twice as long as the right bronchus. The left bronchus passes under the aortic arch. *(Woodburne, p 389)*

51. **The answer is A.** The right lung is divided into the superior, middle, and inferior lobes. The middle lobe of the right lung has two segments, termed lateral and medial. No lobe has superior and inferior segments, although the left lung has superior and inferior lingular divisions. There is no subdivision into lingular and apical, posterior and anterior, or ventral and dorsal segments. *(Gardner et al, p 302)*

52. **The answer is A.** The mediastinum is the interpleuropulmonary space. It is divided into superior, anterior, middle, and posterior mediastina. The superior mediastinum contains the esophagus, trachea, thymus, and great vessels. The anterior mediastinum contains the thymus. The middle mediastinum contains the pericardium, heart, great vessels, and bronchi. The posterior mediastinum contains the esophagus, aorta, splanchnic nerves, and thoracic duct. The only structure of those listed in the question that is not contained in the posterior mediastinum is the thymus or its remnants (in adults). *(Gardner et al, p 279)*

53. **The answer is C.** The cupula of the (cervical) pleura is the dome of the pleural cavity covering the apex of the lung. It is formed by the costal and mediastinal parts of the parietal pleura. It is not thickened or strengthened by the pulmonary ligament, which is a structure found below the root of the lung. *(Gardner et al, pp 293–294)*

54. **The answer is C.** The important relations of the bile duct are as follows. The portal vein, formed behind the neck of the pancreas, ascends behind and to the left of the bile duct. The hepatic artery ascends at the left of the duct in front of the portal vein. The bile duct runs in the free edge of the lesser omentum. The splenic artery arises from the celiac trunk and runs a tortuous course to the left, near the upper border of the body of the pancreas. The right gastroepiploic artery runs in the greater omentum along the greater curvature of the stomach. *(Gardner et al, pp 387,409,415)*

55. **The answer is E.** The major blood supply for the dura is provided by the middle meningeal artery, a branch of the maxillary artery. The ophthalmic artery gives rise to anterior meningeal branches, and the occipital and vertebral arteries provide posterior meningeal branches. *(Carpenter and Sutin, p 1)*

56. **The answer is A.** The pia mater and arachnoid are collectively called the leptomeninges. The meningeal layer gives rise to several septa that divide the cranial cavity into compartments. The largest of these is the sickle-shaped falx cerebri, which extends in the midline from the crista galli to the internal occipital protuberance. The transverse dural septa arising from the superior crest of the petrous portion of the temporal bone is known as the tentorium cerebelli. A small midsagittal septum below the tentorium forms the falx cerebelli; the diaphragma sellae roofs over the pituitary fossa. *(Carpenter and Sutin, p 1)*

57. **The answer is B.** The spinal cord is shorter than the vertebral column in adults. Thus the coccygeal segment of the cord, which is located in the conus medullaris, ultimately is located at about the intervertebral disk between the first and second lumbar vertebrae. *(Heimer, p 47)*

58. **The answer is E.** The inferior olivary nucleus is an important afferent nucleus that projects fibers to the cerebellum. The medial geniculate nucleus is the thalamic nucleus related to the auditory pathways. The other nuclei listed in the question are located in the auditory pathways within the brain stem. *(Heimer, pp 259–270)*

59. **The answer is C.** The following list relates dermatomes with their associated spinal nerves: C-5, shoulder and upper limb; T-1, upper thorax and upper limb; T-10, abdominal wall at the level of the umbilicus; L-1, region of the inguinal ligament; S-1, posterior lower limb and lateral side of the foot. *(Heimer, pp 151–164)*

60. **The answer is D.** The lateral spinothalamic tract conveys pain and temperature sensations. The fasciculus gracilis and fasciculus cuneatus fibers convey conscious proprioceptive and related information. The anterior spinocerebellar tract conveys proprioceptive information that does not reach the conscious level but terminates in the cerebellum. The corticospinal tract is a motor tract. *(Heimer, pp 165–182)*

61. The answer is C. The tactile corpuscles are found in the dermal papillae. The end bulbs vary greatly in dimension and have a wide distribution. The corpuscles of Golgi-Mazzoni are found in the subcutaneous tissue of the fingers. The neuromuscular spindles are widely scattered in the fleshy bellies of skeletal muscles. The pacinian corpuscles are the largest and most widely distributed. *(Carpenter and Sutin, pp 162–164)*

62. The answer is E. The spinothalamic tract is an ascending sensory tract that terminates in the thalamus. The other tracts listed in the question terminate in the spinal cord, as indicated by the suffix "spinal." The fibers in these tracts all impinge on the lower motor neuron or final common pathway. *(Heimer, pp 183–197)*

63. The answer is B. The cartilages of the larynx are the thyroid, cricoid, epiglottic, arytenoid, corniculate, and cuneiform. Only the thyroid, cricoid, and epiglottic cartilages are single and median. They are not ossified before puberty, and the thyroid cartilage begins to ossify around age 20 years in both sexes. They are not responsible for the jugular notch, which is formed by the sternum. The parathyroid and valleculae are not cartilages. *(Gardner et al, pp. 757–761)*

64. The answer is A. The vast majority of the primary afferent neuron cell bodies of the trigeminal system are located within the trigeminal ganglion (semilunar ganglion). A small number of primary afferent (proprioceptive) neurons have cell bodies located within the mesencephalic nucleus of the trigeminal nerve. The axons from the neuronal cell bodies in the ganglion pass into the brain stem to synapse with the sensory nuclei of the trigeminal nerve. *(Heimer, pp 241–243)*

65. The answer is D. The ductus reuniens, which unites the vestibular and cochlear portions of the membranous labyrinth, would by definition contain endolymph, as would the saccule and ampullae of the semicircular canals. The cochlear duct also contains endolymph. Perilymph is present in the space within the osseous labyrinth that surrounds the membranous labyrinth. The vestibular duct (scala vestibuli) thus contains perilymph. *(Heimer, pp 245–247,261–270)*

66. The answer is A. Tumors derived from Schwann's cells usually develop in cranial nerve VIII and are known as acoustic neuromas. Their presence will affect not only the eighth cranial nerve but also adjacent structures, including the seventh cranial nerve (facial), the adjacent pons and middle cerebellar peduncle, the inferior cerebellar peduncle, and closely situated portions of the cerebellum proper, which includes the flocculus. The superior cerebellar peduncle is not in a position to be easily affected by a lesion in the cerebellopontine angle. *(Heimer, pp 257–258)*

67 and 68. The answers are 67-E, 68-A. Fasciculus cuneatus, indicated by the letter Y in the figure that accompanies the question, usually contains fibers originating in the midthoracic, T-6, level and more superior levels. Fasciculus gracilis, indicated by the letter X, contains nerve fibers arising in spinal nerves inferior to the level of T-6. The spatial relationship of the posterior funiculus nerve fibers is such that the most inferiorly originating fibers are located medially and the most cranial are situated laterally. Thus the appropriate sequence from medial to lateral would be sacral, lumbar, thoracic, and cervical. Although trigeminal nerve fibers may be found in the upper cervical cord, they do not lie within the posterior funiculus. *(Heimer, pp 165–182)*

69. The answer is A. The branches of the vagus nerve (cranial nerve X) innervating the larynx are the superior laryngeal nerve, which divides into an internal and an external branch, and the recurrent laryngeal nerve, which terminates as the inferior laryngeal nerve. The inferior laryngeal branch of the recurrent laryngeal nerve innervates most of the intrinsic musculature of the larynx as well as the mucosa inferior to the vocal folds. The external branch of the superior laryngeal nerve innervates the cricothyroid muscle. The internal branch of the superior laryngeal nerve provides the sensory innervation of the laryngeal mucosa superior to the vocal folds. *(Gardner et al, pp 765–767)*

70. The answer is D. The mamillothalamic and mamillotegmental tracts are major efferent pathways carrying fibers from the hypothalamus to the thalamus and brain stem tegmentum, respectively. The medial forebrain bundle is also primarily collections of efferent fibers but does include some afferent fibers to the hypothalmus. The hypothalamohypophyseal tract is the major efferent pathway from the hypothalamus to the pituitary gland. The stria terminalis is a predominantly afferent collection of nerve fibers running from the amygdaloid area to the hypothalamus. *(Heimer, pp 293–307)*

71. The answer is E. The sulcus terminal is the external indication of a well-developed muscular band, the crista terminalis. The upper part of the sulcus terminal is occupied by the sinoatrial node. The conducting system of the adult heart comprises the sinoatrial node, the atrioventricular node, and the atrioventricular bundle, with its two limbs, and the subendocardial plexuses of conducting myofibers. *(Gardner et al, pp 314,319)*

72. **The answer is A.** The anatomic term "infundibulum" denotes a funnel-shaped structure and is used to describe several organs: the ethmoid bone, hypophysis, uterine tubes, and heart. The infundibulum of the heart is identified with the conus arteriosus, that is, the upward or distal extension of the right ventricle into the pulmonary trunk. *(Gardner et al, p 316)*

73. **The answer is C.** The nodule and lunula of the heart are features of the cardiac valves found between (1) the right ventricle and the pulmonary trunk and (2) the left ventricle and the aorta. These are the semilunar valves, located at the roots of the above-mentioned great vessels. Each valve possesses three cusps, and the free edge of each cusp presents a central fibrous tissue thickening, termed the nodule. On each side of the nodule there is a crescentic area, devoid of fibrous tissue, called the lunula (small moon). *(Gardner et al, p 316)*

74. **The answer is C.** The cardiac conduction system is made up of the SA node, three major pathways of atrial muscular bundles, the AV node, the AV bundle (His), the right and left branches, and the Purkinje network. Arteries serve to carry blood away from the heart to various parts of the body. The SA node cannot be supplied by a vein, since the function of the veins is to return blood from various organs to the heart. The SA node is supplied by an atrial branch of the right coronary artery in approximately 60 percent of cases. *(Gardner et al, pp 319–320)*

75. **The answer is A.** The SA node, or pacemaker, is found on the surface of the junction between the superior vena cava and the right atrium, near the sulcus terminalis, and it is crossed by its atrial artery. Therefore, the epicardium or visceral lamina of the pericardium has a much closer relationship with it than with the AV node, located deeply in front of the orifice of the coronary sinus. The right vagus nerve has more control on the SA node than on the AV node. The epicardium contains no Purkinje fibers for conduction purposes. The pars membranacea septi interventricularis cordis is not the upper portion of the interatrial septum either in children or in adults. It is the very small, completely membranous area of the interventricular septum. The AV node is not located either next to the superior vena cava or at the level of the sulcus terminalis but rather is found beneath the endocardium of the right atrium. *(Gardner et al, pp 319–322)*

76. **The answer is D.** The left coronary artery gives off an anterior interventricular branch and the circumflex branch. The right coronary gives rise to the conus artery, nodal artery and posterior interventricular branch. *(Gardner et al, p 322)*

77. **The answer is E.** Lymph nodes polarize infection and disease. An aggregate is a combination of several lymph nodes or nodules. There are several organs (spleen, tonsils) that are composed primarily of lymphatic tissue. Lymph is not produced near the skin, and hematogenic organs produce both WBCs and red blood cells (RBCs). *(Gardner et al, pp 40–41)*

78–81. **The answers are 78-E, 79-A, 80-C, 81-B.** The inferior thyroid artery turns medialward behind the carotid sheath and passes variably behind, in front of, or between strands of the cervical sympathetic trunk. The suprascapular artery passes over the superior transverse ligament of the scapular to reach the supraspinatous fossa. The costacervical trunk divides into the highest intercostal and the deep cervical arteries. The dorsal scapular artery has an intimate relation to the brachial plexus, passing posteriorly through it, most frequently either above or below the middle trunk. *(Woodburne, pp 212–215)*

82–85. **The answers are 82-B, 83-C, 84-A, 85-B.** Muscles of mastication are derived from the 1st branchial arch. The muscles of facial expression arise from the 2nd branchial arch. The 3rd arch gives rise to the stylopharyngeus. The pharyngeal constrictions and intrinsic muscles of the larynx are derived from the 4th and 6th arches. *(Moore, p 184)*

86–87. **The answers are 86-A, 87-D.** The nerves of the arm are the terminal branches of the brachial plexus. These are the axillary, median, ulnar, musculocutaneous, and radial nerves. The axillary nerve is almost entirely a nerve of the shoulder. The ulnar is the largest nerve derived from the medial cord of the brachial plexus. The musculocutaneous pierces the coracobrachialis muscle at its midlength. The radial nerve is the continuation of the posterior cord. The median nerve is distributed to the muscles of the forearm. *(Woodburne, pp 112–116)*

88–92. **The answers are 88-C, 89-A, 90-D, 91-A, 92-A.** Both the SA and AV nodes are specialized myocardium. The SA node is located at the cephalic end of the sulcus terminalis. The right vagal and right sympathetic branches end chiefly in the region of the SA node, and the left vagal and left sympathetic branches terminate chiefly in the region of the AV node. *(Woodburne, pp 386–387)*

93–96.   The answers are 93-C, 94-A, 95-B, 96-D. The obturator nerve is the principal preaxial nerve of the lumbar nerve of the lumbar plexus. It arises from the anterior branches of lumbar nerves 2, 3, and 4. The femoral nerve is a postaxial nerve formed by the posterior branches of the 2nd, 3rd, and 4th lumbar nerves. It gives rise to the cutaneous saphenous branch. The femoral innervates the leg extensors, and the obturator innervates the adductors. *(Woodburne, p 508)*

97–100.   The answers are 97-D, 98-C, 99-A, 100-D. Both the pterygopalatine and submandibular ganglia receive fibers from the superior salivatory nucleus via the intermediate portion of the facial nerve. The pterygopalatine ganglion sends postganglionic fibers to the lacrimal glands. The otic ganglion receives preganglionic fibers from the inferior salivatory nucleus, and the ciliary ganglion receives fibers from the visceral nucleus of the oculomotor nerve. *(Carpenter and Sutin, p 216)*

101.   The answer is B. The deep petrosal nerve is a branch of the internal carotid plexus, the continuation of the cervical sympathetic trunk. The greater petrosal nerve is composed of general visceral efferent fibers for the parasympathetic supply of the lacrimal, nasal, and palatine glands. The chorda tympani branch of the facial nerve carries parasympathetic fibers to the submandibular gland. *(Woodburne, p 278)*

102.   The answer is E (all). The dorsal pancreatic rudiment develops from the wall of the foregut (second portion of the duodenum), whereas the ventral rudiment is a subsidiary diverticulum of the hepatic diverticulum. Through differential growth of the caudal foregut, the ventral rudiment and common bile duct primordium are moved and approach the dorsal rudiment from the embryo's right. As the rudiments fuse, the precursor of the portal vein is caught between them. After the rudiments fuse, the ducts of the dorsal and ventral portions anastomose. The definitive pancreatic duct is composed of dorsal duct contributions in the tail, body, and neck regions of the gland and from the ventral duct contribution in the head region, with the interposed anastomotic section. The "unused" portion of the dorsal duct becomes the accessory pancreatic duct, and the major duct empties into the duodenum with the common bile duct. *(Moore, pp 234–235)*

103.   The answer is C (2,4). The cells of the spiral ganglion receive sensory input from the organ of Corti and thus are related to the auditory system. The hair cells of the crista ampullaris are situated in the semicircular canals, where, through the cupula, they are influenced by relative positional changes in relationships to the endolymph contained within the membranous labyrinth produced by angular or rotational movements. They do not readily respond to linear acceleration, as do the cells in the utricle and saccule. *(Heimer, p 247)*

104.   The answer is B (1,3). The lateral vestibulospinal tract originates in the lateral vestibular nucleus and extends into the spinal cord to influence extensor muscle activity. The superior and medial vestibular nuclei give rise primarily to the medial longitudinal fasciculus, which ascends and descends throughout the brain stem and cervical spinal cord. As it progresses through the brain stem and cord, it connects and coordinates the ocular nuclei and sites of control of cervical muscles to produce conjugate movements of the eyes and appropriate positioning of the head in response to vestibular stimulation. The auditory system does not play a major role in the formation of the medial longitudinal fasciculus but influences the brain stem and spinal cord centers by way of the tectobulbar and tectospinal pathways. *(Heimer, pp 248,249)*

105.   The answer is C (2,4). The blood supply of the pars distalis is derived primarily from the hypophyseal portal system. The primary plexus of this portal system is located in the hypothalamus, whereas the secondary plexus is in the pituitary. The blood within these vessels would contain the hypothalamic peptide-releasing factors. The blood would not contain large amounts of oxytocin, in that this hormone is transmitted intracellularly from the hypothalamus to the posterior pituitary and its related vascular supply. *(Heimer pp 295–307)*

106.   The answer is C (2,4). The fovea centralis is located lateral to the optic disk or nerve head. Although light must pass through the neural retina to reach the receptors of the rod and cone cells, it does not pass through the pigment epithelium, which is located peripheral to the neural retina. Increasing the thickness and thereby the curvature of the lens ("rounding up") increases the refractive power of the lens needed for close vision. *(Heimer, pp 271–286)*

107.   The answer is D (4). The olfactory receptor cells and peripheral processes are located in and developed from the epithelium of the nasal mucosa. The central processes of receptor cells pass through the cribriform plate of the ethmoid bone to terminate in the olfactory bulb. Fibers from the bulb run through the olfactory tract to the olfactory cortex. *(Heimer, pp 287–294)*

108.   The answer is A (1,2,3). Proprioceptive modalities, vibratory sense, and fine touch (two-point discrimination) are conveyed by fibers traveling within the posterior funiculi. These fibers ascend on the same side as they enter as primary sensory fibers. They synapse in either the nucleus gracilis or nucleus cuneatus, and the fibers of the secondary neuron decussate to the opposite side. Primary neurons conveying temperature sense synapse in the dorsal gray horn nuclei at the level of entry. The secondary neuron quickly decussates as it ascends in the spinal cord. *(Heimer, pp 165–182)*

109. **The answer is E (all).** The pontine nuclei relay information to the cerebellum primarily from the cerebral cortex. The vestibular nuclei send fibers to the cerebellum conveying information concerning the position of the head. The nucleus dorsalis of Clarke gives rise to fibers conveying proprioceptive impulses from the lower half of the body to the cerebellum. The inferior olivary nucleus receives information from a wide variety of locations and transmits the information to the cerebellum by means of fibers that are known as the climbing fibers. *(Heimer, pp 211–224)*

110. **The answer is A (1,2,3).** The neocerebellum is primarily concerned with the coordination of muscular activity. A neocerebellum that is not functioning correctly may be reflected in asynergy of movement as characterized by a tremor during movement, inability to correctly gauge distance, and uncoordinated motions. *(Heimer, pp 211–224)*

111. **The answer is B (1,3).** The fasciculus gracilis and fasciculus cuneatus are located in the dorsal funiculi. The spinothalamic and spinocerebellar tracts are located within the lateral funiculi. Therefore, a bullet wound that completely destroys both dorsal funiculi at spinal cord level C-8 would result in a total deficit of sensory modalities conveyed via the fasciculus gracilis and fasciculus cuneatus. *(Heimer, pp 165–182)*

112. **The answer is A (1,2,3).** The spinal nerves related to the midthoracic region of the spinal cord convey sensory fibers and motor fibers to skeletal muscle, as do the spinal nerves related to the rest of the spinal cord. However, the spinal nerves related to the thoracic and upper lumbar portions of the spinal cord also convey the axons of the preganglionic sympathetic neurons, whose cell bodies are located within the intermediolateral cell column of these respective areas. The preganglionic parasympathetic fibers originate in cranial nerve nuclei of the brain stem and the sacral spinal cord. *(Heimer, pp 309–320)*

113. **The answer is C (2,4).** The dorsal mesentery suspends the gastrointestinal tract from the dorsal (posterior) wall of the abdominal cavity. It attaches to the primitive dorsal surface of the gut. The lesser omentum and falciform ligament are regions of the ventral mesentery. The ventral mesentery is a derivative of the septum transversum. *(Moore, pp 229,236–242)*

114. **The answer is B (1,3).** The human placenta is classified as hemochorial in that the maternal blood comes into direct contact with the chorionic derivatives. As pregnancy progresses, the thickness of the cytotrophoblast decreases and ultimately disappears in many areas of the placental villi. Thus, the syncytiotrophoblast and fetal capillary endothelium are always interposed between fetal and maternal blood. *(Moore, pp 14–19)*

115. **The answer is D (4).** The proctodeum is a pit or depression created by the proliferation of mesenchymal tissue surrounding the anal membrane. This pit is covered by epithelium of ectodermal origin and takes the form of a stratified squamous epithelium. The proctodeal portion of the definitive anal canal is the area external to the mucocutaneous junction. The epithelium of the anal canal located internal to the mucocutaneous junction is ultimately derived from cloacal (yolk sac) endoderm and is predominantly columnar in configuration. *(Moore, pp 249–250)*

116. **The answer is C (2,4).** The adrenal (suprarenal) medulla is derived from neural crest tissue, whereas the cortex develops from coelomic epithelium. The medullary cells move into the cortical blastema and become consolidated as a true medulla after degeneration of the fetal cortex. The chromaffin cells of the medulla secrete epinephrine and norepinephrine and are controlled by preganglionic sympathetic neurons. The cells of the zona fasciculata and zona reticularis of the cortex respond to ACTH stimulation. *(Moore, pp 269–271)*

117. **The answer is C (2,4).** The fibers in the hypothalamohypophyseal tract originate in supraoptic and paraventricular nuclei and terminate in the posterior pituitary (neurohypophysis). The cellular products of oxytocin and ADH are bound to a carrier, neurophysin. When found within the neurohypophysis, the secretory product is seen as intracellular vesicles known as Herring bodies. The modified neurons have no major connection with the portal system of the pituitary. *(Heimer, pp 295–307)*

118. **The answer is E (all).** The neurohypophysis is an inferior outgrowth of the floor of the hypothalamus and thus is composed of tissue consisting of modified glial cells (pituicytes) and the axons of neurosecretory cells, whose cell bodies are situated primarily in the supraoptic and paraventricular nuclei. The polypeptide hormones vasopressin (ADH) and oxytocin are produced by the cells in these nuclei, combined with a carrier substance known as neurophysin, and transmitted intracellularly to the neurohypophysis, where the hormones are temporarily stored within the cell terminals. Appropriate stimulation causes release of stored oxytocin, which then enters the blood to stimulate myoepitheleal cells in lactating mammary glands, causing milk to be transported within the duct system of the glands. *(Heimer, pp 21,295–307)*

119. **The answer is B (1,3).** The limb buds appear during the fourth week of development, with the upper limb buds developing first. During later development, the lower limb structures rotate 90 degrees medially, whereas the upper limb structures rotate 90 degrees laterally. Most of the musculature and skeletal elements of the limb develop in sites from the limb mesenchyme. The cranial-caudal and proximal-distal growth gradients are well defined in limb development, the upper limb developing earlier than the lower and the girdle region developing before the digital regions of each limb. *(Moore, pp 366–373)*

120. **The answer is D (4).** The midgut intestinal loop gives rise to most of the small intestine and part of the large intestine. It does not, however, give rise to duodenum oral (proximal) to the hepatopancreatic papillae. The remaining duodenum and initial portion of the jejunum do not participate directly in the umbilical herniation. The proximal limb of the loop is formed from the developing jejunum and ileum, and the caudal limb is formed by a portion of the ileum and the developing ascending colon and most of the transverse colon. A Meckel's diverticulum (yolk stalk derivative) is found at the junction between the cranial and caudal limbs of the loop, and the cecum is thereby found in the caudal limb. Although a total rotational effect of 270 degrees is seen, not all of this takes place in the umbilical cord. Some occurs before the loop enters the cord and some as it returns to the body. The superior mesenteric artery forms the axis of rotation. *(Moore, pp 239–247)*

121. **The answer is C (2,4).** The epithelial components of the pancreas (i.e., acinar cells, islet cells, duct epithelial cells) are derived from the endoderm of the foregut. The connective tissue elements are derived from the splanchnic mesoderm in the area. The tail and body of the pancreas develop from the dorsal pancreatic rudiment, and a portion of the head and uncinate process of the gland develops from the ventral pancreas. Although the definitive pancreatic duct develops from portions of both the dorsal and ventral pancreatic rudiments, it is that portion derived from the ventral rudiments that serves as the terminus of the major duct. *(Moore, pp 234–235)*

122. **The answer is C (2,4).** Development in the embryo follows a general cranial-caudal and proximal-distal sequence. During development of the limbs, some of the mesenchymal cells will aggregate or condense, change to chondroblasts, and produce the cartilaginous precursors of the skeleton. The primary centers of ossification then develop in the region of the future diaphysis of the long bones. *(Moore, pp 366–373)*

123. **The answer is A (1,2,3).** Parasympathetic nerve fibers are located within the oculomotor nerve (cranial nerve III), facial nerve (cranial nerve VII), glossopharyngeal nerve (cranial nerve IX), and vagus nerve (cranial nerve X). The oculomotor, facial, and glossopharyngeal nerves distribute to structures within the head. The vagus nerve fibers are distributed to structures located in the neck, thorax, and abdomen as the nerve innervates the heart, respiratory system, and the major portion of the digestive system. *(Heimer, pp 309–320)*

124. **The answer is A (1,2,3).** Intraarticular structures are found within each of the joints listed in the question. However, the knee joint contains menisci that do not completely compartmentalize the joint but most likely serve to assist in the distribution of synovial fluid. The other three joints listed in the question usually contain a complete intraarticular disk that produces two distinct spaces within the joint. *(Gardner et al, pp 118,152,666)*

125. **The answer is B (1,3).** The second branchial arch derivatives include the muscles of facial expression, a portion of the hyoid bone, the stylohyoid ligament, the styloid process of temporal bone, the stapes, portions of the incus and malleus, and the adjacent temporal bone. The nerve of the second arch is the facial nerve. The first branchial arch gives rise to much of the facial skeleton, the muscles of mastication, and other structures. The trigeminal nerve is the cranial nerve related to the first arch, and Meckel's cartilage is the cartilage of the mandibular process of the arch. *(Moore, pp 179–197)*

126. **The answer is A (1,2,3).** Synovial fluid is produced by the synovial membrane that is a part of the wall or limiting boundary of a synovial joint, a bursa, or synovial tendon sheath. The space within these structures is, in essence, an enlarged intercellular space, and the synovial fluid represents a hydrated form of connective tissue ground substance, predominantly hyaluronic acid. The nucleus pulposus, although semigelatinous in consistency, is not produced by cells of a synovial membrane and thus is not synovial fluid. *(Gardner et al, pp 18–24,535)*

127. **The answer is B (1,3).** The pars distalis of the hypophysis cerebri is composed of cells that have originated from the embryonic oral ectoderm lining the stomodeum. The cells may be classified as chromophils and chromophobes. Acidophilic chromophils produce growth hormone, prolactin, and corticotropin (ACTH). Basophilic chromophils produce thyrotropin (TSH), follicle-stimulating hormone (FSH), luteinizing hormone (LH), and melanocyte-stimulating hormone. The pars distalis cells are regulated by hypothalmic releasing factors that reach the pituitary by way of the tuberoinfundibular tract and the hypophyseal portal system. The neurohypophysis is the site of release for vasopressin (ADH) and oxytocin that are produced in the hypothalamus and transported by way of the hypothalamohypophyseal tract (supraopticohypophyseal tract). *(Heimer, pp 21,295–307)*

BIBLIOGRAPHY

Carpenter MB, Sutin J. *Human Neuroanatomy*. 8th ed. Baltimore: Williams & Wilkins Co; 1983

Gardner E, Gray DS, O'Rahilly R. *Anatomy: A Regional Study of Human Structure*. 5th ed. Philadelphia: WB Saunders Co; 1986

Heimer L. *The Human Brain and Spinal Cord*. New York: Springer-Verlag; 1983

Moore K. *The Developing Human*. 3rd ed. Philadelphia: WB Saunders Co; 1982

Woodburne RT. *Essentials of Human Anatomy*. 8th ed. New York: Oxford University Press; 1988

Subspecialty List: Anatomy

Question Number and Subspecialty

1. Digestive system
2. Urinary system
3. Digestive system
4. Digestive system
5. Heart and great vessels
6. Endocrine system
7. Male genital system
8. Male genital system
9. Peripheral circulation
10. Lymphatic system
11. Respiratory system
12. Musculoskeletal system
13. Peripheral nervous system
14. Female genital system
15. Peripheral nervous system
16. Nervous system
17. Nervous system
18. Nervous system
19. Musculoskeletal system
20. Peripheral circulation
21. Musculoskeletal system
22. Female genital system
23. Female genital system
24. Genital system
25. Male genital system
26. Cardiovascular system
27. Digestive system
28. Digestive system
29. Digestive system
30. Peripheral circulation
31. Peripheral circulation
32. Peripheral circulation
33. Urinary system
34. Female genital system
35. Male genital system
36. Genital system
37. Respiratory system
38. Embryology
    Respiratory system
39. Endocrine system
40. Peripheral circulation
41. Lymphatic system
42. Genital system
43. Female genital system
44. Female genital system
45. Female genital system
46. Male genital system
47. Male genital system
48. Respiratory system
49. Respiratory system
50. Respiratory system
51. Respiratory system
52. Heart and great vessels
53. Respiratory system
54. Digestive system
55. Nervous system
56. Nervous system
57. Nervous system
58. Nervous system
59. Nervous system
60. Nervous system
61. Nervous system
62. Nervous system
63. Respiratory system
64. Nervous system
65. Nervous system
66. Nervous system
67. Nervous system
68. Nervous system
69. Peripheral nervous system
70. Nervous system
71. Cardiovascular system
72. Heart and great vessels
73. Heart and great vessels
74. Heart and great vessels
75. Heart and great vessels
76. Cardiovascular system
77. Lymphatic system
78. Cardiovascular system
79. Cardiovascular system
80. Cardiovascular system
81. Cardiovascular system
82. Embryology
83. Embryology
84. Embryology
85. Embryology
86. Peripheral nervous system

87. Peripheral nervous system
88. Cardiovascular system
89. Cardiovascular system
90. Cardiovascular system
91. Cardiovascular system
92. Cardiovascular system
93. Peripheral nervous system
94. Peripheral nervous system
95. Peripheral nervous system
96. Peripheral nervous system
97. Autonomic nervous system
98. Autonomic nervous system
99. Autonomic nervous system
100. Autonomic nervous system
101. Autonomic nervous system
102. Embryology
     Gastrointestinal system
103. Nervous system
104. Nervous system
105. Nervous system
106. Nervous system
107. Nervous system
108. Nervous system
109. Nervous system

110. Nervous system
111. Nervous system
112. Nervous system
113. Embryology
     Gastrointestinal system
114. Embryology
     Gastrointestinal system
115. Embryology
     Gastrointestinal system
117. Nervous system
118. Nervous system
119. Embryology
120. Embryology
     Digestive system
121. Embryology
     Digestive system
122. Embryology
123. Nervous system
124. Musculoskeletal system
125. Embryology
     Pharynx; branchial arches
126. Musculoskeletal system
127. Nervous system

CHAPTER 2

Physiology
Questions

DIRECTIONS (Questions 128 through 193): Each of
the numbered items or incomplete statements in this
section is followed by answers or by completions of
the statement. Select the ONE lettered answer or
completion that is BEST in each case.

128. The sodium concentration of cerebrospinal fluid
(CSF) is approximately equal to that of plasma,
whereas the potassium concentration of CSF is approximately 40 percent less than that found in plasma. The reason for this discrepancy is that

   (A) CSF is a serum filtrate that is modified by
   the resorptive activity of the choroid plexus
   (B) CSF is a serum filtrate, and potassium is not
   filtered as well as sodium
   (C) CSF is a serum filtrate that is modified by
   the secretory activity of the choroid plexus.
   (D) CSF is a serum filtrate whose potassium
   concentration is depleted by the glial
   potassium sequestration
   (E) none of the above

129. Tremor that is caused by a cerebellar lesion is most
readily differentiated from that caused by loss of
the dopaminergic nigrostriatal tracts in that

   (A) it is present at rest
   (B) it is decreased during activity
   (C) it only occurs during voluntary movements
   (D) its frequency is very regular
   (E) its amplitude remains constant during
   voluntary movements

130. Although both vasopressin (ADH) and aldosterone
significantly contribute to fluid and electrolyte balance, they do not appear to closely regulate blood
volume in the long run. Blood volume is maintained
at near normal levels in diabetes insipidus (absence
of ADH) or Addison's disease (absence of aldosterone) because

   (A) the peripheral renin–angiotensin system is
   stimulated

   (B) salt and water intake are appropriately
   adjusted
   (C) plasma oncotic pressure increases
   (D) sympathetic reflexes decrease glomerular
   filtration
   (E) renal blood flow decreases

131. Under normal conditions, the major mechanism of
body heat loss is

   (A) radiation
   (B) evaporation
   (C) perspiration
   (D) insensible perspiration
   (E) conduction

132. Choreiform movements in humans are most likely
to be associated with degeneration of the

   (A) subthalamic nuclei
   (B) nigrostriatal tracts
   (C) cerebellum
   (D) lateral spinothalamic tracts
   (E) caudate nucleus

133. The stimulation of electrodes implanted in the medial forebrain bundle of experimental animals is
most likely to lead to

   (A) repeated self-stimulation
   (B) rage reactions
   (C) avoidance reactions
   (D) temporary paralysis
   (E) repeated turning movements

134. Many neurons in the basal ganglia are observed to
begin to discharge

   (A) in association with somatosensory stimulation
   (B) at the onset of acoustic stimulation
   (C) before the onset of slow movements
   (D) at a low rate that is independent of motor
   activity
   (E) during visual accommodation

135. The introduction of cold water into one ear may cause giddiness and nausea. The primary cause of this effect of temperature is

   (A) temporary immobilization of otoliths
   (B) decreased movement of ampullar cristae
   (C) increased discharge rate in vestibular afferents
   (D) decreased discharge rate in vestibular afferents
   (E) convection currents in endolymph

136. Reflex sneezing is most likely to be initiated by

   (A) inhibition of olfactory receptor neurons
   (B) stimulation of olfactory receptor neurons
   (C) stimulation of nasal trigeminal nerve endings
   (D) stimulation of gustatory receptors
   (E) stimulation of efferent fibers from olfactory striae

137. Which of the following physiologic responses occurs as the pitch of a sound is increased?

   (A) the frequency of action potentials in auditory nerve fibers increases
   (B) units in the auditory nerve become responsive to a wider range of sound frequencies
   (C) a greater number of hair cells become activated
   (D) the location of maximal basilar membrane displacement moves toward the base of the cochlea
   (E) the latency with which units in the auditory cortex are activated is decreased

138. Stimulation of retinal rod cells with light results in

   (A) increased influx of Na^+ and hyperpolarization
   (B) increased influx of Na^+ and depolarization
   (C) decreased influx of Na^+ and hyperpolarization
   (D) decreased influx of Na^+ and depolarization
   (E) none of the above

139. The peptide substance P may play an important role in primary afferent fibers that conduct responses to noxious stimuli. Sectioning the dorsal roots close to the spinal cord leads to

   (A) increased substance P levels in the substantia gelatinosa
   (B) an increase in substance P in the dorsal root distal to the section
   (C) an increase in substance P in the dorsal root proximal to the section
   (D) a decrease in substance P in dorsal root ganglion cell somata

   (E) an increase in substance P levels in ventral roots

140. The stimulation of nerve endings in the Golgi tendon organs leads directly to

   (A) contraction of intrafusal muscle fibers
   (B) contraction of extrafusal muscle fibers
   (C) reflex inhibition of motor neurons
   (D) increased γ-efferent discharge
   (E) increased activity in group II afferent fibers

141. Which of the following types of receptors would normally show the greatest degree of adaptation?

   (A) muscle spindles
   (B) nociceptors
   (C) touch receptors
   (D) visceral chemoreceptors
   (E) stretch receptors in the lungs

142. A motor neuron receives an excitatory stimulus at its dendritic terminus. In order for that stimulus to result in an action potential, there must be

   (A) electrotonic spread of the resultant hyperpolarization to the axon hillock, where it induces the opening of voltage-gated sodium channels
   (B) electrotonic spread of the resultant depolarization to the soma, where it induces the opening of voltage-gated sodium channels
   (C) electrotonic spread of the resultant hyperpolarization to the soma, where it induces closing of voltage-gated sodium channels
   (D) electrotonic spread of the resultant depolarization to the axon hillock, where it induces opening of voltage-gated sodium channels
   (E) electrotonic spread of the resultant depolarization to the axon hillock, where it induces closing of voltage-gated sodium channels

143. Vagal nerve endings release acetylcholine. The expected effect of stimulating the vagus nerve would be to

   (A) decrease the rate of rhythmicity of the sinoatrial (SA) node by inducing hyperpolarization
   (B) increase conductivity at the atrioventricular (AV) junction by inducing depolarization
   (C) depolarize cells of the SA node by opening potassium channels under the control of the muscarinic acetylcholine receptor
   (D) increase the force of myocardial contractions

(E) decrease the rate of rhythmicity of the SA node by increasing the upward drift in membrane potential caused by sodium leakage

144. Which of the following types of movements occurs in the colon and not in the small intestine?

(A) segmental contractions
(B) mass action contractions
(C) 5 cm/sec peristaltic waves
(D) 20 cm/sec peristaltic waves
(E) peristaltic rushes

145. When the bile duct is blocked, jaundice develops. This jaundice is most likely to be associated with a rise in the plasma concentrations of

(A) glucuronic acid
(B) glucuronyl transferase
(C) free bilirubin
(D) bilirubin glucuronide
(E) urobilinogens

146. Glucagon is secreted by the alpha cells of the pancreatic islets. Which of the following is most likely to induce glucagon secretion?

(A) low serum concentrations of amino acids
(B) low serum concentrations of glucose
(C) high serum concentrations of glucose
(D) secretion of somatostatin by the delta cells
(E) sympathetic stimulation

147. Vitamin B_{12} is required for a number of metabolic processes. Which of the following lesions would not lead to a deficiency of this vitamin?

(A) chronic gastritis resulting in achlorhydria
(B) autoimmune destruction of gastric parietal cells
(C) surgical resection of the jejunum
(D) surgical resection of the ileum
(E) total gastrectomy

148. The major fate of triglycerides within cells of the intestinal mucosa is

(A) hydrolysis to 2-monoglycerides and free fatty acids
(B) incorporation into chylomicrons, followed by exocytosis
(C) incorporation into micelles in conjunction with bile salts
(D) passive diffusion into portal blood
(E) hydrolysis to glycerol and free fatty acids

149. When measuring skeletal muscle tension that develops during isometric contractions, it is observed that

(A) total tension is inversely proportional to the length of the fiber
(B) total tension increases monotonically with the length of the fiber
(C) active tension increases monotonically with the length of the fiber
(D) active tension first increases then decreases with the length of the fiber
(E) passive tension first increases then decreases with the length of the fiber

150. A neuronal soma has a resting membrane potential of −65 mV. Opening potassium channels in the neuronal membrane will most likely cause

(A) depolarization to about −30 mV
(B) hyperpolarization to about −86 mV
(C) initiation of an action potential
(D) no change in membrane potential
(E) depolarization to about +61 mV

151. Electrical synapses conduct electricity directly from one cell to the next. The subcellular structure that mediates this process is the

(A) tight junction
(B) desmosome
(C) zonula adherens
(D) adhesion plaque
(E) gap junction

152. Which of the following statements most accurately describes the response of a cell to a decrease in the conductance of the cell membrane to chloride ions?

(A) the cell will hyperpolarize if its membrane potential is positive with respect to the equilibrium potential for chloride ions
(B) the cell will depolarize if its membrane potential is positive with respect to the equilibrium potential for chloride ions
(C) the cell will hyperpolarize if the external chloride concentration is greater than the internal chloride concentration
(D) the cell will hyperpolarize if the external chloride concentration is less than the internal chloride concentration
(E) no change in membrane potential will occur if the external and internal chloride ion concentrations are equal

153. The drug captopril prevents the action of angiotensin-converting enzyme (ACE). Its clinical usefulness, therefore, is

(A) as an antihypertensive because it prevents renin secretion

(B) as an antihypertensive because it prevents the action of renin on angiotensinogen

(C) as an antihypertensive, since ACE converts the inactive angiotensin I to the active angiotensin II

(D) as a pressor, since ACE converts the active angiotensin I to the inactive angiotensin II

(E) as a pressor, since the action of ACE prevents angiotensin's stimulation of aldosterone secretion

154. Miniature end-plate potentials that can be recorded from a muscle fiber are believed to represent

(A) the postsynaptic action of a single neurotransmitter molecule released from the presynaptic terminal

(B) the opening of a single receptor-ion channel in the muscle membrane

(C) the opening of multiple ion channels in the muscle membrane because of the spontaneous release of a small amount of transmitter

(D) the spontaneous opening of ion channels in the muscle membrane in the absence of presynaptically released transmitter

(E) the opening of multiple ion channels in the postsynaptic membrane in response to a single presynaptic action potential

155. A lesion that produces partial or total blindness but that spares the pupillary light response is most likely to be located in the

(A) optic nerve

(B) optic chiasm

(C) optic tract

(D) pretectal area

(E) geniculocalcarine tract

156. All of the following might be expected to occur in an animal whose bile duct has been ligated EXCEPT

(A) total inhibition of cholesterol absorption

(B) total inhibition of monoglyceride absorption

(C) decreased triglyceride hydrolysis

(D) decreased free fatty acid absorption

(E) none of the above

157. If an electrode that records the activity of neuronal units were placed in the spiral ganglion, it would be most likely to detect

(A) afferent impulses from inner hair cells of the cochlea

(B) afferent impulses from outer hair cells of the cochlea

(C) afferent impulses from the utricle

(D) afferent impulses from the semicircular canals

(E) efferent impulses to inner hair cells of the cochlea

158. If a person suffered a stab injury and air entered the intrapleural space (pneumothorax), the most likely response would be for the

(A) lung to expand outward and the chest wall to spring inward

(B) lung to expand outward and the chest wall to spring outward

(C) lung to collapse inward and the chest wall to collapse inward

(D) lung to collapse inward and the chest wall to spring outward

(E) lung volume to be unaffected and chest wall to spring outward

159. Normally, O_2 transfer is perfusion limited—that is, the amount of O_2 taken up is a function of pulmonary blood flow. All of the following may, however, favor diffusion limitation of transfer of O_2 from alveolus to pulmonary capillary blood EXCEPT

(A) increased extravascular lung water

(B) breathing hypoxic gas mixture

(C) interstitial fibrosis

(D) increased ventilatory rate

(E) strenuous exercise

160. All of the following statements accurately describe the interaction of respiratory centers in the CNS and their effect on respiration EXCEPT that

(A) sectioning the brain stem above the pons, near the inferior colliculus of the midbrain, does not alter respiration in animals

(B) the apneustic and pneumotaxic centers of the pons are not necessary for maintenance of the basic rhythm of respiration

(C) transection above the apneustic center results in prolonged inspiration and very short expiration

(D) prolonged inspiration and very short expiration may be exacerbated by transection of the afferent fibers of the vagus and glossopharyngeal nerves

(E) the medullary rhythmicity center is a discrete group of neurons whose rhythmicity is abolished when the brain is transected above and below this area

161. There is very little protein in the glomerular filtrate. This is because

    (A) all serum proteins are too large to fit through the glomerular pores
    (B) of the positive charges lining the pores, which repel serum proteins
    (C) of the combination of pore size and negative charges lining the pores
    (D) of active reabsorption of filtered protein by glomerular epithlial cells
    (E) none of the above

162. The extra energy required for a burst of vigorous physical activity lasting between 10 and 20 sec comes from

    (A) the breakdown of glycogen to lactic acid
    (B) the breakdown of adenosine triphosphate (ATP) in muscle cells
    (C) the breakdown of creatine phosphate
    (D) oxidative reactions
    (E) gluconeogenesis

163. All of the following are true statements regarding mechanisms of sweating EXCEPT that

    (A) acclimatization to hot weather includes increased sweating with increased concentration of sodium chloride (NaCl)
    (B) stimulation of the preoptic area of the anterior hypothalamus excites sweating
    (C) atropine will decrease the rate of sweating by inhibition of postganglionic cholinergic fibers to sweat glands
    (D) aldosterone decreases concentration of Na^+ in sweat by increasing reabsorption of Na^+ in the sweat gland
    (E) profuse sweating can seriously affect electrolyte balance

Questions 164 and 165

The figure below represents a pressure–volume loop of the left ventricle for a single cardiac cycle.

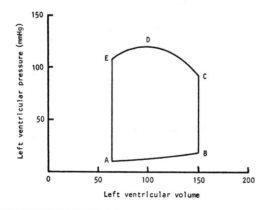

164. The point in the figure at which the aortic valve opens is

    (A) point A
    (B) point B
    (C) point C
    (D) point D
    (E) point E

165. According to the figure above, if aortic pressure is maintained at constant level, a sudden transfusion of blood will result in

    (A) a shift in B to the left
    (B) a shift in B to the right
    (C) a shift in C to the left
    (D) a decrease in the area inscribed by $\overline{ABCDE}$
    (E) a decrease in segment $\overline{CDE}$

166. A major difference between the heart muscle and skeletal muscle is that

    (A) only cardiac cells are made up of sarcomeres
    (B) the sliding filament hypothesis explains only skeletal muscle contraction
    (C) length–tension relationship in the heart does not depict an optimum length
    (D) graded contraction occurs only in the skeletal muscles
    (E) only skeletal muscle has both thick and thin filaments

167. The figure below represents the effect of drug A on mean systemic blood pressure (BP), both before and after the administration of drug B. These drugs are most likely

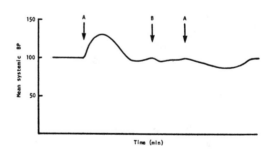

	DRUG A	DRUG B
(A)	acetylcholine	atropine
(B)	histamine	diphenhydramine (H_1 blocker)
(C)	epinephrine	propranolol (β blocker)
(D)	norepinephrine	propranolol (β blocker)
(E)	epinephrine	phenoxybenzamine

168. The pituitary hormone follicle-stimulating hormone (FSH) differs from ACTH in that FSH

(A) is sensitive to proteolysis
(B) is secreted by the intermediate lobe
(C) is a single-peptide chain
(D) is a glycoprotein
(E) regulates the function of another endocrine gland

169. Insulin stimulates facilitated diffusion of glucose into cells of all of the following tissues EXCEPT

(A) fat
(B) lymphatic
(C) muscle
(D) brain
(E) none of the above

170. Which of the following is a strong stimulus to the secretion of growth hormone?

(A) insulinlike growth factor I
(B) rapid-eye-movement (REM) sleep
(C) nerve growth factor
(D) glucagon
(E) free fatty acids

171. All of the following statements concerning CO_2 transport are true EXCEPT that

(A) compared to O_2, dissolved CO_2 plays a significant role in its transport
(B) the bulk of CO_2 transport involves reversible combination of CO_2 with water in red blood cells (RBCs)
(C) CO_2 is rapidly converted to bicarbonate ions in plasma
(D) chloride ions diffuse into RBCs
(E) CO_2 combines with terminal amine groups, and these carbamino compounds are important in CO_2 unloading

172. The cellular volume of human erythrocytes will decrease when

(A) they are suspended in a medium whose osmotic strength is 300 mOsm and that has a sodium concentration of 140 mmol/L
(B) the cells' sodium pump is inhibited with ouabain
(C) they are suspended in a medium whose osmotic strength is 200 mOsm
(D) they are suspended in a medium whose osmotic strength is 450 mOsm
(E) they are suspended in a medium whose osmotic strength is 300 mOsm and that has a sodium concentration of 100 mmol/L

173. In chronic renal insufficiency (glomerulonephritis, pyelonephritis, renal vascular disease), there is a net functional loss of nephrons. If we assume that production of urea and creatinine is constant and that the patient is in a steady state, a 50 percent decrease in the normal glomerular filtration rate (GFR) will

(A) not affect plasma creatinine
(B) decrease plasma urea concentration
(C) greatly increase plasma Na+
(D) increase the percent of filtered Na+ excreted
(E) significantly decrease plasma K+

174. Before inspiration, alveolar pressure (PA) is atmospheric and intrapleural pressure (Ppl) is −5 cm H_2O. At the end of an inspiration in a healthy person, with the glottis open, these readings would be

(A) PA of +2, Ppl of −8 cm H_2O
(B) PA of −2, Ppl of −8 cm H_2O
(C) PA of 0, Ppl of +5 cm H_2O
(D) PA of 0, Ppl of −5 cm H_2O
(E) PA of 0, Ppl of −8 cm H_2O

175. If alveolar ventilation is halved (while breathing room air and if CO_2 production remains unchanged), then

(A) alveolar CO_2 pressure (P_{ACO_2}) will be halved
(B) arterial O_2 pressure (P_{aO_2}) will double
(C) arterial CO_2 pressure (P_{aCO_2}) will double
(D) alveolar O_2 pressure (P_{AO_2}) will double
(E) P_{aO_2} will not change

176. Bronchoalveolar segments of the lung with low ventilation/perfusion ratios may collapse when 100 percent O_2 is inhaled for 1 hr because

(A) pulmonary surfactant is inactivated
(B) O_2 toxicity causes alveolar edema
(C) CO_2 elimination is greater than normal
(D) interstitial edema around small airways causes airway closure
(E) gas is removed by blood faster than it enters the unit by ventilation

177. A patient has a plasma volume of 4 L, extracellular fluid (ECF) volume of 20 L, and intracellular volume of 30 L. If the patient is hyponatremic, to raise plasma Na+ by 10 mmol/kg water would require administration of

(A) 40 mmol of NaCl
(B) 200 mmol of NaCl
(C) 300 mmol of NaCl
(D) 500 mmol of NaCl
(E) 1000 mmol of NaCl

178. A patient is admitted to the hospital with a respiratory acidosis. The patient's renal excretion of potassium would be expected to

(A) rise, since acid and potassium excretion are coupled

(B) rise, since acidosis is a stimulus to renin secretion by the juxtaglomerular apparatus

(C) rise, since acidosis increases the affinity of the aldosterone receptor for aldosterone

(D) fall, since the filtered load of potassium to the tubules falls in acidosis

(E) fall, since tubular secretion of potassium is inversely coupled to acid secretion

179. If the cabin of an airplane is pressurized to an equivalent altitude of 10,000 ft (barometric pressure of 523 mm Hg), the PA_{O_2} in a healthy person compared with his or her predicted PA_{O_2} at sea level will

(A) decrease to < 100 mm Hg because the fraction of inspired air that is O_2 (FI_{O_2}) will be < 0.21

(B) not change because PA_{CO_2} will decrease because of hyperventilation

(C) not change because the cabin is pressurized

(D) decrease to < 100 mm Hg even though the FI_{O_2} is still around 0.2

(E) remain approximately the same because water vapor pressure is low at high altitude

180. In a normal person, Pa_{O_2} is slightly less than PA_{O_2} primarily because of

(A) shunted blood

(B) significant diffusion gradients

(C) reaction time of O_2 with hemoglobin

(D) unloading of CO_2

(E) none of the above

181. The slowest conduction rate is found in which of the following cardiac pathways?

(A) from the sinoatrial (SA) node to the atrioventricular (AV) node

(B) in the AV node

(C) in the bundle of His

(D) in the Purkinje fibers

(E) in the ventricular muscle

182. Radiolabeled inulin is most useful for the determination of which of the following body fluid volumes?

(A) plasma volume

(B) total blood volume

(C) interstitial fluid volume

(D) extracellular fluid (ECF) volume

(E) intracellular fluid volume

183. The anatomic dead space in an individual with a tidal volume of 500 ml is 125 ml when determined by plotting nitrogen concentration vs. expired volume after a single inspiration of 100 percent O_2 (Fowler's method). If the patient's lungs are healthy and the Pa_{CO_2} is 40 mm Hg, the mixed expired CO_2 tension (PE_{CO_2}) should be about

(A) 0 mm Hg

(B) 10 mm Hg

(C) 20 mm Hg

(D) 30 mm Hg

(E) 40 mm Hg

184. A patient is given 100 percent O_2 to breathe, and arterial blood gases are determined. A Pa_{O_2} of 125 mm Hg is associated with

(A) diffusion abnormality

(B) ventilation/perfusion inequality

(C) anatomic right-to-left shunting

(D) the normal response

(E) profound hypoventilation

185. All of the following statements concerning the regulation of respiration are true EXCEPT that

(A) the increase in pulmonary ventilation is linearly related to end-tidal Pa_{CO_2}

(B) the main stimulus to increase ventilation comes from central chemoreceptors

(C) arterial hypoxemia potentiates the ventilatory drive to elevations in Pa_{CO_2}

(D) central chemoreceptors respond to increases in local H^+ ion concentration or decreases in local Pa_{O_2}

(E) an increase in the work of breathing may be associated with a decreased ventilatory response to CO_2

186. In a normal kidney, with a low filtration coefficient, a large increase in glomerular filtration rate (GFR) may be expected to occur

(A) on afferent arteriolar constriction

(B) with strong sympathetic stimulation of the kidney

(C) after modest increases in renal blood flow

(D) with an increase in systemic arterial pressure

(E) on constriction of efferent arterioles

Questions 187 and 188

The figure below is a schematic diagram of renal clearance. In this diagram, Px is plasma concentration, Cx is plasma clearance, Ux is urine concentration, and V̇ is urine flow.

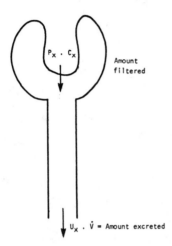

187. If Px = 20 mg/100 ml, V̇ = 1 ml/min, Ux = 25 mg/ml, renal blood flow is 500 ml/min, and glomerular filtration fraction is 0.25, then substance x is

(A) glucose
(B) inulin
(C) *p*-aminohippurate (PAH)
(D) actively reabsorbed
(E) actively secreted

188. In the figure above, Px = 1 mg/100 ml, V̇ = 1 ml/min, and Ux = 6 mg/ml. If these data were obtained from a healthy adult male under normal physiologic conditions, with a glomerular filtration rate (GFR) of 125 ml/min, then x is most likely to be

(A) inulin
(B) Na+
(C) glucose
(D) *p*-aminohippurate (PAH)
(E) none of the above

189. Head injuries can lead to a syndrome in which the hormone vasopressin (ADH) is secreted at abnormally high levels. Patients manifesting the symptoms of the syndrome of inappropriate ADH secretion (SIADH) would be expected to have:

(A) low serum sodium due to the dilutional effect of ADH-induced water retention in the collecting tubules
(B) low serum sodium due to a direct inhibitory effect of ADH on distal tubular sodium resorption

(C) no change in serum sodium, since the dilutional effect of ADH-induced water retention is balanced by a direct stimulatory effect of ADH on distal tubular sodium resorption
(D) high serum sodium due to the direct stimulatory effect of ADH on distal tubular sodium resorption
(E) high serum sodium due to the conconcentrating effect of ADH-induced water excretion in the collecting tubules

190. All of the following statements regarding physiologic adjustments to exercise are true EXCEPT that

(A) alveolar ventilation increases because of an increase in tidal volume and respiratory rate
(B) cardiac output increases with an increase in heart rate and stroke volume
(C) body temperature falls because of increased evaporative heat loss
(D) arteriolar vasodilation occurs in working muscle, with an accompanying vasoconstriction in skin and viscera
(E) the oxyhemoglobin dissociation curve shifts to the right, enhancing O_2 use

191. If O_2 consumption (measured by analysis of mixed expired gas) is 300 ml/min, arterial O_2 content is 20 ml/100 ml blood, pulmonary arterial O_2 content is 15 ml/100 ml blood, and heart rate is 60/min, what is the stroke volume?

(A) 1 ml
(B) 10 ml
(C) 60 ml
(D) 100 ml
(E) 200 ml

192. All of the following statements about the fetal circulation are true EXCEPT that

(A) a significant portion of inferior vena cava flow is shunted through the foramen ovale to the left
(B) the major portion of right ventricular output passes through the ductus arteriosus to the aorta
(C) Po_2 of fetal blood leaving the placenta is slightly greater than maternal mixed venous Po_2
(D) the presence of fetal hemoglobin shifts the oxyhemoglobin dissociation to the left
(E) the liver, heart, and head of the fetus receive the most highly O_2-saturated blood

193. The resistance to blood flow in the cerebral circulation of humans will increase when

(A) Pa_{O_2} decreases to < 50 mm Hg

(B) an individual inhales a gas mixture enriched with CO_2

(C) an individual's hematocrit is decreased to < 0.30 by isovolemic exchange transfusion

(D) systemic arterial pressure increases from 100 to 130 mm Hg

(E) an individual suffers an epileptic seizure

DIRECTIONS (Questions 194 through 207): Each group of items in this section consists of lettered headings followed by a set of numbered words or phrases. For each numbered word or phrase, select the ONE lettered heading that is most closely associated with it. Each lettered heading may be selected once, more than once, or not at all.

Questions 194 through 196

For each condition listed, choose the set of arterial blood gas values with which it is most likely associated.

(A) Pa_{CO_2} decreased, pH normal

(B) Pa_{CO_2} increased, pH increased

(C) Pa_{CO_2} increased, pH normal

(D) Pa_{CO_2} decreased, pH increased

(E) Pa_{CO_2} normal, pH decreased

194. Compensated metabolic acidosis

195. Hyperventilation

196. Uncompensated hypoventilation

Questions 197 through 199

For each cell type in the visual system, choose the visual stimulus that is likely to bring about the largest change in the firing rate of the cell.

(A) a small stationary spot or annulus

(B) a small moving spot or annulus

(C) a stationary bar in a specific orientation

(D) a moving bar in a specific orientation

(E) a moving bar in any orientation

197. Retinal ganglion cells

198. Lateral geniculate neurons

199. Simple cells of the visual cortex

Questions 200 through 204

For each of the electroencephalographic (EEG) patterns named below, select the phase of sleep most likely to be associated with it.

(A) alpha waves

(B) beta waves

(C) theta waves

(D) delta waves

(E) low voltage punctuated by occasional sleep spindles

200. Rapid eye movement (REM) sleep

201. Light sleep (first stage of slow wave sleep)

202. Deep sleep (stage 4 of slow wave sleep)

203. Alert wakefulness

204. Quiet wakefulness

Questions 205 through 207

For each process listed below, choose the hormone that is most likely to directly stimulate it.

(A) estradiol

(B) estriol

(C) luteinizing hormone (LH)

(D) follicle-stimulating hormone (FSH)

(E) inhibin

205. Induction of LH surge

206. Ovulation

207. Stimulate Sertoli cells to convert spermatids to sperm

DIRECTIONS (Questions 208 through 214): Each group of items in this section consists of lettered headings followed by a set of numbered words or phrases. For each numbered word or phrase, select

A if the item is associated with (A) <u>only</u>,
B if the item is associated with (B) <u>only</u>,
C if the item is associated with <u>both</u> (A) <u>and</u> (B),
D if the item is associated with <u>neither</u> (A) <u>nor</u> (B).

Questions 208 and 209

Blood flow through an artery is given by the formula $Q = (P_{in} - P_{out})/R$ where Q is flow, P_{in} is inflow pressure, P_{out} is outflow pressure, and R is vascular resistance. Vascular resistance is given by $R = 8\eta L/(\pi r^4)$ where η is blood viscosity, L is vascular length, and r is vessel radius.

(A) increased blood flow through an arterial segment
(B) decreased vascular resistance
(C) both
(D) neither

208. Low hematocrit

209. Vasodilation

Questions 210 and 211

The figure below represents the pressure–flow curves of a cylindrical tube with steady, laminar flow of newtonian fluid. Flow may be described by Poiseuille's law as follows:

$$\dot{Q} = \pi r^4 (P_{in} - P_{out}) / 8\eta L$$

where $\dot{Q}$ is flow, P_{in} is inflow pressure, P_{out} is outflow pressure, η is viscosity, L is tube length, and r is radius.

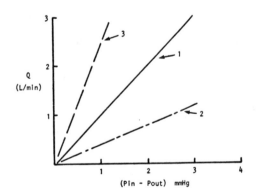

(A) radius decreased
(B) viscosity increased
(C) both
(D) neither

210. Condition 1 to condition 2

211. Condition 1 to condition 3

Questions 212 through 214

(A) increased HCO_3 in pancreatic juice
(B) increased enzymes in pancreatic juice
(C) both
(D) neither

212. Response to cholecystokinin (CCK)

213. Response to secretin

214. Response to food in the duodenum

DIRECTIONS (Questions 215 through 254): For each of the items in this section, <u>ONE</u> or <u>MORE</u> of the numbered options is correct. Choose the answer

A if only <u>1, 2, and 3</u> are correct,
B if only <u>1 and 3</u> are correct,
C if only <u>2 and 4</u> are correct,
D if only <u>4</u> is correct,
E if <u>all</u> are correct.

215. In the figure below, the rates of glucose filtration, reabsorption, and urinary loss are plotted vs. plasma glucose concentration for a constant glomerular filtration rate (GFR). If the above measurements were made at steady state, then

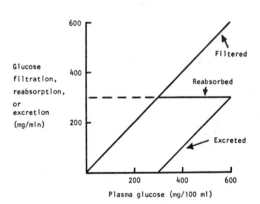

(1) glucose appears in the urine when plasma glucose is < 200 mg/100 ml
(2) plasma glucose is not reabsorbed until levels are > 300 mg/100 ml
(3) 50 percent of glucose that enters the glomerulus is excreted when plasma glucose is > 300 mg/100 ml
(4) GFR is 100 ml/min, and transport maximum for glucose is 300 mg/min

216. A patient is on a ventilator with a tidal volume of 800 ml at a rate of 10/min. The patient's anatomic dead space is 150 ml, and the ventilator's dead space is 250 ml. Which of the following will increase the patient's alveolar ventilation by 50 percent?

    (1) decreasing the ventilator's dead space from 250 to 50 ml
    (2) increasing the tidal volume of the ventilator by 50 percent to 1,200 ml
    (3) increasing the rate by 50 percent
    (4) increasing the rate by 100 percent and decreasing the tidal volume by 50 percent

217. The O_2 dissociation curve is shifted to the right by

    (1) an increase in body temperature
    (2) a decrease in pH
    (3) an increase in diphosphoglycerate
    (4) a decrease in Pa_{CO_2}

218. The normal hemoglobin–oxygen dissociation curve

    (1) reflects cooperative oxygen binding
    (2) is shifted to the left by low pH
    (3) is shifted to the right by 2,3-DPG
    (4) is the same shape as the myoglobin–oxygen dissociation curve

219. Which of the following statements may correctly describe the respiratory quotient (RQ), which is the ratio of CO_2 produced to the O_2 consumed in metabolism?

    (1) RQ is < 1.0, since most of the nonprotein respiratory exchange is in oxidation of fat
    (2) measurement of RQ is an indirect method for calculating energy metabolism
    (3) RQ may be > 1.0 during strenuous exercise
    (4) in persons who fast, RQ will gradually increase during hard work as the proportion of carbohydrates used for fuel increases

220. An action potential recorded from a ventricular myocardial cell differs from that of a sinoatrial (SA) nodal cell, which will

    (1) have a more negative resting membrane potential
    (2) show steady depolarization during phase 4
    (3) have a more rapid phase 3 repolarization
    (4) lack a plateau (phase 2)

221. Pulmonary arterial BP is normally low (mean of 15 mm Hg). It may increase by 10 to 15 mm Hg or more when

    (1) a normal person exercises

    (2) a person enters the hospital with moderate congestive heart failure
    (3) an otherwise normal person has one lung removed because of bronchial carcinoma
    (4) a person suddenly arrives at a high altitude

222. In normal individuals, cerebral blood flow will increase when

    (1) an individual inhales a gas mixture containing 5 to 7% CO_2
    (2) mean arterial pressure is elevated from 90 mm Hg to 120 mm Hg via injection of angiotensin I
    (3) an individual inhales a gas mixture with an F_{IO_2} of 0.10
    (4) an individual increases his ventilatory rate while breathing 100% O_2

223. Which of the following changes may result in an increase in net filtration of fluid?

    (1) venous hypertension due to cardiac failure
    (2) proteinuria due to nephrosis
    (3) lymphatic obstruction due to filariasis
    (4) arteriolar dilatation secondary to allergic reactions

224. In a patient on a mechanical ventilator, maintenance of 15 cm H_2O positive airway pressure at the end of expiration may

    (1) increase pulmonary vascular resistance by decreasing lung volume
    (2) decrease cardiac output by increasing the afterload of the right ventricle
    (3) decrease functional residual capacity
    (4) decrease cardiac output by increasing intrathoracic pressure

225. Hypercalcemia (elevation of serum calcium level) causes a number of physiologic changes related to calcium's effects on excitable and contractile tissues. These changes include:

    (1) diarrhea
    (2) lengthening of the heart's QT interval
    (3) tetany
    (4) hypoexcitable reflexes

226. A strong withdrawal reflex is associated with

    (1) afterdischarge in motor neurons
    (2) polysynaptic pathways
    (3) nociceptive stimuli
    (4) extension of the opposite limb

SUMMARY OF DIRECTIONS				
A	B	C	D	E
1, 2, 3 only	1, 3 only	2, 4 only	4 only	All are correct

227. Pain arising in the viscera is correctly described as

(1) conducted toward the brain in the lateral spinothalamic tract

(2) causing reflex excitation of related skeletal musculature

(3) often referred to a related somatic structure

(4) more intense than somatic pain because of the greater density of pain receptors in viscera

228. The symptoms of a growth hormone-secreting pituitary tumor might be expected to include

(1) increased fat deposition

(2) acromegaly

(3) high serum glucagon levels

(4) hyperglycemia

229. Desynchronization of the electroencephalogram (EEG) may be produced by

(1) stimulation of the reticular formation

(2) sensory stimuli

(3) stimulation of nonspecific projection nuclei in the thalamus

(4) stimulation of sensory relay nuclei in the thalamus

230. Emesis may be initiated by

(1) irritation of the GI mucosa

(2) activation of chemoreceptors in the subfornical organ

(3) activation of chemoreceptors in the area postrema

(4) activation of chemoreceptors in the organum vasculosum of the lamina terminalis

231. Elevated levels of thyroid hormone can be expected to

(1) increase heart rate

(2) markedly increase mean arterial pressure

(3) stimulate gluconeogenesis

(4) cause constipation

232. Insulin deficiency can lead to a number of severe metabolic consequences. These might be expected to include

(1) high levels of serum ketones

(2) high levels of serum glucose

(3) high serum levels of amino acids

(4) decreased delivery of glucose to the brain

233. Products of cells in the adrenal medulla that are secreted in response to preganglionic stimulation, include

(1) Met-enkephalin

(2) dopamine

(3) adenosine triphosphate (ATP)

(4) aldosterone

234. Effects of adrenalectomy that can be directly attributed to the loss of circulating glucocorticoids include

(1) attenuation of the response of vascular smooth muscle to catecholamines

(2) elevation of blood glucose levels

(3) impaired excretion of water

(4) inhibition of ACTH release

235. Regions of the adrenal gland that are most likely to show rapid signs of atrophy shortly after hypophysectomy include the

(1) zona fasciculata

(2) zona glomerulosa

(3) zona reticularis

(4) adrenal medulla

236. Responses that may occur when a person moves from a supine to an erect position are correctly described by which of the following statements?

(1) reflex venoconstriction is primarily responsible for maintaining systemic arterial pressure

(2) hypotension and fainting may occur during pharmacologic sympathetic blockade

(3) muscle contraction in the legs helps propel blood toward the heart

(4) Cerebral veins tend to collapse

237. Cerebellar Purkinje cells may be directly excited by

(1) neurons in the inferior olive

(2) neurons in the pontine nuclei

(3) cerebellar granule cells

(4) cerebellar basket cells

238. The depolarizing phase of an action potential in a nerve cell is caused by

(1) an increase in the permeability of the membrane to sodium ions

(2) the entry of sodium ions into the cell through an electrogenic sodium pump

(3) the passive movement of sodium ions down their electrochemical gradient

(4) an increase in the permeability of the membrane to potassium ions

239. Light impinging on retinal rod cells will result in

(1) increased levels of neurotransmitters being released by rod cells

(2) excitation of all of the bipolar cells

(3) excitation of bipolar cells by amacrine cells

(4) alteration of the spontaneous rate of ganglion cell firing

240. The blood–brain barrier is accurately described as

(1) freely permeable to ionized compounds

(2) primarily at the endothelial cells, which are joined by tight junctions

(3) impermeable to lipid-soluble substances

(4) temporarily disrupted by intra-arterial injections of hyperosmotic solutions

241. The electrogenic Na^+, K^+ pump in neurons is known to

(1) prevent the buildup of internal sodium ions that could develop after the occurrence of many action potentials

(2) prevent the buildup of internal potassium ions that could occur after multiple action potentials

(3) cause the membrane potential to hyperpolarize following an elevation of internal sodium ions

(4) provide the repolarizing phase of an action potential

242. Which of the following may occur during the relative refractory period that follows an action potential?

(1) all sodium channels are inactivated

(2) an action potential may be elicited by a larger than usual stimulating current

(3) potassium channels are largely inactivated

(4) some potassium channels that opened during the action potential still remain open

243. Renin secretion from the juxtaglomerular cells is likely to be stimulated by

(1) increased activity of the sympathetic nervous system

(2) sodium depletion

(3) prostaglandins

(4) increased BP

244. Vascular smooth muscle is stimulated to contract by

(1) angiotensin II

(2) prostaglandin E

(3) vasopressin (ADH)

(4) bradykinin

245. Steps in the contraction and relaxation of skeletal muscle that directly require adenosine triphosphate (ATP) include

(1) calcium–troponin C interaction

(2) calcium movement into sarcoplasmic reticulum

(3) spread of the action potential into the T-tubule system

(4) actin–myosin interaction

246. Which of the following statements may correctly characterize properties of cardiac muscle?

(1) the T-tubule system is located at the Z lines

(2) a transient influx of extracellular calcium ion contributes to contraction

(3) individual cells are electrically coupled

(4) peak contraction occurs during an action potential

247. Glucose uptake by the intestinal brush border depends on the presence of

(1) intracellular potassium

(2) an alkaline lumenal pH

(3) insulin

(4) luminal sodium

248. Several hormones exert effects on the gastric parietal cells. Histamine's effects include:

(1) synergistic action with gastrin and acetylcholine

(2) increased parietal cell oxygen consumption

(3) increased parietal cell chloride secretion

(4) stimulation of gastrin release from G cells

SUMMARY OF DIRECTIONS				
A	**B**	**C**	**D**	**E**
1, 2, 3 only	1, 3 only	2, 4 only	4 only	All are correct

249. In the figure below, absolute lung volume is plotted vs. measured intrathoracic esophageal pressures in a normal person and in a person of similar weight and height but suspected of having lung disease. The figure shows that

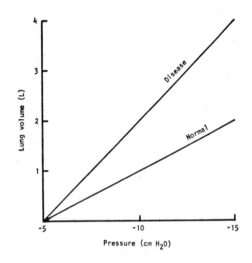

(1) the compliance of the normal lung is 0.2 L/cm H_2O

(2) the compliance of the diseased lung is greater than that of the normal lung

(3) at a lung volume of 2 L, the elastic recoil of the diseased lung is less than that of the normal lung

(4) at a lung volume of 2 L, the elastic recoil of the normal lung is 10 cm H_2O

250. Which of the following statements may correctly describe the coupling of excitation and contraction in the heart?

(1) increases in extracellular K^+ may cause cardiac arrest in diastole

(2) absence of Na^+ prevents the heart from beating

(3) free intracellular Ca^{2+} is primarily responsible for the state of myocardial contractility

(4) relaxation occurs when free Ca^{2+} is taken up by the sarcoplasmic reticulum or bound to the cell membrane

251. A loop diuretic, such as furosemide, works in part by blocking absorption of Cl^- and Na^+ in the ascending limb of Henle's loop. Urine output is increased manyfold because of

(1) increased delivery of Na^+ to distal tubules, causing osmotic diuresis in distal and collecting tubes

(2) depressed removal of K^+ in the distal tubules

(3) decreased concentration of materials in medullary interstitial fluid

(4) depressed secretion of H^+ in the distal tubules

252. The adjustment to working in a hot environment may be facilitated by

(1) providing adequate water and NaCl

(2) dehumidifying the environment

(3) gradually increasing the work load

(4) providing antipyretics

253. Tonic activity in the muscles of the lower esophageal sphincter is believed to

(1) prevent the entry of gastric contents into the esophagus

(2) be relaxed by gastrin

(3) be relaxed by swallowing

(4) propel ingested food along the esophagus

254. Which of the following may occur during alveolar hypoventilation in normal individuals?

(1) the quantity of sodium bicarbonate in the extracellular fluid (ECF) increases

(2) plasma pH tends to decrease

(3) urinary excretion of $H_2PO_4^-$ increases

(4) urinary excretion of $NH_4^+Cl^-$ increases

Answers and Explanations

128. The answer is E. The CSF is not a serum filtrate. The ionic and proteinaceous composition of the CSF is caused by active transport (secretion and resorption) by the epithelial cells of the choroid plexus. These cells actively pump sodium into the CSF. Water and chloride passively follow the active sodium transport. Potassium is not actively transported into the CSF and, in fact, is resorbed to some extent by the choroid plexus. *(Guyton, p 375)*

129. The answer is C. The cerebellum is generally considered to play an important role in the coordination and smoothing out of voluntary movements. Intention tremor, which may be observed in cerebellar disease, is absent at rest but appears at the onset of voluntary movements. This aspect of the tremors readily differentiates them from those observed with the degeneration of the nigrostriatal dopaminergic tracts in Parkinson's disease, which produces tremors that are present at rest. The amplitude of oscillations caused by cerebellar deficits is not generally constant throughout a voluntary movement. *(Ganong, pp 181–184)*

130. The answer is B. In both diabetes insipidus and Addison's disease, appropriate water and salt intake will adequately compensate for the potential excess volume loss. If access to appropriate intake is prevented, however, tremendous volume loss will occur. All of the other changes listed in the question would tend to maintain blood volume, but all are either short-term effects or the result of extreme stimuli, such as hemorrhage or intense sympathetic activity. *(Guyton, pp 431–433)*

131. The answer is A. A wide variety of environmental conditions provoke several mechanisms to come into play to maintain body temperature by balancing heat production and heat loss. The loss of heat via infrared rays (radiation) accounts for more than 60 percent of the normal heat loss. Conduction of heat to objects or to air (i.e., convection) accounts for 15 percent, and evaporation accounts for about 25 percent. Sweating is an important form of heat loss and is regulated by various body mechanisms. Insensible perspiration through the skin and lungs, although important, remains relatively constant despite environmental changes and thus does not provide a major mechanism to regulate body temperature. *(Guyton, pp 851–852)*

132. The answer is E. Huntington's disease in humans is characterized by the degeneration of the caudate nuclei. This is associated with the appearance of disorganized, choreiform movements. Damage to other regions of the nervous system involved in the control of movements may produce other forms of movement disorders. For example, damage to the subthalamic nuclei may result in sudden, intense, and involuntary movements, termed ballistic movements. Degeneration of the nigrostriatal dopaminergic system characterizes Parkinson's disease, which is associated with akinesia and tremor. Lesions of the cerebellum may result in the incoordination of voluntary movements, termed ataxia. The spinothalamic tracts convey sensory information to the thalamus, and their loss does not produce choreiform movements. *(Ganong, pp 178–179)*

133. The answer is A. Experiments have been performed in which stimulating electrodes were implanted in certain regions of the nervous system of rats and the animals were allowed to control the stimulus by pressing a bar that triggered the application of the stimulating current. Electrodes implanted in the medial forebrain bundle, as well as in areas of the frontal cortex, caudate nucleus, ventral tegmentum, and the septal nuclei, frequently led to repeated self-stimulation by the animals. The neural circuits that subserve this self-stimulation behavior have been considered to constitute an endogenous reward system within the brain. Rage reactions and avoidance reactions may be induced by stimulation of other parts of the CNS, such as regions of the hypothalamus. Temporary paralysis or repeated turning movements are not normally observed on stimulation of the medial forebrain bundle. *(Ganong, pp 196–198)*

134. The answer is C. The basal ganglia constitute part of the extrapyramidal system concerned with the control of movement. Many neurobiologists believe that the basal ganglia play an important role in the initiation of voluntary movement. Consistent with such a notion is the experimental observation that unit activity in the basal ganglia is associated with movements and that many units start to fire before the onset of slow, sustained movements. Basal ganglia units are less likely to discharge during rapid movements. The discharge of units in basal ganglia has not been linked to somatosensory stimulation, acoustic stimulation, or visual accommodation. *(Ganong, pp 168–169)*

135. The answer is E. Water that is either higher or lower than body temperature and that is introduced into the external auditory meatus may set up convection currents within the endolymph of the inner ear. These currents may result in the stimulation of the semicircular canals by causing movements of the ampullar cristae. This, in turn, may result in vertigo and nausea. Decreased movement or immobilization of the otoliths or of the ampullar cristae is not caused by such changes in temperature. Furthermore, changes in the discharge rate of vestibular afferents, which must occur with caloric stimulation, are most likely to be caused by the changes in the activity of the receptors rather than being a direct response of the afferents to changes in temperature. *(Ganong, p 139)*

136. The answer is C. The olfactory mucous membranes are rich in trigeminal nerve endings, which may respond to nasal irritants and initiate a variety of reflex reactions that include sneezing and lacrimation. Neither olfactory nor gustatory receptors nor the efferent pathways to the olfactory bulb are believed to be involved in the initiation of such reflex responses. The activation of trigeminal nerve endings by certain olfactory stimuli may, however, contribute to the characteristics of certain odors. *(Ganong, p 152)*

137. The answer is D. The primary change in the cochlea that registers an increase in the frequency of a sound wave is a change in the position of maximal displacement of the basilar membrane. A sound of low pitch produces the greatest displacement toward the apex of the cochlea and produces the greatest activation of hair cells at that location. As the pitch is increased, the position of greatest displacement moves closer to the base of the cochlea. Increases in the number of hair cells that are activated and in the frequency of discharge of units in the auditory nerve fibers, together with an increase in range of frequencies to which such units respond, are all more likely to be observed in response to increases in the intensity of a sound stimulus rather than to increases in pitch. In auditory

cortex, sound frequencies are organized topographically so that a change in pitch may be represented by a change in the location of activated cortical units. A change in the latency with which cortical units are activated would not be expected, however. *(Ganong, pp 140–145)*

138. The answer is C. Light-induced decomposition of rhodopsin results in closure of sodium channels. This results in decreased Na$^+$ influx and a consequent hyperpolarization of the membrane potential. *(Guyton, p 715)*

139. The answer is B. Much evidence has accumulated that certain dorsal root ganglion cells synthesize substance P. This peptide is carried, by axoplasmic transport, to both the central and peripheral branches of these sensory neurons. Centrally, most of these substance P-containing processes end in the substantia gelatinosa, and a variety of experimental approaches have led to the hypothesis that substance P is the transmitter used by the sensory cells that mediate responses to pain. Sectioning the dorsal roots results in a fall in substance P levels in the substantia gelatinosa and in the dorsal roots proximal to the section. The peptide, however, continues to be manufactured in the dorsal root ganglion cells and to be transported along the branches of the cells, leading to a buildup of substance P distal to the section. Sectioning the dorsal roots does not produce an increase in substance P concentration in the ventral roots. *(Takahashi and Otsuka)*

140. The answer is C. The stimulation of receptors in the Golgi tendon organs leads to the inverse stretch reflex. This reflex is responsible for the relaxation that is observed when a muscle is subjected to a strong stretch. Impulses from the organs travel in type Ib fibers to the spinal cord, where they activate inhibitory interneurons. These in turn suppress the activity of motor neurons and therefore lead to the relaxation of the extrafusal muscle fibers attached to the tendons. The activity in group II afferent fibers, the γ-efferent discharge rate, and the state of contraction of intrafusal fibers control the stretch reflex, which is distinct from the inverse stretch reflex mediated by the Golgi tendon organs. *(Ganong, pp 103–104)*

141. The answer is C. When a constantly maintained stimulus is applied to a receptor cell, the firing rate in the sensory nerve fibers may remain approximately constant during the time that the stimulus is present. Such a response may be termed a tonic receptor response. Alternatively, a stimulus may produce a bout of action potentials whose frequency declines markedly as the stimulus is maintained. This is known as a phasic response, and the decline or cessation of firing is called adaptation. Muscle spindles, pain receptors (nociceptors), visceral chemoreceptors, and stretch receptors in the lungs generally show little adaptation. Cutaneous touch receptors, on the other hand, are characterized by strong adaptation to a maintained stimulus. *(Ganong, pp 76–79)*

142. The answer is D. The excitatory stimulation at the dendritic terminus results in a depolarization, which spreads electronically toward the soma. The concentration of voltage-gated sodium channels is highest at the axon hillock. If it is of sufficient magnitude, the depolarization results in the opening of these sodium channels and the initiation of an action potential. *(Guyton, p 555)*

143. The answer is A. Acetylcholine released by the vagal nerve stimulates muscarinic receptors in the cells of the SA node, resulting in the opening of potassium channels and, consequently, in hyperpolarization. It, therefore, takes longer for sodium leakage to cause the membrane potentials of these cells to reach the threshold required for an action potential. The rate of rhythmicity is thus decreased. A similar hyperpolarization of the fibers at the AV junction decreases conduction of atrial impulses to the ventrical. *(Guyton, p 170)*

144. The answer is B. Segmental contractions appear as alternating regions of contraction and relaxation within both the small intestine and the colon. Peristaltic waves also may occur at a variety of rates in both regions and are responsible for the movement of the contents of the small intestine toward the colon and those of the colon toward the rectum. Peristaltic rushes are intense intestinal peristaltic waves that are not normally observed unless a blockage occurs within the intestine. Mass action contractions, which are only observed in the colon, are due to the simultaneous contraction of colon smooth muscle over a large area. *(Ganong, pp 431–432)*

145. The answer is D. Within the liver, bilirubin is conjugated to glucuronic acid through the action of the enzyme glucuronyl transferase. Although some bilirubin glucuronide that is formed in the liver may enter the blood, most of it is transported to the bile canaliculi, from where it may enter the bile ducts and then the duodenum. When bile ducts are blocked, bilirubin glucuronide levels in the blood increase and produce symptoms of jaundice. Jaundice may, however, also develop under a variety of conditions in which the blood concentrations of free, unconjugated bilirubin are elevated. *(Ganong, p 426)*

146. The answer is B. Hypoglycemia is the most potent stimulus for glucagon secretion. High serum levels of amino acids (especially alanine and arginine)

also will induce glucagon release. Somatostatin inhibits glucagon secretion. *(Guyton, pp 931–932)*

147. The answer is C. Absorption of vitamin B_{12} requires that it form a complex with intrinsic factor, which is secreted by the parietal cells of the stomach. Destruction of these cells thus results in a vitamin B_{12} deficiency. The vitamin B_{12}–intrinsic factor complex is absorbed in the ileum. Thus, surgical resection of the ileum will also produce a deficiency. *(Guyton, p 799)*

148. The answer is B. Within mucosal cells, the major source of triglycerides is the acylation of 2-monoglycerides, which enter the cells by diffusion across their luminal membranes. The triglycerides, together with cholesterol, cholesteryl esters, phospholipids, and proteins, then form chylomicrons. These are released to the extracellular space by exocytosis, after which they enter the lymphatic system. *(Ganong, pp 401–404)*

149. The answer is D. The total tension that is developed on stimulating a muscle isometrically is the sum of the passive tension of the unstimulated muscle and the active tension exerted by stimulation. The passive tension increases monotonically with the length of the fiber. Active tension, however, increases up to the resting length of the fiber and then declines as the length is increased further. The total tension therefore also shows first an increase and then a decrease as a fiber is lengthened. *(Ganong, p 56)*

150. The answer is B. Increasing the membrane's conductance to potassium will result in the membrane potential approaching the value dictated by the potassium Nernst potential, which is about −86 mV. *(Guyton, p 556)*

151. The answer is E. Gap junctions form channels that join the cytoplasmic compartments of two adjoining cells, thus allowing electrical current to flow between then. *(Guyton, p 549)*

152. The answer is B. Although electrogenic pumps may contribute to the membrane potential of certain cells, the major determinants of membrane potential are the external and internal concentrations of permeant ions and their relative permeabilities in the membrane. Increasing the conductance for an ion causes the membrane potential to approach the equilibrium potential for that ion. Conversely, decreasing the conductance causes the membrane potential to move away from the equilibrium potential for that ion. Thus a decrease in the conductance of a membrane to chloride ions causes the cell to depolarize—that is, become more positive—if the membrane potential is positive with respect to the chloride equilibrium potential. *(Kandel and Schwartz, pp 39–41)*

153. The answer is C. ACE cleaves the inactive angiotensin I (which is produced by the action of renin on angiotensinogen) to the active angiotensin II. Angiotensin II is a powerful vasoconstrictor and also induces decreased renal excretion of salt and water through its stimulation of aldosterone secretion. These actions of angiotensin II tend to raise blood pressure. Therefore, inhibition of the action of ACE has an antihypertensive effect. *(Guyton, p 254)*

154. The answer is C. The transmitter at the muscle end-plate, acetylcholine, may be released spontaneously in small packets or quanta, without the presynaptic terminal's being invaded by an action potential. These quanta are believed to represent the contents of single transmitter vesicles. Release of acetylcholine activates multiple ion channels in the muscle to produce a miniature end-plate potential. *(Ganong, pp 81–82)*

155. The answer is E. The constriction of the pupil of the eye in response to light is mediated by a pathway that travels from the retina through the optic nerves, the optic chiasm, and the optic tracts. Lesions in these areas are, therefore, likely to impair this reflex. The pathway leaves the optic tracts anterior to the lateral geniculate to enter the pretectal area. Lesions in this area would, therefore, also prevent normal functioning of the reflex. A lesion of the geniculocalcarine tracts, which convey visual information from the lateral geniculate bodies to the occipital cortex, would cause partial or total blindness in humans but would not, however, affect the pupillary reflex. *(Ganong, pp 121–122)*

156. The answer is B. Bile acid micelles serve a ferrying function in the intestine, carrying free fatty acids, monoglycerides, and cholesterol to the epithelial cells, where they are absorbed. The bile acid micelles also accelerate triglyceride digestion by sequestering the products of the reversible digestion reactions. Bile acid ferrying is absolutely necessary for cholesterol absorption. In contrast, the absence of bile acids that would follow bile duct ligation would reduce monoglyceride and free fatty acid absorption by only approximately 50 percent. *(Guyton, pp 788–789,795)*

157. The answer is A. The spiral ganglion contains neurons whose processes project from both the inner and outer hair cells of the cochlea to the cochlear nuclei. Although there are more than five times as many outer hair cells in the cochlea as there are inner hair cells, more than 90 percent of the neurons within the spiral ganglion receive inputs from the less numerous inner hair cells.

Efferent activity to hair cells is primarily generated by neurons in the olivary nucleus. Vestibular information from the semicircular canals and the utricle is relayed via the vestibular ganglion. *(Ganong, pp 139–140)*

158. The answer is D. The response to a stab wound that punctures the lung demonstrates the elasticity of the lung and chest wall. The tendency of the lung to collapse is normally balanced by the tendency of the chest wall to spring out. Thus intrapleural pressures are subatmospheric. Introduction of air in this space allows the lung to collapse and the chest wall to spring out. *(West, 1979, p 99)*

159. The answer is D. Normally, O_2 is transferred from air spaces to blood via a perfusion-limited process. Thus, O_2 moves across the alveolar–capillary membrane by a process of simple diffusion, and the amount of gas taken up depends entirely on the amount of blood flow. Processes that impair diffusion of O_2 transform the normal relationship to a diffusion-limited process. Thus if the O_2 must move a greater distance because of a thickened barrier, as would occur with increased extravascular lung water or cell components (interstitial fibrosis), the diffusion process is limited. Furthermore, decreasing the driving passage (by lowering inspired O_2 concentrations or decreasing the residence time of blood in the lungs), as occurs with strenuous exercise, may also alter the normal relationship. Increasing the ventilatory rate will not have this effect and will only serve to maintain a high gradient of O_2 from air to blood. *(West, 1979, pp 23–25)*

160. The answer is E. The respiratory center of the CNS consists of a diffuse group of neurons whose inherent activity persists even after all known afferent stimuli have been eliminated. Although sectioning the brain and observing respiratory changes are a useful approach to locating important central areas of respiratory regulation, this approach interferes with many complex pathways that may interact. Nonetheless, transectioning of the brain above the pons has little effect. An apneustic center can be identified in the pons. Transection above the center results in prolonged inspiration and short expiration. Apparently, a pneumotaxic center in the upper pons modulates this effect along with vagal impulses. The medullary center is capable of initiating and maintaining sequences of respiration. *(Comroe, p 26)*

161. The answer is C. Glomerular pores have a diameter of approximately 8 nm. Albumin, the smallest serum protein (with a molecular weight of 69,000) has a diameter of approximately 6 nm. Albumin is prevented from passing through the pores by electrostatic repulsion, since the pores are lined by negative charges, and albumin, like most serum proteins, is itself negatively charged. *(Guyton, p 398)*

162. The answer is A. Energy can be derived from either aerobic or anaerobic sources. Although aerobic oxidative processes can provide a significant amount of energy, these processes are too slow to provide all of the energy required. Although stores of ATP and creatinine phosphate are present in muscle, they provide sufficient energy for only very brief periods of exercise. Deaminated proteins may undergo gluconeogenesis, in which they are converted to glucose or glycogen. This pathway is not normally used for strenuous exercise. The breakdown of glycogen to lactic acid provides sufficient energy rapidly enough to support brief periods of strenuous exercise. The depletion of glycogen and production of lactic acid contribute to an energy debt, which is repaid via oxidative metabolism in the period after exercise. *(Guyton, pp 842–843)*

163. The answer is A. Sweating is a function of eccrine glands that are innervated with sympathetic postganglionic cholinergic fibers, and thus atropine will depress the rate of sweating. Stimulation of the preoptic area of the anterior hypothalamus will stimulate sweating. Normal sweat is low in Na+ and Cl− because reabsorptive mechanisms are in part regulated by circulating aldosterone. Serious fluid electrolyte imbalance may occur if sodium chloride (NaCl) is not properly reabsorbed. Acclimatization to hot weather involves increased sweat production with decreased concentration of NaCl, thus allowing appropriate heat balance with electrolyte conservation. *(Guyton, pp 852–853)*

164. The answer is C. In the figure that accompanies the question, diastolic filling of the left ventricle starts at A and terminates at B (mitral valve closes). Depolarization of the ventricles causes contraction of the ventricle. This contraction causes an abrupt increase in ventricular pressure with no change in ventricular volumes ($\overline{BC}$), since the aortic valve remains closed. Opening of the aortic valve at point C marks onset of the ejection phase, and thereafter ventricular volume falls rapidly ($\overline{CD}$) and then somewhat more slowly ($\overline{DE}$). Closure of the aortic valve (E) occurs at the end of systole. At this point, pressure in the aorta is greater than that in the ventricles, blood flow is reversed in the aorta, and the aortic valve closes. In an aortic pressure curve, this is depicted by the isovolumetric relaxation curve, where ventricular pressure decreases rapidly with no change in ventricular volumes. *(Berne and Levy, p 92)*

165. The answer is B. An increase in filling by transfusion of blood will, at constant aortic pressure, increase the end-diastolic pressure (point B in the figure that accompanies the question). By the Frank-

Starling law of the heart, an increase in filling will be accompanied by an increase in stroke volume. Thus C will be shifted to the right and $\overline{CDE}$ will increase. The area inside the curve represents stroke work and would be expected to be increased with an increase in cardiac output. *(Berne and Levy, p 92)*

166. The answer is D. The heart is a functional syncyctium, since a wave of depolarization causes the entire myocardium to contract when a suprathreshold stimulus is applied. In skeletal muscle, graded contraction can occur and is a function of the number of muscle fibers that are stimulated. Although there are other differences, both cell types consist of sarcomeres with thick (myosin) and thin (actin) filaments. Similar length–tension curves for both cell types have been demonstrated, with optimal sarcomere length characteristic of both. Although still a hypothesis, the sliding filament theory appears to adequately describe muscle mechanics of both the heart and skeletal muscles. At rest, the thin actin filaments are separated but overlap the thick myosin filaments. During stimulation, the actin filaments are pulled inward among myosin filaments, resulting in muscle contraction. *(Berne and Levy, pp 72–76; Guyton, pp 122,131–132)*

167. The answer is E. Epinephrine has both α- and β-receptor effects. The α effect causes a rise in systemic BP. By blocking this α effect with phenoxybenzamine, the β effect is unmasked, which is usually a moderate decrease in systemic BP. Histamine usually depresses systemic BP, as might acetylcholine. Occasionally, high doses of acetylcholine increase BP because of stimulation of the adrenal gland and release of epinephrine. However, atropine would not antagonize this effect. β blockade will enhance the effect of both epinephrine and norepinephrine. *(Berne and Levy, p 217)*

168. The answer is D. Both FSH and ACTH have a primary peptide structure and are therefore subject to degradation by proteolytic enzymes. FSH, however, belongs to that group of pituitary hormones that contain carbohydrates in their structure and are made up of two different protein subunits. Other glycoproteins in this group are thyroid-stimulating hormone (TSH) and luteinizing hormone (LH). ACTH, on the other hand, is a single-polypeptide chain. Both FSH and ACTH regulate the functions of other endocrine glands. *(Ganong, pp 204–206)*

169. The answer is D. Insulin action stimulates the activation or membrane insertion of glucose carriers in most of its target tissues. These glucose carriers greatly enhance the permeability of the cell membrane to glucose, thus allowing glucose to flow passively down its concentration gradient into the cytoplasm. Glucose uptake is not stimulated by insulin in liver and brain. *(Guyton, p 926)*

170. **The answer is D.** A variety of stimuli are able to elicit an increase in the release of growth hormone, including elevations in the plasma concentration of glucagon. Growth hormone acts by increasing the circulating levels of certain growth factors. Among growth factors that have been described are insulinlike growth factor I and nerve growth factor, although the identity and actions of the growth factors controlled by growth hormone have not been fully elucidated. Although an increase in the rate of growth hormone secretion occurs at the onset of sleep, episodes of REM sleep are associated with a decrease in the secretion of this hormone. The release of growth hormone is also enhanced by fasting and by exercise and may be inhibited by glucose and free fatty acids. *(Ganong, pp 204–206)*

171. **The answer is C.** The solubility of CO_2 in blood is 20 times that of O_2, and thus a small (5 percent) but considerable portion of CO_2 is dissolved in blood. More importantly, almost 10 percent of the total CO_2 transported is in the dissolved form. The bulk of CO_2 transport involves its reversible combination with water. This occurs rapidly enough because of the action of carbonic anhydrase, an enzyme located inside RBCs. As bicarbonate ion diffuses out of RBCs, chloride ions diffuse in according to Gibbs-Donnan equilibrium. Combination of CO_2 with amine groups, especially those of hemoglobin, also accounts for a considerable portion of CO_2 transport (30 percent). *(West, 1979, pp 74–75)*

172. **The answer is D.** The normal osmolality of plasma is approximately 300 mOsm. In order to maintain a stable intracellular volume, therefore, cells such as erythrocytes work to maintain an intracellular osmolarity of about 300 mOsm. Placing red blood cells in a medium with an osmotic strength of 450 mOsm will result in net water loss and consequent cell shrinkage, since the cell membrane is permeable to water, and the osmotic driving force will cause water to flow from the more dilute to the more concentrated compartment. The cell volume will not be affected by the ionic composition of the extracellular medium as long as its ionic strength is 300 mOsm. Inhibiting the sodium pump will result in an increase in intracellular sodium, with a resultant increase in the osmotic strength of the intracellular fluid and will thus cause the cells to swell. *(Guyton, pp 94–98)*

173. **The answer is D.** Such substances as creatinine (almost exclusively excreted by glomerular filtration) and urea (some reabsorption) have no adaptive mechanisms to regulate plasma levels. Thus a significant decrease in GFR results in significant increases in plasma creatinine and urea (if production of both species is constant). This is because the amount excreted ($U_x \cdot \dot{V}$) equals the amount produced. Furthermore, $U_x \cdot \dot{V}$ equals $GFR \cdot P_x$. If GFR decreases, P_x increases. However, both Na^+ and K^+ need to be closely regulated. Thus as GFR decreases in disease, the percentage of either Na^+ or K^+ excreted increases in order to maintain a normal amount of Na^+ or K^+ excretion. In kidney disease, some unknown natriuretic and kaliuretic substance may be responsible for this adaptive mechanism. *(Mountcastle, pp 1211–1215)*

174. **The answer is E.** At any time in the respiratory cycle, when the glottis is open and no air is moving, P_A is equal to atmospheric pressure, or 9 cm H_2O. Inspiration is accomplished by a decrease in P_{pl} such that it is most subatmospheric at end-inspiration. The increase in thoracic volume lowers P_{pl}, and the elastic recoil of the lung (surface tension, tissue forces) determines the magnitude of the decrease. During expiration, P_A is > 0 and P_{pl} returns toward -5 cm H_2O in this case. With a forced expiratory maneuver, P_{pl} can be > 0 cm H_2O. *(West, 1979, p 103)*

175. **The answer is C.** The relationship between alveolar ventilation ($\dot{V}_A$) and alveolar CO_2 pressure (P_{ACO_2}) is represented as

$$\dot{V}_A = \frac{\dot{V}_{CO_2}}{P_{ACO_2}} \times K$$

where K is a constant such that $P_{ACO_2} = F_{ECO_2} \times K$. ($F_{ECO_2}$ is the fraction of expired CO_2.) Since $\dot{V}_{CO_2}$ is constant, P_{ACO_2} will double if $\dot{V}_A$ is halved. In normal persons, P_{ACO_2} is virtually identical to arterial CO_2 pressure (P_{aCO_2}). Unless inspired air is enriched with O_2, arterial O_2 pressure (P_{aO_2}) and alveolar O_2 pressure (P_{AO_2}) will decrease. *(West, 1979, pp 17,54)*

176. **The answer is E.** When ventilation/perfusion ($\dot{V}_A/\dot{Q}$) inspired ratios become very low, an unstable situation occurs. At the point beyond which all the gas is removed by blood, very little gas is available for expiration from this bronchoalveolar segment. A critical point then arises, and the unit tends to collapse. Neither O_2 toxicity nor surfactant inactivation would be expected to occur in this brief period of time. Although interstitial edema may occur, this would more likely produce trapped air segments than collapsed alveoli. CO_2 elimination will eventually decrease to zero as the unit collapses. *(West, 1981, pp 184–186)*

177. **The answer is D.** A NaCl increase of 10 mmol/kg of body water is equivalent to an increase of 20 mOsm/kg body water, since NaCl rapidly ionizes. In the patient described in the question, whole body

water is 20 L + 30 L, or 50 L. Thus, 50 L × 20 mOsm/L = 1,000 mOsm of solute. Since 500 mmol of NaCl is equal to 1,000 mOsm of NaCl, 500 mmol of NaCl is necessary for therapy. *(Mountcastle, p 1156)*

178. The answer is E. Secretion of acid and of potassium by the renal tubule are inversely related. Thus, increased excretion of protons will result in decreased secretion (or increased retention) of potassium ions, with the result that the body's potassium store rises. *(Davenport, 1974, p 81)*

179. The answer is D. Even though the cabin of the airplane described in the question is pressurized, the barometric pressure decreased to 523 mm Hg. Thus, the $F_{I}O_2$ remains the same (0.21) but inspired P_{O_2} decreases, since it is the product of $F_{I}O_2$ and barometric pressure. Water vapor pressure remains at 47 mm Hg as long as body temperature is normal, and thus P_{O_2} of humidified alveolar air must be less than that at sea level. Although a decrease in P_{ACO_2} (due to some hyperventilation) may slightly enhance P_{AO_2} and the rate of P_{AO_2} loss to body metabolism may decrease, neither is sufficient to prevent the decrease in P_{AO_2} due to the drop in barometric pressure. *(West, 1979, p 128)*

180. The answer is A. Shunted blood is blood that bypasses ventilated parts of the lung and directly enters the arterial circulation. In normal persons, this is largely due to mixing of arterial blood with bronchial venous and some myocardial venous blood, which drains into the left heart. Diffusion, although finite, is usually immeasurably small, as is reaction velocity with hemoglobin. *(West, 1979, p 54)*

181. The answer is B. Under normal circumstances, depolarization is initiated in the SA node and then propagates to the AV node. From there, action potentials are propagated through the bundle of His and through the Purkinje system to the ventricular muscle. Conduction in the AV node is slower than conduction either from the SA node to the AV node or from the AV node to ventricular muscle. The AV nodal delay is typically of the order of 100 msec. *(Ganong, p 459)*

182. The answer is D. Inulin is an inert carbohydrate that fails to enter cells but readily enters extracellular space. It is therefore most useful in the determination of the ECF volume. If the plasma volume has been determined by some other method, the interstitial fluid volume may be calculated as the difference between the extracellular and plasma volumes. *(Ganong, pp 1–2)*

183. The answer is D. Bohr's equation states that

$$\dot{V}_D/\dot{V}_T = (P_{ACO_2} - P_{ECO_2})/P_{ACO_2}$$

where P_{ECO_2} is mixed expired CO_2. In a normal person, P_{ACO_2} is virtually identical to P_{ACO_2}. Thus

$$\dot{V}_D/\dot{V}_T = (P_{ACO_2} - P_{ECO_2})/P_{ACO_2}$$

Since by Fowler's method, $\dot{V}_D/\dot{V}_T = 0.25$ in the patient described in the question, the $(P_{ACO_2} - P_{ECO_2})/P_{ACO_2} = 0.25$ (40 − P_{ECO_2})/40 = 0.25. Therefore P_{ECO_2} = 30 mm Hg. If considerable inequality of blood flow and ventilation were present, P_{ECO_2} could be much less than 30 mm Hg, and the patient's physiologic dead space would exceed the anatomic dead space. *(West, 1979, p 20)*

184. The answer is C. In an ideal lung, breathing 100 percent O_2 should increase P_{AO_2} to P_{AO_2} (approximately 670 mm Hg). In abnormalities related to diffusion impairment or hypoventilation, the driving pressure, or P_{AO_2}, is still sufficiently high to raise P_{AO_2} to almost alveolar levels. In $\dot{V}/\dot{Q}$ abnormalities, P_{AO_2} will differ from communicating air spaces only by differences in P_{ACO_2}. Thus P_{AO_2} will be high in all counts. In true anatomic right-to-left shunts, such as atrial septal defects, hypoxemia will not be greatly relieved by breathing 100 percent O_2. The small increase in P_{AO_2} is due mostly to dissolved O_2. Right-to-left shunts differ from other pulmonary diseases associated with impaired gas exchange in that desaturated blood directly enters the arterial circulation, and at the upper part of the O_2 dissociation curve, a small decrease in content is accompanied by a large decrease in P_{AO_2}. *(West, 1979, pp 56–57)*

185. The answer is D. Hypoxemia is an important stimulus to ventilatory drive but derives all its effects via stimulation of peripheral, *not* central, chemoreceptors. In humans, the most important regulating factor with respect to ventilation is the P_{ACO_2}. Ventilation increases linearly with a rise in P_{AO_2}. Although some of the response to CO_2 may be attributed to peripheral chemoreceptors, the largest percentage is the result of stimulation of central chemoreceptors. The effect of CO_2 presumably is via increase in H^+ in the cerebrospinal fluid (CSF) and cerebral extracellular fluid (ECF). Arterial hypoxemia will potentiate this effect, both by increasing the response to CO_2 and by reducing the level at which this response occurs. Increased work of breathing will reduce this ventilatory drive by depressing the effector organs involved. *(West, 1979, pp 121–124)*

186. The answer is E. GFR is equal to the product of filtration pressure and a filtration coefficient. The glomerular capillary pressure is approximately 60 mm Hg and will *decrease* with afferent arteriolar vasoconstriction or *increase* with efferent arteriolar vasoconstriction. The hydraulic pressure in Bowman's capsule is approximately 18 mm Hg. The colloid osmotic pressure entering the capsule is 28 mm Hg and rises 20 to 25 percent as protein-free plasma is filtered. Alterations in these forces will produce expected changes in filtration. An increase in renal blood flow in a glomerulus with low filtration coefficient will produce only modest increases in GFR. This is because a low filtration coefficient causes fluid to be reabsorbed at the efferent artery, and colloid osmotic pressure promptly rises. Sympathetic stimulation will cause afferent vasoconstriction and thus lower plasma hydraulic pressure. A rise in blood pressure may be expected to increase GFR, but the kidney autoregulates and afferent vasoconstriction maintains GFR. *(Guyton, pp 399–400)*

187. **The answer is B.** Plasma clearance, or Cx, $(ml/min) = (x \cdot \dot{V})/Px$. In the example that accompanies the question, $Cx = (25 \text{ mg/ml}) \times 1 \text{ ml/min}/(20 \text{ mg/100 ml}) = 125 \text{ ml/min}$. If renal blood flow is 500 ml/min and glomerular filtration fraction is 0.25, then the glomerular filtration rate (GFR) is 125 ml/min. If Cx = GFR, then substance x is neither reabsorbed nor secreted and may be inulin or perhaps creatinine. Glucose is normally totally reabsorbed, and PAH is actively secreted. *(Mountcastle, p 1175)*

188. **The answer is D.** Plasma clearance of substance x in the question is represented as

$$\frac{(6 \text{ mg/ml}) \times (1 \text{ ml/min})}{1 \text{ mg/100 ml}} = \frac{600 \text{ ml}}{\text{min}}$$

If the GFR = 125 mL/min, then 600 mL/min is a reasonable value for effective renal plasma flow (ERPF). PAH is a substance that freely crosses the glomerular membrane, but unlike inulin, it is secreted into the tubules by tubular epithelium. A value of 600 mL/min is a reasonable normal value for ERPF. Actual flow is somewhat higher, since extraction of PAH is not complete (< 85 percent). Plasma clearance of Na^+ in a normal subject is orders of magnitude less than the GFR, and in normal individuals there is no clearance of glucose. *(Mountcastle, p 1175)*

189. **The answer is A.** ADH acts on the collecting tubules of the kidney to induce water retention. Inappropriately high levels of ADH, as are achieved in SIADH, result in the renal retention of free water, which consequently exerts a dilutional effect on serum ion concentrations. Thus, serum sodium can fall dramatically in SIADH. ADH does not exert any direct effect on the renal handling of sodium. *(Guyton, p 895)*

190. **The answer is C.** Strenuous exercise provides a good example of how various physiologic adjustments operate and are integrated. Although the un-

derlying mechanisms are in large part unknown, it is clear that alveolar ventilation and cardiac output both increase. Regional blood flow is altered so that active muscles have increased blood flow and less active, nonessential areas, such as the skin and viscera, have temporally decreased blood flow. O_2 use is enhanced by decreases in tissue Po_2 in exercising muscle, as well as a shift to the right of the oxyhemoglobin dissociation curve due to increases in H^+, temperature, and CO_2. The body temperature rises, although sweating mechanisms are significantly increased. *(Mountcastle, pp 1401–1411)*

191. **The answer is D.** The Fick principle is derived by applying the law of conservation of mass and states that

$$\dot{V}o_2 = \dot{Q}(Cao_2 - C\overline{v}o_2)$$

where $\dot{V}o_2$ is O_2 consumption, $\dot{Q}$ is cardiac output, and Cao_2 and $C\overline{v}o_2$ are arterial and mixed venous O_2 content, respectively.

Thus,

$$\dot{Q} = \frac{Vo_2}{(Cao_2 - C\overline{v}o_2)}; \quad \dot{Q} = \frac{300 \text{ ml/min}}{(20-15)\text{ml}/100 \text{ ml}} = \frac{6,000 \text{ ml}}{\text{min}}$$

Stroke volume × heart rate = cardiac output.

$$\text{Stroke volume} = \frac{\text{Cardiac output}}{\text{heart rate}} = \frac{6,000 \text{ ml/min}}{60/\text{min}} = 100 \text{ ml}.$$

(Berne and Levy, p 183)

192. **The answer is C.** The high rate of blood flow at the placenta and the significant resistance of the placenta to diffusion of O_2 result in blood in the umbilical vein that has a lower Po_2 (30 mm Hg) than maternal mixed venous blood. However, the shift in fetal oxyhemoglobin concentration and the Bohr effect all increase the transport of O_2 to fetal tissues. A number of significant differences in circulating patterns are present in the fetus, including shunting of blood across a patent foramen ovale and ductus arteriosus. The net effect of these shunts in the presence of high fetal pulmonary vascular resistance is very low fetal pulmonary blood flow. At birth, these patterns normally are quickly changed to ex utero patterns with high pulmonary perfusion. Since the liver is supplied by umbilical venous blood and the heart and head receive blood before it has mixed with significant amounts of desaturated blood, these important organs receive blood that is relatively high in saturated oxyhemoglobin. *(Berne and Levy, pp 248–250)*

193. **The answer is D.** Cerebral blood flow will increase when Pao_2 is decreased to > 50 mm Hg or when $Paco_2$ increases above normal. A decrease in viscosity will also increase cerebral blood flow. Cerebral blood flow is closely linked to brain parenchymal metabolism, and intense activity during a seizure will result in large, widespread increases in blood flow. Since resistance is equal to the ratio of pressure/flow, the factors listed that increase flow are likely to *decrease* vascular resistance. In addition, the brain autoregulates, and consequently an increase in blood pressure is offset by an *increase* in local vascular resistance to maintain constant cerebral blood flow. *(Berne and Levy, pp 233–235)*

194–196. The answers are 194-A, 195-D, 196-B. Metabolic acidosis as a result of diabetes mellitus, hypoxemia, or other factors causes HCO_3^- to fall and lower the pH. The increased H^+ ions increase the ventilatory rate by their actions on peripheral chemoreceptors, thus lowering the $Paco_2$ and returning the pH toward normal values.

Hyperventilation will decrease $Paco_2$ ($\dot{V}A = [\dot{V} co_2 \times K]/Paco_2$) and thus increase $(Hco_3^-)/Paco_2$, thereby elevating pH.

Hypoventilation due to overdosage of drugs or CNS pathology results in an increase in $Paco_2$. When there is no renal compensation, the pH will decrease. Increased $Paco_2$ and normal pH might be encountered during respiratory compensation for metabolic alkalosis. Normal $Paco_2$ and decreased pH are most likely to occur during metabolic acidosis without respiratory compensation. *(West, 1979, pp 79–84)*

197–199. The answers are 197-A, 198-A, 199-C. Retinal ganglion cells relay visual information from the retina to other regions of the brain after it has been processed by the retinal network containing the photoreceptors and the horizontal, bipolar, and amacrine cells. The optimal stimulus for a retinal ganglion cell is typically a stationary spot or annulus of light in its circular receptive field. Two types of cell responses may be observed. A ganglion cell may be excited by a spot of light at the center of its receptive field and inhibited by an annulus of light that surrounds the center (an on-center cell). Conversely, inhibition by a central spot of light and excitation by the surrounding annulus may be observed (an off-center cell). Moving stimuli are not optimal for retinal ganglion cells. A stationary bar in any orientation within its receptive field also will generally evoke a brisk response in a retinal ganglion cell. Such a stimulus is not considered optimal, however, because it simultaneously activates both the center and, to a lesser extent, the surrounding area of the receptive field.

The response properties of neurons in the lateral geniculate are for the most part similar to those of retinal ganglion cells, the optimal stimulus also being a small stationary spot or annulus. For this reason, the lateral geniculate is widely considered

to be a relay station that faithfully transmits information from the retina to the cortex, with little internal processing of visual information.

In contrast to cells in the retina and the lateral geniculate, the optimal stimulus for the simple cells that are found in layer III of the visual cortex is a stationary bar. To obtain a maximal response, the bar must be held at a specific orientation in the receptive field of the cell. Changes in the orientation of the bar away from this position cause the response to decline. The optimal orientation varies from cell to cell, but neurons within a cortical column tend to respond to the same orientation. The ability to provide a maximal response to moving visual stimuli, such as a bar that is moving across the visual field, is characteristic of complex cells of the visual cortex. *(Ganong, pp 130–134)*

200–204. The answers are 200-B, 201-E, 202-D, 203-B, 204-A. In the first stage of slow wave sleep, which is associated with very light sleep, the EEG pattern shows very low voltage waves punctuated by occasional bursts of alpha activity, called sleep spindles. As sleep progresses, frequency of the EEG waveform decreases until it is approximately 2 to 3 cycles per second. This pattern, called delta waves, is characteristic of the deep sleep of slow wave stage 4. Alert wakefulness and REM sleep are both characterized by beta waves, which indicate a high degree of brain activity. Quiet wakefulness is associated with alpha waves. *(Guyton, pp 669–672)*

205–207. The answers are 205-A, 206-C, 207-D. Although the early maturation of an ovarian follicle is dependent on the presence of FSH, ovulation is induced by a surge of LH. Although estrogen usually has a negative feedback effect on LH and FSH secretion, the LH surge seems to be a response to elevated estrogen levels. In concert with FSH, LH induces rapid follicular swelling. LH also acts directly on the granulosa cells to cause them to decrease estrogen production as well as to initiate production of small amounts of progesterone. These changes lead to ovulation. FSH is required for Sertoli cells to mediate the development of spermatids into mature sperm. *(Guyton, pp 956,971,977–978)*

208–209. The answers are 208-C, 209-C. Blood flow is inversely proportional to vascular resistance, and vascular resistance is directly proportional to blood viscosity. A low hematocrit, therefore, that decreases blood viscosity will both decrease resistance and increase flow. Similarly, since resistance is inversely proportional to the fourth power of vessel radius, vasodilation alone will both decrease resistance and increase flow. *(Guyton, pp 208–213; Smith and Kampine, pp 16–31)*

210–211.   The answers are 210-C, 211-D. In the example given in the question, if $\dot{Q} = \pi r^4 (P_{in} - P_{out})/8\eta L$ and $\dot{Q} = (P_{in} - P_{out})/R$ (by analogy to Ohm's law), where R is resistance, then $R = 8\eta L/\pi r^4$.

The slope, $\dot{Q}/(P_{in} - P_{out})$, decreased in condition 2 to condition 1; thus R increased. An increase in resistance could be due to either a decrease in radius or increase in viscosity.

The slope, $\dot{Q}/(P_{in} - P_{out})$, increased in condition 3 compared with condition 1; thus R decreased. Neither an increase in viscosity nor a decrease in radius would cause this type of change. *(Berne and Levy, p 58)*

212–214.   The answers are 212-B, 213-A, 214-B. CCK is released in response to the presence of food in the duodenum. It induces secretion of pancreatic zymogens from pancreatic acinar cells. Acid in the duodenum is a potent stimulus for secretin release. This hormone results in copius HCO_3 secretion by the pancreatic duct cells, which serves to neutralize the acid delivered in stomach content, thus protecting the intestinal mucosa from the damaging effects of low pH. *(Guyton, p 780)*

215.   The answer is D (4). The data presented in the question indicate that the clearance of glucose into the filtrate was the slope of the filtered curve (i.e., 100 ml/min). In this idealized case, this is the GFR, since glucose is totally filtered. The reabsorption transport maximum occurs at the plateau of the curve, which is 300 mg/min in this case. Plasma glucose is totally absorbed up to 200 mg/100 ml, at which point a threshold emerges and glucose appears in the urine. When plasma glucose exceeds 300 mg/100 ml, excretion of glucose is quantitative. *(Mountcastle, p 1177)*

216.   The answer is B (1,3). Alveolar ventilation ($\dot{V}_A$) is expressed as $\dot{V}_A = \dot{V}_E - \dot{V}_D$, where $\dot{V}_E$ is expired total ventilation and $\dot{V}_D$ is dead space ventilation. $\dot{V}_A = n(V_T - V_D)$, where n is respiratory rate, V_T is tidal volume, and V_D is dead space volume. In the example given, V_D equals anatomic dead space + ventilator dead space. Therefore, $\dot{V}_A = 10/min \cdot [800 \text{ ml} - (150 + 250)] = 4$ L/min. $\dot{V}_A$ can be increased to 6 L/min by lowering ventilator dead space to 50 ml or increasing the rate by 50 percent to 15/min. Increasing tidal volume by 50 percent will increase $\dot{V}_A$ by more than 50 percent. Doubling the rate and halving the tidal volume will not provide significant alveolar ventilation under these circumstances ($\dot{V}_A = 0$). It is possible that at higher ventilatory rates, adequate gas exchange can occur even when V_T is less than dead space volume (i.e., high-frequency ventilation). However, at this modest rate, we would not expect this to occur. *(West, 1979, pp 19–21,164)*

217.   The answer is A (1,2,3). A rise in body temperature, a fall in pH, and a rise in diphosphoglycerate are all known to shift the O_2 dissociation curve to the right. This shift means that more O_2 may be unloaded at a given Pa_{O_2} and thus enhance delivery of O_2 to a given bed. A rise in Pa_{CO_2}, not a fall in Pa_{CO_2} will also shift the curve to the right, predominantly via the action of CO_2 on pH (Bohr effect). *(West, 1979, p 73)*

218.   The answer is B (1,3). The sigmoid shape of the hemoglobin–oxygen dissociation curve reflects the cooperative binding of four oxygen molecules to each hemoglobin tetramer. Although myoglobin is very similar to hemoglobin, it does not form tetramers. The binding of oxygen to myoglobin monomers is represented by a rectangular hyperbola. As a result, the oxygen affinity of myoglobin is higher than that of hemoglobin at low oxygen tensions. Thus, muscle myoglobin can effectively scavenge O_2 from circulating hemoglobin. Both low pH and 2,3-DPG shift the hemoglobin–oxygen dissociation curve to the right, resulting in lower percentage saturations for given oxygen tensions. These effects increase the ability of hemoglobin to dump oxygen in the tissues. *(Ganong, pp 529–532)*

219.   The answer is A (1,2,3). The RQ ratio is a simple, easy, cheap, indirect calorimetric measure of whole body metabolism. The RQ of carbohydrate metabolism is 1.0, fat is 0.7, and protein is 0.8. In an average diet, RQ is about 0.8. When a well-nourished person exercises, carbohydrate use increases and so does RQ. However, when a person fasts and then exercises, RQ *decreases* because of an increased use of fat for energy. In a normal person during strenuous exercise, CO_2 production rises faster than O_2 consumption, since lactic acid is formed and affects the bicarbonate buffer system. *(Mountcastle, pp 1394–1400)*

220.   The answer is C (2,4). SA nodal cells are typical pacemaker cells. Their pacemaking activity chiefly underlies the automaticity and rhythmicity of cardiac tissue. Their action potential is distinctly different from that of nonautomatic cells, such as myocardial ventricular cells. Principal differences are a slow, steady depolarization (due to reduction in outward K^+ current) during phase 4 and lack of plateau. The resting membrane potential is not as negative as that of ventricular cells, and repolarization is slower, not faster, in SA nodal cells. *(Berne and Levy, pp 20–21)*

221. The answer is C (2,4). Pulmonary arterial BP (Ppa) and vascular resistance are considerably lower than their respective systemic values. There are also unique mechanical effects of lung volume, airways, and left atrial pressure as well as P_{CO_2} on this bed. Thus, elevations in left atrial pressure during congestive heart failure would be expected to result in an increase in Ppa if cardiac output were not affected too greatly. Alveolar hypoxia usually causes an increase in Ppa in most experimental animals and in humans. Thus, high altitude would be expected to initially produce pulmonary vasoconstriction in most subjects. Interestingly, the lungs may accommodate a large increase in cardiac output, such as is encountered in exercise, without increasing Ppa. Furthermore, after pneumonectomy, the intact lung may accommodate the preoperative cardiac output without an increase in Ppa. The latter two observations presumably are caused by a high reserve of unperfused capillaries or distention of already perfused capillaries in the normal lung, or both. *(West, 1979, pp 131–133)*

222. The answer is C (2,4). Regulation of cerebral blood flow is the result of interaction of local metabolic factors and possibly other neurohumoral factors. The effect is (1) to maintain overall cerebral perfusion and provide for relatively constant extravascular fluid volume in the brain and cerebral metabolism and (2) apparently to match blood flow and delivery of substrates to the local metabolism in a closely regulated regional fashion. Of the many stimuli that will increase cerebral blood flow, hypercapnia and hypoxemia are well described in experimental animals and humans. Furthermore, the brain autoregulates very well. Thus, changes in perfusion pressure from approximately 60 to 160 mm Hg do not significantly alter cerebral blood flow. Since angiotensin I (and its vasoconstrictor product, angiotensin II) do not cross the blood–brain barrier, neither systemic hypertension nor any local metabolic effects should alter cerebral blood flow. Both lowering of CO_2 and elevation of Pa_{O_2} are stimuli for cerebral vasoconstriction. *(Berne and Levy, pp 234–238)*

223. The answer is E (all). Fluid filtration is in large part a result of physical forces acting at the capillary and was described by Starling as represented by the following equation:

$$\text{Fluid movement} = K\left[(Pc + \pi i) - (Pi + \pi p)\right]$$

where Pc is capillary hydrostatic pressure, Pi is interstitial fluid hydrostatic pressure, πp is plasma protein oncotic pressure, πi is interstitial fluid oncotic pressure, and K is filtration constant for the capillary membrane. Normally, a small net positive fluid movement is present, and excess fluid and proteins are removed via lymphatic vessels. If venous pressure increases because of cardiac failure, Pc may increase. If protein is lost in the urine because of nephrosis, πp decreases. If lymphatics are obstructed with parasites, πi will increase, since lymphatics are the major thoroughfare for movement of proteins in the interstitial spaces. If arteriolar vasodilatation occurs with allergy, perhaps because of histamine release, then Pc will increase. All of these changes will tend to increase the net movement of fluid according to the Frank-Starling law. *(Guyton, pp 375–378)*

224. The answer is C (2,4). Although positive end-expiratory pressure (PEEP) appears useful in improving arterial oxygenation (probably by increasing the surface area for gas exchange), it has a number of potential limitations in intensely ill patients. Of primary concern is the possible decrease in cardiac output. PEEP will raise intrathoracic pressure and thus right atrial pressure. Since cardiac output is determined by the pressure gradient from peripheral veins to thorax, this gradient will be reduced if no compensatory mechanisms occur. Furthermore, PEEP expands the lungs and thus increases pulmonary vascular resistance, especially in small vessels. This tends to increase the afterload on the right ventricle, which can affect cardiac function in both ventricles in very complex ways. *(West, 1979, pp 193,199)*

225. The answer is D (4). Hypercalcemia leads to a general depression of the activity of excitable tissues. Its symptoms, therefore, include hypoexcitable reflexes, constipation (because of depressed contractility of gastrointestinal musculature), and weakness. Hypercalcemia also results in a shortened QT interval. *(Guyton, p 940)*

226. The answer is E (all). A withdrawal reflex may be triggered by noxious stimuli to the skin or to underlying tissue in a limb. Afferent input to the spinal cord engages polysynaptic pathways and produces the muscle contractions that result in withdrawal of the stimulated limb. The strong stimulation that produces a withdrawal reflex may result in long-lasting repetitive firing in the motor neurons that mediate the reflex. Such prolonged firing, which outlasts the duration of the stimulus itself, is termed an afterdischarge. The stimulation also may result in extension of the opposite limb, termed the crossed extensor response. *(Ganong, pp 105–106)*

227. The answer is A (1,2,3). Viscera generally contain a lower density of pain receptors than does skin, although the intensity of pain produced from viscera may be great. Impulses generated by the pain receptors are propagated centrally through sympathetic or parasympathetic nerves. Impulses entering the spinal cord ascend to the thalamus via the lateral spinothalamic tract. In common with deep somatic pain, the onset of visceral pain may result in the reflex excitation of a somatic structure, such as, for example, the abdominal wall. As with deep somatic pain, visceral pain may be referred to a somatic structure, usually one with which the affected organ was associated during embryologic development. (Ganong, pp 114–117)

228. The answer is C (2,4). Acromegaly is the hallmark of growth hormone-secreting tumors. The elevated levels of growth hormone lead to the growth of membranous bones and soft tissues, resulting in the characteristic jutting jaw, exagerated brow ridges, and enlarged feet and hands. Growth hormone secretion also leads to elevated serum glucose levels and release of fatty acids from fat stores. In light of the elevated serum glucose levels (and the possibility of elevated somatostatin secretion in the face of high growth hormone levels), serum glucagon would not be elevated and might be expected to be depressed. (Guyton, pp 887–893)

229. The answer is A (1,2,3). Desynchronization of the EEG is the onset of fast low-amplitude electrical activity and is generally associated with arousal. Desynchronization is also observed during paradoxical sleep. Sensory stimuli are generally able to produce arousal with desynchronization of the EEG, and this effect may be mimicked by peripheral stimulation of sensory pathways and stimulation of the nonspecific projection nuclei of the thalamus. Stimulation of specific sensory nuclei in the thalamus or of their projection areas in the cortex, however, usually fails to produce desynchronization. The phenomenon of desynchronization is believed to be primarily controlled by the activity of neurons in the reticular formation, which receive input from sensory systems. Stimulation at this site may also produce arousal and its associated EEG desynchronization. (Ganong, pp 162–163)

230. The answer is B (1,3). When the mucosa of the upper gastrointestinal tract is irritated, impulses generated in sympathetic afferents are conveyed to neurons in the medulla oblongata, which initiate the vomiting reflex. The area of integration in the medulla that receives such impulses also receives input from chemosensitive cells associated with the nearby area postrema, one of the circumventricular organs. Lesions of the area postrema prevent vomiting in response to emetic agents in the plasma. Such findings indicate that the area postrema is the principal chemoreceptor region for activating the vomiting reflex and that other circumventricular organs, such as the organum vasculosum of the lamina terminalis and the subfornical organ, do not play a major role in vomiting induced by bloodborne agents. (Ganong, pp 191–192)

231. The answer is B (1,3). Thyroid hormone stimulates increased heart rate. It can also lead to vasodilatation and an increase in stroke volume. Thus, cardiac output rises, although there is no significant change in mean arterial blood pressure. The concomitant vasodilatation and increase in stroke volume can, however, lead to a rise in pulse pressure (i.e., systolic blood pressure minus diastolic blood pressure). Thyroid hormone increases gastrointestinal motility and secretion, potentially resulting in diarrhea. (Guyton, pp 901–902)

232. The answer is A (1,2,3). In the absence of insulin, glucose uptake by most tissues is markedly decreased, and glycogen deposition is inhibited. Thus, serum glucose levels rise. The absence of insulin also results in increased catabolism of protein and decreased protein synthesis, resulting in elevated serum amino acid levels. Insulin deficiency results in the breakdown of fat to form free fatty acids, which are metabolized in the liver into ketones. High circulating ketones are, therefore, also associated with the absence of insulin. Since glucose uptake by the brain is not insulin dependent, it is not decreased in insulin deficiency. (Guyton, pp 925–929)

233. The answer is A (1,2,3). The major secretory products of the adrenal medulla are epinephrine and norepinephrine. Their precursor, dopamine, is also released. Dopamine secreted from the adrenal medulla may account for about half of the dopamine in the plasma. The catecholamines are packaged into granules in cells of the adrenal medulla along with high concentrations of ATP, which is also released on stimulation. The opiate peptide Met-enkephalin is another product of the adrenal medulla that is released into the circulation. The mineralocorticoid aldosterone is synthesized and released by cells in the adrenal cortex. (Ganong, pp 305–306)

234. The answer is B (1,3). Effects of adrenalectomy that can be directly attributed to the loss of circulating glucocorticoids are those effects that can be reversed by the administration of glucocorticoids. After adrenalectomy, vascular smooth muscle may progressively cease to respond to the sympathetic transmitters epinephrine and norepinephrine. This results in the dilatation of capillaries, and eventually their permeability is markedly enhanced. Adrenalectomy also results in a severe slowing of the rate at which a water load is excreted. Both of these effects are reversed by glucocorticoids. Although glucocorticoids control glucose metabolism, blood glucose levels do not rise in the absence of glucocorticoids but may, under circumstances such as fasting, decrease markedly.

Similarly, the effect of glucocorticoids on ACTH secretion from the anterior pituitary is to suppress release, and adrenalectomy results in an enhancement, rather than an inhibition, of secretion. *(Ganong, p 320)*

235. The answer is B (1,3). The adrenal medulla is little affected by hypophysectomy. The adrenal cortex, composed of three layers (zona glomerulosa, zona fasciculata, and zona reticularis), however, responds to ACTH released by the anterior pituitary and is significantly altered by hypophysectomy. The outer zona glomerulosa is the site at which new cells of the adrenal cortex are formed. It is also the primary locus of the synthesis of aldosterone, a mineralocorticoid whose synthesis is controlled not only by ACTH but also by other factors, such as circulating angiotensin II. The synthesis of steroids in the inner zona fasciculata and zona reticularis is primarily under the control of the pituitary, and hypophysectomy rapidly results in signs of atrophy in these two zones, without immediate changes in the outer zona glomerulosa. Prolonged pituitary deficit, however, also results in signs of degeneration in the zona glomerulosa. *(Ganong, pp 302–303)*

236. The answer is A (1,2,3). Reflex responses and mechanical effects related to extravascular pressure normally ensure maintenance of systemic arterial pressure and adequate perfusion as a normal person moves from the sitting to the erect position. In this postural change, an effective column of fluid will produce hydrostatic gradients such that venous pressure in the legs may be 70 to 100 mm Hg higher than in the standing position. Likewise, intravascular pressures in structures above the right atrium will decrease, in some instances by as much as 30 to 40 mm Hg. However, baroreceptor-mediated venoconstriction and extravascular compression of leg veins propel blood toward the heart, thereby maintaining circulating volume, venous return, and cardiac output. The venoconstriction depends on intact sympathetic reflex pathways. In the brain, transmural pressure would decrease by 30 to 40 mm Hg, and cerebral veins would collapse if it were not for the fact that the vessels are in a closed cranium. Since the cerebral veins are within incompressible tissue in a closed vault, the predicted fall in pressure also occurs in the surrounding tissues, thereby maintaining transmural pressure of cerebral veins greater than atmospheric pressure. *(Mountcastle, p 1039)*

237. The answer is B (1,3). Neurons in the inferior olivary nuclei are the source of the climbing fiber input to the cerebellum. Climbing fibers synapse directly on the dendritic branches of the Purkinje cells and generate excitatory input to these cells. The second source of excitation is from granule cells, in the cerebellar cortex, whose axons extend to the molecular layer. Here they bifurcate and extend, in parallel with the axons from other granule cells, to make multiple excitatory synapses with the dendrites of Purkinje cells. Basket cells within the cerebellar cortex also receive input from the parallel fibers, but their activity produces inhibition of Purkinje cells. Neurons in the pontine nuclei project to the cerebellar cortex, but their axons do not directly excite the Purkinje cells. *(Ganong, pp 182–183)*

238. The answer is B (1,3). The depolarizing phase of an action potential in a nerve cell is caused by an increase in the permeability of the nerve cell membrane to sodium ions. As the sodium channel in the membrane is sensitive to the voltage across the membrane, a depolarization of the cell, from its resting potential, causes the channel to open and, therefore, to increase the permeability to sodium ions. Sodium ions then flow passively down their electrochemical gradient and into the cell, thereby generating the depolarizing phase of the action potential. *(Ganong, pp 37–40)*

239. The answer is D (4). Stimulation of rod cells results in hyperpolarization and decreased release of rod neurotransmitters. Depolarizing bipolar cells are stimulated by this decreased secretion, whereas hyperpolarizing bipolar cells are inhibited by this same effect. Amacrine cells are excited by the discharges of bipolar cells and, in turn, stimulate ganglion cells. Stimulated ganglion cells then alter their rate of spontaneous firing (~5 per second) in a manner reflecting the excitatory or inhibitory nature of the stimulus. *(Guyton, pp 720–722)*

240. The answer is C (2,4). The blood–brain barrier is primarily attributable to the interendothelial cell tight junctions. This unusually high-resistance endothelium acts as an extended plasma membrane, restricting polar, ionized, charged, or high-molecular-weight substances from entering the brain. Lipid-soluble substances can cross the blood–brain barrier readily. Although the exact mechanism is unknown, hyperosmotic solutions can temporarily disrupt the barrier and may provide a potential technique for introducing drugs into the CNS. *(Mountcastle, p 1229)*

241. The answer is B (1,3). The Na^+, K^+ pump is a membrane protein that uses adenosine triphosphate (ATP) to pump sodium ions out of a cell and to pump potassium ions in. The pump is stimulated by an elevation of internal sodium ions. For every three sodium ions that are pumped out, two potassium ions are pumped in. Activity of the pump, therefore, produces current flow that may hyperpolarize the cell. This hyperpolarization, however, does not contribute to the form of an action potential. *(Ganong, pp 237–239)*

242. **The answer is C (2,4).** During the relative refractory period, sodium channels that suffered inactivation during the preceding action potential have, to some extent, recovered from activation. A proportion of the potassium channels that opened during the action potential, however, may still be open. This accounts for the greater stimulating current that must be applied to elicit an action potential during the relative refractory period. *(Kandel and Schwartz, pp 59–60)*

243. **The answer is A (1,2,3).** The secretion of renin from the kidneys is regulated by a wide variety of factors. The juxtaglomerular cells, which contain renin within secretory granules, are located along the afferent arterioles to the glomeruli. Any stimulus that causes a fall in intra-arteriolar pressure will evoke renin release from these cells. An increase in BP, therefore, results in the inhibition of renin release. The secretion of renin is also affected by the rate of electrolyte transport across the nearby macula densa cells, such that a diminution in the amounts of sodium and chloride ions reaching these cells causes increased secretion of renin from the juxtaglomerular cells. Prostaglandins stimulate renin release, whereas drugs such as indomethacin (which inhibit prostaglandin synthesis) inhibit release. Circulating catecholamines, as well as activity in the renal sympathetic nerves, also stimulate renin release. *(Ganong, pp 390–392)*

244. **The answer is B (1,3).** Angiotensin II and ADH are potent vasoconstrictors, whereas prostaglandin E (as well as most other prostaglandins) and bradykinin exert a vasodilatory effect. *(Guyton, pp 241–242)*

245. **The answer is C (2,4).** The spread of an action potential is caused by a depolarization-induced increase in the permeability of the membrane to sodium ions, which then enter the cell. This process itself does not directly use ATP, although ATP-dependent pumps generate the sodium concentration gradient across the cell membrane. The binding of calcium ions to troponin C, which initiates contraction, also does not require ATP. The formation and breakage of bonds between actin and myosin molecules, which result in shortening of the muscle, are, however, accompanied by the hydrolysis of ATP. This is catalyzed by an ATPase in the heads of the myosin molecules. The pumping of calcium ions into the sarcoplasmic reticulum during relaxation is carried out by an ATP-dependent calcium pump. *(Ganong, pp 237–239)*

246. **The answer is E (all).** In cardiac muscle, the T system is located at the Z lines. This is in contrast to skeletal muscle, in which the T system is found at the junction of the A bands and I bands. The long duration of cardiac action potential (200 msec or more) is largely due to the slow, inward calcium current that is expressed during the plateau phase of the actin potentials. The calcium that enters during this phase contributes to the contractile response, which endures for about 300 msec. Peak contraction, however, occurs toward the end of the plateau phase of the action potential. *(Ganong, pp 60–64)*

247. **The answer is D (4).** Intestinal glucose uptake is mediated by a cotransport system in the epithelial brush border that couples the import of lumenal glucose and sodium. The lumen-to-cytoplasm sodium gradient (which is maintained by the Na,K-ATPase, or sodium pump, which keeps intracellular sodium low) can thus drive the rapid import of glucose against its concentration gradient. *(Davenport, 1978, pp 98–100)*

248. **The answer is A (1,2,3).** Histamine acts synergistically with gastrin and acetylcholine to stimulate parietal cell proton and chloride secretion, which is associated with an increase in parietal cell oxygen consumption. Gastrin release from G cells is stimulated by local neural reflexes that are triggered by the presence of food products in the stomach lumen. *(Davenport, 1978, pp 45–55)*

249. **The answer is A (1,2,3).** Compliance is the change in volume per unit change in pressure. In the normal lung,

$$\text{Compliance} = 2L/[(-5) - (-15)] = 0.2 \text{ L/cm H}_2\text{O}$$

The steeper slope representing the diseased lung in the figure that accompanies the question is indicative of an increased compliance. The elastic recoil of the lung is the pressure surrounding the lung to maintain a given volume (or to oppose the tendency of the lung to collapse). It is equal and opposite to the intrapleural pressure (estimated here by intrathoracic esophageal pressure). In the diseased lung, it is 10 cm H_2O (at 2 L), which is < 15 cm H_2O at 2 L in the normal lung. The recoil pressure of the normal lung at 2 L is 15 cm H_2O, not 10 cm H_2O. *(Murray, pp 81–82)*

250. **The answer is E (all).** The concentration of cations affects cardiac functioning, and the importance of these ions on excitation–contraction coupling has been demonstrated in isolated perfused hearts. Ultimately, the ionic basis of coupling of excitation and contraction resides in free intracellular Ca^{2+}. However, supraphysiologic levels of K^+ may arrest the heart in diastole, and lack of Na^+ will prevent an isolated perfused heart from beating. Contraction occurs as a result of entry of Ca^+ from interstitial fluid (especially T tubules), and relaxation occurs by the removal of Ca^{2+} from the myoplasm by the sarcoplasmic reticulum. *(Berne and Levy, p 82)*

251. The answer is B (1,3). Loop diuretics operate in part as described in the question. An increased amount of Na^+ is presented to the distal and collecting tubules, and water reabsorption is in part prevented. Furthermore, the medullary interstitial fluid osmolality is depressed, reducing the concentrating mechanism of the kidney. Both K^+ and H^+ are removed in amounts above normal because of increased Na^+ reaching the tubules. These agents may, therefore, depress K^+ levels. *(Guyton, pp 459–460)*

252. The answer is A (1,2,3). Heat stroke and circulatory collapse may occur if work in a hot environment is undertaken without adequate precautions. Humidity exacerbates this potential, and thus dehumidifying the environment, if possible, is useful. Access to water and salt is critical to maintain body fluids and electrolytes. Acclimatization is critical and appears to enhance sweating ability as well as reabsorption of NaCl. Although antipyretics are useful in preventing damage to the body from excessively high body temperature, there is no evidence to suggest that they facilitate adjustment when used on a continuous basis. Indeed, these agents may produce abnormalities in thermoregulation. *(Guyton, p 859)*

253. The answer is B (1,3). The muscles of the lower esophageal sphincter differ from those of the remainder of the esophagus in that they are tonically active. Swallowing results in the relaxation of this tonic activity. This in turn allows food that has already been propelled along the esophagus to enter the stomach. There is evidence to suggest that the relaxation of the lower esophageal sphincter is brought about by vasoactive intestinal peptide (VIP)-containing neurons. High levels of gastrin may increase the tone of these muscles, but the physiologic importance of this effect is not clear. *(Ganong, pp 415–416)*

254. The answer is E (all). Alveolar hypoventilation will increase extracellular CO_2. The regulation of H^+ secretion in the renal tubular system is a function of extracellular CO_2 concentration. CO_2 diffuses into the proximal tubular epithelium and reacts with water to form carbonic acid, which itself rapidly dissociates to H^+ and HCO_3^-. The H^+ is actively transported into the tubular fluid, where it combines with bicarbonate to form carbonic acid. The tubular carbonic acid dissociates, and CO_2 enters the epithelial cell, where it ultimately dissociates to HCO_3^-. This HCO_3^- is reabsorbed into the ECF. H^+ transport is gradient limited, and to facilitate the excretion of H^+, it is buffered in tubular fluid with phosphate and ammonia buffer systems. The net effect is a decrease in plasma pH due to the presence of increased CO_2, and hence carbonic acid, in the ECF which is partially compensated by renal acid excretion. Increased renal acid excretion is associated with excretion of H_2PO_4 and NH_4Cl. *(Guyton, pp 442–448)*

BIBLIOGRAPHY

Berne RM, Levy MN. *Cardiovascular Physiology.* 4th ed. St. Louis: CV Mosby Co; 1981.

Comroe JH. *Physiology of Respiration.* 2nd ed. Chicago: Year Book Medical Publishers, Inc; 1974.

Davenport HW. *The ABC of Acid-Base Chemistry.* 6th ed. Chicago: University of Chicago Press; 1974.

Davenport HW. *A Digest of Digestion.* 2nd ed. Chicago: Year Book Medical Publishers, Inc; 1978.

Ganong WF. *Review of Medical Physiology.* 14th ed. Los Altos, Calif: Lange Medical Publications; 1989.

Guyton AC. *Textbook of Medical Physiology.* 7th ed. Philadelphia: WB Saunders Co; 1986.

Kandel ER, Schwartz JH, eds. *Principles of Neural Science.* New York: Elsevier/North-Holland; 1981.

Mountcastle VB. *Medical Physiology.* 14th ed. St. Louis: CV Mosby Co; 1980.

Murray J. *The Normal Lung.* Philadelphia: WB Saunders Co; 1976.

Smith JJ, Kampine JP. *Circulatory Physiology—The Essentials.* 2nd ed. Baltimore: Williams & Wilkins Co; 1984.

Takahashi T, Otsuka M. Regional distribution of substance P in the spinal cord and nerve roots of the cat and the effect of dorsal root section. Brain Res. April 1975; 1–11.

West JB. *Respiratory Physiology—The Essentials.* 2nd ed. Baltimore: Williams & Wilkins Co; 1979.

West JB. *Pulmonary Pathophysiology—The Essentials.* 2nd ed. Baltimore: Williams & Wilkins Co; 1981.

Subspecialty List: Physiology

216. Pulmonary gas exchange
217. Blood gas transport
218. Blood gas transport
219. Exercise
220. Cardiac electrophysiology
221. Circulation in specific organs
222. Circulation in specific organs
223. Capillary exchange
224. Circulation in specific organs
225. General physiology
226. Nervous system
227. Sensory mechanisms
228. Endocrinology
229. Nervous system
230. Nervous system
231. Endocrinology
232. Endocrinology
233. Endocrinology
234. Endocrinology
235. Endocrinology
236. Cardiovascular regulation
237. Nervous system
238. General physiology
239. Special senses
240. Body fluids
241. General physiology
242. General physiology
243. Fluid balance
244. General physiology
245. General physiology
246. General physiology
247. Gastrointestinal
248. Gastrointestinal
249. Mechanics of breathing
250. Cardiac cycle
251. Excretory function
252. Temperature
253. Gastrointestinal
254. Body fluids

CHAPTER 3

Biochemistry
Questions

DIRECTIONS (Questions 255 through 305): Each of the numbered items or incomplete statements in this section is followed by answers or by completions of the statement. Select the ONE lettered answer or completion that is BEST in each case.

255. Free purine and pyrimidine bases and nucleosides can be converted to the corresponding nucleoside 5'-monophosphate via salvage pathways. These pathways are important for conversion of certain antimetabolites that are employed for chemotherapy. Which of the following antimetabolites would require salvage for proper function?

    (A) azaserine
    (B) methotrexate
    (C) 5-fluorouracil
    (D) allopurinol
    (E) none of the above

256. In muscle tissue, acetoacetate can be converted to acetoacetyl-CoA by the following reaction:

    Acetoacetate + coenzyme A + ATP → acetoacetyl-CoA + ADP + P_i

    How many moles of ATP (net) can be derived by muscle on conversion of 1 mol of acetoacetate to CO_2 and water?

    (A) 11
    (B) 12
    (C) 22
    (D) 23
    (E) 24

257. Lactate that is released into the circulation can be converted back to glucose in

    (A) liver
    (B) heart muscle
    (C) erythrocytes
    (D) adipose tissue
    (E) brain

258. All of the following are involved in movement of CO_2 from peripheral tissues to the lungs EXCEPT

    (A) carbamate
    (B) carbonic anhydrase
    (C) CO_2 bound to the iron of hemoglobin (Hb)
    (D) bicarbonate
    (E) dissolved CO_2

259. All of the following are true for smooth muscle, cardiac muscle, skeletal muscle, and macrophages EXCEPT that they

    (A) contain actin
    (B) respond to nervous stimulation
    (C) contain myosin
    (D) have a cytoskeleton
    (E) use ATP for contraction

260. The standard free-energy change ($\Delta G^{\circ\prime}$) for the hydrolysis of phosphoenolpyruvate is −14.8 kcal/mol and that for ATP hydrolysis to ADP and orthophosphate (P_i) is −7.3 kcal/mol. For the production of phosphoenolpyruvate by the reaction

    ATP + pyruvate $\rightleftharpoons$ phosphoenolpyruvate + ADP + P_i the $\Delta G^{\circ\prime}$ is

    (A) + 7.5 kcal/mol
    (B) − 7.5 kcal/mol
    (C) +22.1 kcal/mol
    (D) −22.1 kcal/mol
    (E) −14.8 kcal/mol

261. The carbohydrate employed in the biosynthesis of nucleic acids is made in which of the following pathways?

    (A) glycolysis
    (B) gluconeogenesis
    (C) urea cycle
    (D) citric acid cycle
    (E) pentose phosphate pathway

262. What is the pH of a buffer solution containing 0.05 mol/L KH_2PO_4 and 0.15 mol/L K_2HPO_4? The pK_1 of phosphoric acid is 1.96 and pK_2 is 6.8.

(A) 4.38
(B) 6.35
(C) 6.80
(D) 7.28
(E) 8.76

263. The ATPase activity required for muscle contraction is located in

(A) myosin
(B) troponin
(C) myokinase
(D) sarcoplasmic reticulum
(E) actin

264. All of the following are allosteric effectors regulating the glycolytic pathway EXCEPT

(A) glucose 6-phosphate
(B) ATP
(C) fructose 6-phosphate
(D) citrate
(E) AMP

265. Which of the following saccharides enters glycolysis at the level of three-carbon intermediates?

(A) lactose
(B) mannose
(C) galactose
(D) maltose
(E) fructose

266. The primary positive control of gluconeogenesis is exerted by

(A) high acetyl-CoA levels
(B) high citrate levels
(C) low citrate levels
(D) low ATP levels
(E) high ATP levels

267. All of the following are involved in the cascade of events leading to glycogenolysis in skeletal muscle EXCEPT

(A) adenylate cyclase
(B) phosphorylase kinase
(C) phosphorylase
(D) protein kinase
(E) glucagon

268. Fluorouracil is a drug that is used in the chemotherapy of several solid tumors. The mechanism of action of fluorouracil is

(A) it is an inhibitor of ribonucleotide reductase
(B) it is an inhibitor of thymidylate synthase
(C) it is an inhibitor of thymidine kinase
(D) it is an inhibitor of de novo pyrimidine biosynthesis
(E) it is an inhibitor of de novo purine biosynthesis

269. For determination of the K_m of an enzyme, it is necessary to know

(A) the molecular weight of the enzyme
(B) the initial velocity of the enzyme-catalyzed reaction at several different substrate concentrations
(C) the turnover number of the enzyme
(D) the equilibrium constant of the enzyme-catalyzed reaction
(E) the initial velocity of the enzyme-catalyzed reaction at several different enzyme concentrations

270. Which of the following is the single most important force in stabilizing protein tertiary structure?

(A) peptide bonds
(B) disulfide bonds
(C) hydrogen bonds
(D) polar interactions
(E) hydrophobic interactions

271. The $\Delta G^{\circ\prime}$ for the sum of the reactions leading to the activation and transfer of amino acids to tRNA is close to zero.

$$Amino\ acid + ATP + tRNA + H_2O \rightleftharpoons aminoacyl\text{-}tRNA + AMP + 2\ P_i$$

The synthesis of aminoacyl-tRNA is driven by

(A) hydrolysis of pyrophosphate (PP_i)
(B) aminoacyl-tRNA synthetase
(C) hydrolysis of ATP
(D) formation of the phosphate ester of aminoacyl-tRNA
(E) formation of the phosphate ester of an intermediate aminoacyl-AMP

272. Since liver glucokinase has a K_m of 10 mmol/L and muscle hexokinase has a K_m of 100 μmol/L, it may be assumed that

(A) the liver sequesters glucose more avidly than does muscle

(B) hexokinase has a greater affinity for glucose

(C) glucokinase is more widely distributed

(D) glucokinase has a greater affinity for phosphorylation of glucose

(E) muscle releases glucose more easily than does liver

273. All of the following statements concerning the activation of free fatty acids prior to β oxidation are true EXCEPT that

(A) only long-chain fatty acids are activated

(B) activation occurs within the mitochondrial matrix

(C) activation occurs outside the mitochondrial matrix

(D) the carboxyl groups of fatty acids form thioester linkages with CoA

(E) the activation reaction is made irreversible by the hydrolysis of PP_i

274. The key regulatory enzyme of fatty acid synthesis is

(A) citrate cleavage enzyme

(B) ATP citrate lyase

(C) acetyl-CoA carboxylase

(D) malonyl-CoA decarboxylase

(E) malonyl transacylase

275. All of the following reaction sequences in cholesterol biosynthesis are unique to cholesterol biosynthesis EXCEPT the

(A) formation of 3-hydroxy-3-methylglutaryl CoA from acetyl-CoA

(B) demethylation of lanosterol

(C) cyclization of squalene to form lanosterol

(D) formation of mevalonic acid from 3-hydroxy-3-methylglutaryl-CoA

(E) formation of isoprenoid isomers from mevalonic acid

276. The major site of regulation of cholesterol synthesis is

(A) cyclization of squalene to lanosterol

(B) 3-hydroxy-3-methylglutaryl-CoA synthase

(C) 3-hydroxy-3-methylglutaryl-CoA lyase

(D) 3-hydroxy-3-methylglutaryl-CoA reductase

(E) synthesis of squalene from isoprenoid isomers

277. All of the following are phosphoglycerides found in plasma membranes of mammalian cells EXCEPT

(A) phosphatidyl ethanolamine

(B) sphingomyelin

(C) phosphatidyl inositol

(D) phosphatidyl serine

(E) lecithin

278. In adipocytes, a lack of glucose is known to

(A) cause an inhibition of lipolysis

(B) result in glycerol 3-phosphate synthesis

(C) lead to an inhibition of triacylglycerol synthesis

(D) allow gluconeogenesis to proceed

(E) inhibit ketogenesis

279. Which of the following occurs in the lipidosis known as Tay-Sachs disease?

(A) synthesis of a specific ganglioside is excessive

(B) xanthomas due to cholesterol deposition are observed

(C) phosphoglycerides accumulate in the brain

(D) ganglioside GM_2 is not catabolized by lysosomal enzymes

(E) synthesis of a specific ganglioside is decreased

280. In diabetes, the increased production of ketone bodies is primarily a result of

(A) elevated acetyl-CoA levels in skeletal muscle

(B) a substantially increased rate of fatty acid oxidation by hepatocytes

(C) increased gluconeogenesis

(D) decreased cyclic AMP levels in adipocytes

(E) an increase in the rate of the citric acid cycle

Questions 281 through 283

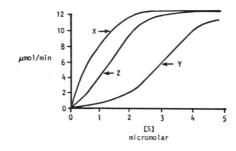

281. Assuming that curve Z represents the plot of an allosteric enzyme with no additions, curve X represents

(A) an allosteric enzyme with a positive modulator

(B) a noncompetitively inhibited enzyme

(C) an allosteric enzyme with an increased K_m

(D) an allosteric enzyme with a negative modulator

(E) an irreversibly inhibited enzyme

282. Assuming that all of the curves shown represent the same allosteric enzyme under different conditions, in going from left to right

    (A) the Vmax is increased
    (B) cooperative binding of substrate is decreasing
    (C) the concentration of a negative modulator is increasing
    (D) the K_m is decreasing
    (E) the concentration of a needed cofactor is increasing

283. The K_m for curve Y is

    (A) 2 μmol/min
    (B) 3 μmol/L
    (C) 5 μmol/L
    (D) 12 μmol/min
    (E) not available in the data given

284. An overdose of insulin in diabetic persons leads to

    (A) hypoglycemia
    (B) glucosuria
    (C) ketonuria
    (D) hyperglycemia
    (E) ketonemia

285. The pituitary prohormone pro-opiocortin is the precursor of all of the following hormones EXCEPT

    (A) thyroid-stimulating hormone (TSH)
    (B) melanocyte-stimulating hormone (MSH)
    (C) adrenocorticotropin (ACTH)
    (D) β-endorphin
    (E) γ-lipotropin

286. Consumption of raw eggs, which contain the protein avidin, could lead to a deficiency resulting in

    (A) an inhibition of decarboxylation reactions
    (B) an inability to form acetylcholine
    (C) a decrease in CoA formation
    (D) an increase in transaminations
    (E) an inhibition of carboxylation reactions

287. Both glutamate transaminase and alanine transaminase require a prosthetic group derived from

    (A) vitamin B_6 (pyridoxine)
    (B) vitamin B_1 (thiamine)
    (C) vitamin B_{12} (cobalamin)
    (D) vitamin B_2 (riboflavin)
    (E) biotin

288. The active form of the cofactor required for oxidative decarboxylation reactions is

    (A) thiamine monophosphate
    (B) thiamine
    (C) thiamine pyrophosphate
    (D) thiamine triphosphate
    (E) hydroxyethyl thiamine prophosphate

289. Which of the following is quantitatively the major contributor to routine clinical measurements of circulating plasma cholesterol concentrations?

    (A) chylomicrons
    (B) low-density lipoproteins (LDLs)
    (C) high-density lipoproteins (HDLs)
    (D) intermediate-density lipoproteins (IDLs)
    (E) very low density lipoproteins (VLDLs)

290. A deficiency in the enzyme galactose 1-phosphate uridyl transferase results in

    (A) low levels of glucose 1-phosphate
    (B) high levels of uridine diphosphate (UDP)-glucose
    (C) high levels of UDP-galactose
    (D) high levels of blood galactose
    (E) high levels of blood glucose

291. Liver conversion of bilirubin to the hydrophilic form secreted in bile involves

    (A) decarboxylation
    (B) conjugation with glucuronic acid
    (C) the reduced form of nicotinamine adenine dinucleotide phosphate (NADPH)-dependent reduction to biliverdin
    (D) conjugation with glycine
    (E) esterification with taurine

292. Activated core oligosaccharides that are transferred to the asparagine of proteins are carried by

    (A) guanosine diphosphate (GDP)-mannose
    (B) N-acetylglucosamine
    (C) dolichol phosphate
    (D) N-acetylgalactosamine
    (E) UDP-glucose

293. All of the following statements concerning fatty acid synthesis are true EXCEPT that

    (A) a decarboxylation takes place
    (B) the reductant is NADPH
    (C) most of the intermediates are bonded to CoA
    (D) a carboxylation takes place
    (E) the reactions occur in the cytosol

294. Which of the following is considered to be rate limiting in detoxification of ethanol in alcoholic individuals?

(A) the oxidized form of nicotinamide adenine dinucleotide (NAD+)

(B) the oxidized form of flavin adenine dinucleotide (FAD)

(C) the oxidized form of nicotinamide adenine dinucleotide phosphate (NADP+)

(D) alcohol dehydrogenase

(E) acetaldehyde dehydrogenase

295. Concerning the malate-aspartate shuttle, all of the following are correct EXCEPT that

(A) the shuttle is bidirectional with respect to electron transfer between cytosol and mitochondria

(B) both cytosolic and mitochondrial NADH serve as electron transporters

(C) two ATP are formed for each pair of electrons transferred from cytosolic NADH to mitochondrial electron transport

(D) oxaloacetate is an intermediate

(E) α-ketoglutarate is an intermediate

296. The steps of the pathway for β oxidation of palmitic acid differ from those of the biosynthetic pathway in all of the following respects EXCEPT

(A) acyl group carrier

(B) pyridine nucleotide specificity

(C) effect of citrate

(D) β-hydroxyacyl intermediate

(E) intracellular location

297. Which of the following reactions is the major oxidation reaction of energy metabolism in erythrocytes?

(A) NADPH $\rightleftharpoons$ NADP+

(B) FADH $\rightleftharpoons$ FAD

(C) dihydroxyacetone phosphate + NADH $\rightleftharpoons$ glycerol 3-phosphate + NAD+

(D) pyruvate + NADH $\rightleftharpoons$ lactate + NAD+

(E) acetaldehyde + NADH $\rightleftharpoons$ ethanol + NAD+

298. The affinity of Hb for O_2 is increased by

(A) the formation of salt bridges in Hb

(B) the cross-linking of the β-chains of Hb

(C) lowering of pH

(D) decreases in 2,3-diphosphoglycerate (DPG)

(E) increases in the partial pressure of CO_2

299. An inherited metabolic disorder of carbohydrate metabolism characterized by higher than normal levels of glycolytic intermediates in most cells and a low O_2 affinity of erythrocyte Hb is the result of a deficiency in

(A) pyruvate kinase

(B) hexokinase

(C) aldolase

(D) phosphofructokinase

(E) glucokinase

300. The increased intracellular concentrations of 5-phosphoribosyl-1-pryophosphate (PRPP) and urate in the genetic hyperuricemia called the Lesch-Nyhan syndrome is most likely a consequence of

(A) allopurinol inhibition of xanthine formation

(B) increased purine synthesis

(C) elevated synthesis of hypoxanthine

(D) deficiency of hypoxanthine-guanine phosphoribosyltransferase (HGPRT)

(E) elevated PRPP synthetase activity

301. Although complete blocks of any step of the urea cycle are incompatible with life, inherited partial enzymatic defects have been diagnosed. Mental retardation, episodic vomiting, and lethargy are caused by the diseases. The biochemical hallmark of almost all of these deficiencies is

(A) high blood levels of ammonia

(B) excess accumulation of urea

(C) decreases in aspartate concentrations

(D) gout

(E) increases in the amount of α-ketoglutarate

302. All of the following are feedback inhibitors of either purine or pyrimidine synthesis EXCEPT

(A) adenosine monophosphate (AMP)

(B) thymidine monophosphate (TMP)

(C) guanosine monophosphate (GMP)

(D) uridine monophosphate (UMP)

(E) cytidine triphosphate (CTP)

303. In the presence of a poison that uncouples oxidative phosphorylation, what would be the net energy yield of the complete oxidation of 1 mol equivalent of glucose in muscle?

(A) 1 mol equivalent ATP

(B) 2 mol equivalent ATP

(C) 3 mol equivalent ATP

(D) 4 mol equivalent ATP

(E) 5 mol equivalent ATP

304. In the complete oxidation of glucose by muscle cells, the phosphorus/O_2 ratio is

(A) 2

(B) 3

(C) 4

(D) 36

(E) 38

305. Which of the following steps is common to both gluconeogenesis and glycolysis?

(A) fructose 6-phosphate to glucose 6-phosphate
(B) pyruvate to oxaloacetate
(C) glucose 6-phosphate to glucose
(D) fructose 1,6-diphosphate to fructose 6-phosphate
(E) oxaloacetate to phosphoenolpyruvate

DIRECTIONS (Questions 306 through 308): Each group of items in this section consists of lettered headings followed by a set of numbered words or phrases. For each numbered word or phrase, select the ONE lettered heading that is most closely associated with it. Each lettered heading may be selected once, more than once, or not at all.

Questions 306 through 308

For each item described, select the letter in the figure with which it is associated.

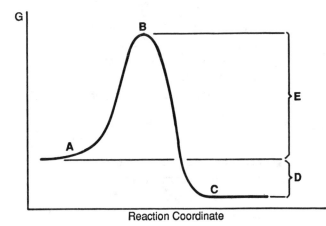

Reaction Coordinate

306. Transition state

307. Energy of activation for the reaction

308. ΔG for the reaction

Questions 309 through 311

For each of the citric acid cycle reactions shown, indicate the statement that applies.

(A) requires a flavoprotein enzyme
(B) requires coenzyme A
(C) requires ATP
(D) yields GTP
(E) yields CO_2

309. Isocitrate → α-ketoglutarate

310. Succinyl-CoA → succinate

311. Succinate → fumarate

Questions 312 through 315

For each reaction described below, choose the enzyme with which it is associated.

(A) glycogen phosphorylase
(B) glycogen synthase
(C) glucose 6-phosphate dehydrogenase
(D) glucokinase
(E) glucose 6-phosphatase

312. Catalyzes a reaction in which inorganic phosphate is a substrate

313. Catalyzes a reaction in which ATP is a substrate

314. Catalyzes a reaction in which UDP-glucose is a substrate

315. Catalyzes a reaction in which glucose is a product

Questions 316 through 319

For each description below, choose the amino acid with which it is associated.

(A) serine
(B) glutamine
(C) glutamate
(D) aspartate
(E) asparagine

316. The common intermediate for the entry of several amino acids into the citric acid cycle

317. A major source of carbon for the one-carbon pool

318. Can be formed by the one-step transamination of an intermediate of the citric acid cycle

319. One-step transamination of it forms a citric acid cycle intermediate

Questions 320 through 322

For each description below, choose the substance with which it is associated.

(A) hydroxyproline
(B) O-phosphoserine
(C) γ-carboxyglutamate
(D) D-valine
(E) cystine

320. Is present in large amounts in keratin

321. Occurs in prothrombin

322. Can be found in collagen

Questions 323 and 324

For each description below, choose the structure with which it is associated.

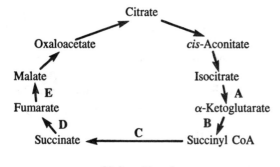

323. Found only in DNA

324. Forms dimers on exposure of DNA to ultraviolet light

Questions 325 and 326

For each step described in the citric acid cycle, choose the lettered point on the diagram with which it is associated.

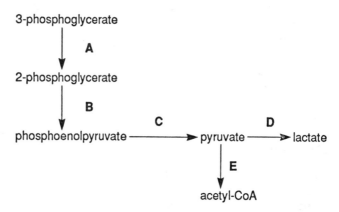

Citric acid cycle.

325. Step at which flavin nucleotide is reduced

326. Step at which substrate level phosphorylation occurs

Questions 327 and 328

For each description below, choose the correct enzyme based on the data in the table.

Enzyme	K_m (M)	k_{cat} (sec^{-1})
(A) chymotrypsin	5×10^{-3}	100
(B) lysozyme	6×10^{-6}	0.5
(C) carbonic anhydrase	8×10^{-3}	600,000
(D) penicillinase	5×10^{-5}	2,000
(E) tyrosyl-tRNA synthetase	1×10^{-5}	40

327. The enzyme with the greatest affinity for its substrate

328. The enzyme with the greatest catalytic efficiency

Questions 329 and 330

For each description below, choose the lettered point in the pathway with which it is associated.

```
3-phosphoglycerate
        |
        | A
        ↓
2-phosphoglycerate
        |
        | B
        ↓
                    C              D
phosphoenolpyruvate ──────→ pyruvate ──────→ lactate
                                |
                                | E
                                ↓
                           acetyl-CoA
```

329. ATP is formed by substrate level phosphorylation

330. Requires NADH

DIRECTIONS (Questions 331 through 333): Each group of items in this section consists of lettered headings followed by a set of numbered words or phrases. For each numbered word or phrase, select

A if the item is associated with (A)only,
B if the item is associated with (B) only,
C if the item is associated with both (A) and (B),
D if the item is associated with neither (A) nor (B).

Questions 331 through 333

Within each of the reaction pathways shown below

(A) ATP is consumed
(B) ATP is generated
(C) both
(D) neither

331. Glycogen → fructose 6-phosphate

332. Fructose 6-phosphate → glyceraldehyde 3-phosphate

333. Glyceraldehyde 3-phosphate → pyruvate

Questions 334 through 336

(A) protein synthesis
(B) RNA synthesis
(C) both
(D) neither

334. Dactinomycin is an inhibitor

335. Tetracycline is an inhibitor

336. Methotrexate is an inhibitor

Questions 337 through 339

(A) transcription in eukaryotes
(B) transcription in prokaryotes
(C) both
(D) neither

337. Occurs in a 3′ to 5′ direction

338. Is inhibited by α-amanitin

339. Begins at specific sequences on the DNA template

Questions 340 through 342

(A) HDLs
(B) LDLs
(C) both
(D) neither

340. Contain primarily triacylglycerides

341. Transport cholesterol from peripheral tissues to the liver

342. Transport cholesterol to peripheral tissues

Questions 343 through 345

(A) mitochondrial electron transport
(B) mitochondrial oxidative phosphorylation dependent on oxidation of succinate
(C) both
(D) neither

343. Inhibited by dinitrophenol

344. Inhibited by rotenone

345. Inhibited by antimycin A

Questions 346 and 347

(A) phosphatidyl choline or sphingomyelin
(B) anion channel protein
(C) both
(D) neither

346. Major constituent of myelin

347. Major constituent of RBC membrane

DIRECTIONS (Questions 348 through 381): For each of the items in this section, ONE or MORE of the numbered options is correct. Choose the answer

A if only 1, 2 and 3 are correct,
B if only 1 and 3 are correct,
C if only 2 and 4 are correct,
D if only 4 is correct,
E if all are correct.

348. The biosynthesis of saturated fatty acids is

(1) localized in the cytoplasm
(2) decreased when the fatty acid concentration is elevated
(3) controlled by the rate of the reaction catalyzed by acetyl-CoA carboxylase
(4) increased when the levels of citric acid cycle intermediates are elevated

349. Which of the following features may characterize sickle cell anemia?

(1) sickling occurs when there is a high concentration of the deoxygenated form of Hb S
(2) a single amino acid in the β chain is altered

(3) the solubility of deoxygenated Hb S is abnormally low

(4) Hb S has an abnormal electrophoretic mobility

350. Which of the following statements may correctly describe vertebrate skeletal muscle?

(1) thin filaments contain actin, tropomyosin, and troponin

(2) calcium ions inhibit contraction

(3) nerve excitation triggers the release of calcium from sarcoplasmic reticulum

(4) creatine kinase catalyzes the transfer of a phosphate group from ATP to creatine to form phosphocreatine during active muscle contraction

351. Hydrogen ion concentration in solution is expressed as pH, which can be determined by

(1) $- \log \dfrac{[\text{base}]}{[\text{acid}]}$

(2) $- \log [\text{H}^+]$

(3) $1/\log [\text{H}^+]$

(4) $\text{p}K + \log \dfrac{[\text{base}]}{[\text{acid}]}$

352. UDP-glucose is required for the

(1) synthesis of glucose 6-phosphate

(2) synthesis of glycogen

(3) debranching of glycogen

(4) use of galactose

353. The symptomatic end result of the biochemical defect of which of the following diseases allows detection without chemical analysis?

(1) albinism

(2) alkaptonuria

(3) maple syrup urine disease

(4) phenylketonuria (PKU)

354. Major products of the pentose phosphate pathway include

(1) NADPH

(2) six-carbon sugars

(3) five-carbon sugars

(4) NADH

355. GDPCP is an analog of guanosine triphosphate (GTP) that cannot be hydrolyzed to GDP. Which of the following may be expected to occur if GDPCP replaces GTP in a protein-synthesizing system?

(1) binding of aminoacyl-tRNA to ribosomes will be inhibited

(2) polypeptide chain initiation will be inhibited

(3) polypeptide chain elongation will be inhibited

(4) peptidyl transferase activity will be inhibited

356. The accumulation of an oxygen debt during strenuous physical exercise may be accompanied by increases in

(1) NAD^+ in muscle

(2) lactate in blood

(3) ATP in muscle

(4) pyruvate in blood

357. Glycogen synthase is an enzyme that

(1) requires UDP-glucose as a substrate

(2) is only active in the phosphorylated form

(3) is found in glycogen particles

(4) is inactivated by phosphorylase kinase

358. Antibiotic inhibitors of transcription include

(1) streptomycin

(2) actinomycin

(3) puromycin

(4) rifamycin

359. Carnitine, a zwitterionic compound derived from lysine, is involved in fatty acid metabolism. It is

(1) required for absorption of long-chain fatty acids from the intestine

(2) a component of bile salts

(3) a component of CoA

(4) required for transport of long-chain fatty acids into mitochondria

360. In addition to the enzymes needed for the β oxidation of saturated fatty acids, the oxidation of unsaturated fatty acids also requires

(1) isomerase

(2) reductase

(3) epimerase

(4) dehydratase

361. The synthesis of all of the steroid hormones involves

(1) mono-oxygenases (mixed-function oxygenases)

(2) molecular O_2

(3) pregnenolone

(4) NADPH

SUMMARY OF DIRECTIONS				
A	**B**	**C**	**D**	**E**
1, 2, 3 only	1, 3 only	2, 4 only	4 only	All are correct

362. Which of the following factors are important in the control of de novo purine biosynthesis?

(1) stimulation of the conversion of IMP to AMP by GTP

(2) stimulation of the conversion of IMP to GMP by ATP

(3) availability of 5-phosphoribosyl-1-pyrophosphate (PRPP)

(4) inhibition of the enzyme PRPP amidotransferase by GMP

363. Which of the following enzyme abnormalities would be expected to lead to hyperuricemia?

(1) glucose 6-phosphatase deficiency (von Gierke's disease)

(2) elevated PRPP synthetase activity

(3) hypoxanthine-guanine phosphoribosyltransferase (HGPRT) deficiency (Lesch-Nyhan syndrome)

(4) purine nucleoside phosphorylase deficiency

364. Reduced glutathione is known to

(1) react with hydrogen peroxide to detoxify cells

(2) maintain the disulfide bridges of proteins in a reduced state

(3) regenerate from the oxidized form in RBCs by reacting with electrons donated from NADPH to FAD

(4) regenerate from the oxidized state by electrons donated from NADH

365. In the presence of arsenate, which of the following may occur during glycolysis?

(1) 1,3-DPG is formed

(2) NADH is formed

(3) P_i reacts with glyceraldehyde 3-phosphate

(4) 3-phosphoglycerate is formed

366. Which of the following can be synthesized from diacylglyceride in one step?

(1) phosphatidyl ethanolamine

(2) phosphatidyl choline

(3) triacylglyceride

(4) lysophosphatidic acid

367. In mitochondria, both cyanide and carbon monoxide inhibit

(1) oxidative phosphorylation

(2) electron transport

(3) proton gradient formation

(4) the consumption of molecular O_2

368. Electron transfer to or from NAD^+ in the respiratory chain directly involves

(1) cytochrome c

(2) FMN

(3) cytochrome c_1

(4) NADH dehydrogenase

369. The figure below displays the effect of ATP addition on the activity of phosphofructokinase. This information indicates that

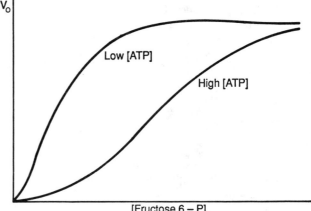

(1) there is cooperative binding of the substrate, fructose 6-phosphate, to the enzyme in the presence of ATP

(2) ATP decreases the apparent Vmax of the reaction

(3) ATP increases the apparent K_m of the enzyme

(4) ATP activates the enzyme

370. Cytochrome P_{450} may be correctly described as

(1) directly reducing molecular O_2

(2) a microsomal electron transport cytochrome

(3) simultaneously forming water and hydroxylating organic substrates

(4) being found in superoxide dismutase

371. Some characteristics of eukaryotic chromosome structure include

(1) the repeating unit of chromatin structure is the nucleosome

(2) histones are large acidic proteins that are components of nucleosomes

(3) some small sequences in the eukaryotic chromosome may be repeated as many as 1 million times

(4) RNA is an integral component of the nucleosome core

372. Which of the following reagents are employed for the determination of the N-terminal amino acid in proteins?

(1) ninhydrin

(2) phenylisothiocyanate

(3) cyanogen bromide

(4) fluorodinitrobenzene (FDNB)

373. Restriction endonucleases

(1) recognize specific palindromic sequences in DNA

(2) are produced by bacteria to protect against transformation by foreign DNA

(3) cleave both strands of DNA at specific sites

(4) do not degrade the host cell's DNA because the recognition site is methylated

374. Electrons from NADH formed in the cytosol of muscle cells can

(1) be transferred into mitochondria as glycerol 3-phosphate

(2) be carried as FADH in mitochondria

(3) enter electron transport at the level of coenzyme Q

(4) be carried as dihydroxyacetone phosphate in mitochondria

375. Which of the following events may occur in the citric acid cycle?

(1) the carbon atoms of acetyl-CoA are lost as CO_2

(2) two NAD^+ molecules are reduced in each round

(3) four water molecules are consumed in each round

(4) one FAD molecule is reduced in each round

376. The liver is the only body organ that is capable of

(1) urea formation

(2) ganglioside synthesis

(3) bile acid synthesis

(4) medium-chain fatty acid catabolism

377. The amino acid tyrosine is the precursor of

(1) histamine

(2) epinephrine

(3) serotonin

(4) thyroxine

378. Which of the following cofactors or their derivatives must be present for the conversion of pyruvate to acetyl-CoA?

(1) NAD^+

(2) FAD

(3) thiamine

(4) lipoic acid

379. The disease pellagra can be prevented by a dietary sufficiency of

(1) riboflavin

(2) tryptophan

(3) thiamine

(4) niacin (nicotinic acid)

380. Which of the following statements may correctly describe the receptors of hormones using cyclic AMP as a second messenger?

(1) only one protein is responsible for both interaction with the hormone and production of cyclic AMP

(2) a G protein is intermediate between the receptor protein and the catalytic protein

(3) binding of hormone to the receptor releases a catalytic subunit

(4) the receptor protein is separate from the catalytic protein

381. Which of the following may be classified as covalently modulated enzymes?

(1) pepsin

(2) glycogen synthase

(3) chymotrypsin

(4) aspartate transcarbamoylase

Answers and Explanations

255. The answer is C. Two distinct pathways for nucleotide biosynthesis exist in most cells. In the de novo pathway, nucleotides are synthesized from smaller precursor molecules, such as amino acids, CO_2, and ammonia. Free nucleic acid bases or nucleosides are not produced as intermediates in this pathway. These latter compounds, however, may be used for the synthesis of nucleotides via the salvage pathways. Free bases and nucleosides become available either through nucleic acid breakdown or diet. Thymidylate can be synthesized in two steps from thymine via the salvage pathways. Thymine is first converted to thymidine by the enzyme thymidine phosphorylase and then to thymidylate by the action of thymidine kinase. 5-Fluorodeoxyuridylate is a potent inhibitor of thymidylate synthase, the enzyme responsible for de novo thymidylate biosynthesis. Inhibition of this enzyme will have a major effect on DNA synthesis, since thymidylate is a precursor employed specifically for DNA synthesis. Cells cannot take up charged compounds, such as nucleotides, from the surrounding environment, and, therefore, the base fluorouracil must be administered rather than fluorodeoxyuridylate. In order to inhibit thymidylate synthase, the fluorouracil must be converted to its corresponding nucleotide by the salvage pathway. *(Stryer, pp 613–616)*

256. The answer is D. Under certain conditions (e.g., fasting) acetyl-CoA derived from fatty acid oxidation is diverted from use in the citric acid cycle and employed instead for the formation of acetoacetate and 3-hydroxybutyrate. These compounds are referred to as ketone bodies. The major site of acetoacetate production is the liver, but it can diffuse into the blood, where it can be taken by peripheral tissue. In muscle, a thiokinase enzyme uses 1 mol of ATP to convert acetoacetate to acetoacetyl-CoA. Once produced, acetoacetyl-CoA is cleaved by thiolase to yield 2 mol of acetyl-CoA, which is metabolized via the citric acid cycle to produce 12 mol of ATP/mol of acetyl-CoA. Subtracting the 1 mol of ATP employed in the initial formation of acetoacetyl CoA gives a net production of 23 mol of ATP. *(Stryer, pp 478–480)*

257. The answer is A. Under anaerobic conditions (e.g., intense exercise), the production of pyruvate via glycolysis exceeds its oxidation by the citric acid cycle. This results in the synthesis of lactate by muscle. Lactate diffuses into the bloodstream and is taken up by liver, where it is oxidized back to pyruvate. The latter is converted to glucose in liver via gluconeogenesis. *(Stryer, pp 444–445)*

258. The answer is C. In the interior of peripheral tissues, the concentration of CO_2 is high, and the relative O_2 tension is low. As a consequence, O_2 is unloaded from Hb, and CO_2 is taken up. Although some CO_2 is transported as a dissolved gas, most CO_2 is transported as bicarbonate. Bicarbonate is formed by the action of carbonic anhydrase within red blood cells.

$$CO_2 + H_2O \rightleftharpoons HCO_3^- + H^+$$

In addition, CO_2 is carried by Hb as carbamino derivatives. The un-ionized α-amino groups of Hb react reversibly with CO_2.

$$CO_2 + R - NH_2 \rightleftharpoons R - NHCOO^- + H^+$$

The charged carbamates form salt bridges that stabilize the T form of Hb and lower its O_2 affinity. Unlike O_2, CO_2 does not bind to the iron of the heme group. *(Stryer, p 162)*

259. The answer is B. All contractile cells contain actin and myosin. In nonmuscle cells, such as macrophages, the contractile elements are important for mobility and shape changes. The mechanisms of contraction seem to be similar, using ATP hydrolysis as a driving force. In all cell types, the cytoskeletons are composed of the contractile filaments. In nonmuscle cells, the cytoskeleton is composed mainly of actin polymerized into a latticework of microfilaments approximately 70 nm thick. Unlike muscle cells, the contraction of non-muscle cells does not seem to be governed by nervous stimulation. *(Stryer, pp 936–938)*

260. The answer is A. During glycolysis, pyruvate is synthesized from phosphoenolpyruvate with the concomitant production of ATP from ADP. The equilibrium of this reaction lies far to the left for the reaction as written.

$$ATP + pyruvate \rightleftharpoons phosphoenolpyruvate + ADP + P_i$$

The standard free-energy change ($\Delta G^{\circ\prime}$) for the hydrolysis of ATP is -7.3 kcal/mol, whereas the $\Delta G^{\circ\prime}$ for the phosphorylation of pyruvate to phosphoenolpyruvate is $+14.8$ kcal/mol (the opposite of the $\Delta G^{\circ\prime}$ for the hydrolysis of phosphoenolpyruvate). Thus, the calculated $\Delta G^{\circ\prime}$ for the thermodynamically unfavorable production of phosphoenolpyruvate is $+7.5$ kcal/mol. *(Stryer, p 316)*

261. The answer is E. The carbohydrate moieties in RNA and DNA are ribose and deoxyribose, respectively. A major product of the pentose phosphate pathway is ribose 5-phosphate. The latter is converted to 5-phosphoribosyl-1-pyrophosphate (PRPP), which serves as the donor of ribose in the biosynthesis of nucleotides. *(Stryer, pp 427–430,602–608)*

262. The answer is D. Phosphoric acid, H_3PO_4, contains three ionizable hydrogen atoms as indicated in the following equation.

$$H_3PO_4 \rightarrow H_2PO_4^- \rightarrow HPO_4^{2-} \rightarrow PO_4^{3-}$$

pK_2 is the relevant pKa to use in calculating the pH of the solution in this problem because the dissociation involves $H_2PO_4^-$ and HPO_4^{2-}. The pH can be determined by the Henderson-Hasselbalch equation.

$$pH = pKa + \log [salt]/[acid] = 6.8 + \log 0.15/0.05 = 6.8 + \log 3 = 7.28$$

(Stryer, pp 41–42)

263. The answer is A. Myosin contains the ATPase activity that hydrolyzes ATP and allows contraction to proceed. The binding of actin to myosin enhances the ATPase activity of myosin. In fact, actin alternatively binds to myosin and is released from myosin as ATP is hydrolyzed. This reaction requires Mg^{2+} and is the driving force of contraction. Although troponin is not directly involved in the ATPase reaction, it binds calcium released by the sarcoplasmic reticulum and in doing so allows conformational changes in tropomyosin and actin to occur, permitting contraction. Myokinase cata-

lyzes the formation of ATP and AMP from two molecules of ADP. *(Stryer, pp 930–932)*

264. The answer is C. The allosteric regulatory enzymes of glycolysis are hexokinase, phosphofructokinase, and pyruvate kinase. Of these, phosphofructokinase is the key regulatory enzyme. A high-energy charge or the presence of sufficient citric acid cycle precursors causes the inhibition of phosphofructokinase via accumulation of the negative effectors ATP and citrate. ADP and AMP are positive effectors of phosphofructokinase. Accumulation of glucose 6-phosphate inhibits hexokinase. Pyruvate kinase is inhibited by high ATP levels. Fructose 6-phosphate, the substrate of phosphofructokinase, is not an effector. *(Stryer, pp 359–362)*

265. The answer is E. Of the monosaccharides and disaccharides listed in the question, only fructose enters the glycolytic pathway at the level of three-carbon intermediates. Fructokinase catalyzes the phosphorylation of fructose by ATP to fructose 1-phosphate, which is then cleaved to glyceraldehyde and dihydroxyacetone phosphate by aldolase. The glyceraldehyde is phosphorylated to glyceraldehyde 3-phosphate. Thus, two intermediates of glycolysis are formed from one molecule of fructose. In contrast, galactose and mannose enter glycolysis at the level of glucose 1-phosphate and fructose 6-phosphate, respectively. The breakdown products of maltose (i.e., glucose) and lactose (i.e., glucose and galactose) enter glycolysis at the level of six-carbon sugars. *(Stryer, pp 357–359)*

266. · **The answer is A.** The first step in gluconeogenesis is the formation of oxaloacetate from pyruvate. The enzyme controlling this step is pyruvate carboxylase, an allosteric enzyme that does not function in the absence of its primary effector, acetyl-CoA, or a closely related acyl-CoA. Thus, a high level of acetyl-CoA signals the need for more oxaloacetate. If there is a surplus of ATP, oxaloacetate will be used for gluconeogenesis. Under conditions of low ATP, oxaloacetate will be consumed in the citric acid cycle. Citrate is the primary negative effector of glycolysis and the primary positive effector of fatty acid synthesis. *(Stryer, p 441)*

267. The answer is E. In skeletal muscle, the hormone epinephrine or the neurotransmitter norepinephrine binds to sarcolemma receptors and activates adenylate cyclase. Glucagon, which causes similar effects in the liver, is not specific for muscle. Activated adenylate cyclase forms cyclic AMP from ATP. Cyclic AMP activates protein kinase, which in turn activates phosphorylase kinase. Phosphorylase kinase activates phosphorylase, converting it from the inactive *b* form to the activated *a* form. Both the phosphorylase kinase and phosphorylase itself are activated by phosphorylation mechanisms. Activated glycogen phosphorylase hydrolyzes glycogen, sequentially cleaving off glucose units as glucose 1-phosphate. *(Stryer, pp 462–464)*

268. **The answer is B.** Thymidylate (TMP) is synthesized by methylation of deoxyuridylate (dUMP) at the five-carbon in a reaction catalyzed by thymidylate synthase. TMP is the only precursor for DNA synthesis that is produced separately from the major biosynthetic pathways for purine and pyrimidine ribonucleotides. For this reason, reactions required for TMP biosynthesis are specific targets for drugs that will inhibit DNA synthesis. 5-Fluorouracil is a modified uracil that contains a fluorine attached to the five-carbon. It binds to thymidylate synthase because it is a structural analog of dUMP and forms a covalent complex with the enzyme. This results in complete inactivation of thymidylate synthase. Cells that are rapidly proliferating, such as tumor cells, carry out high levels of DNA synthesis. They, therefore, require larger amounts of TMP than normal cells and, for this reason, are more susceptible to the action of fluorouracil. *(Stryer, pp 614–616)*

269. **The answer is B.** The Michaelis constant (K_m) is determined by measuring the rate of the reaction in the presence of a fixed concentration of enzyme and varying concentrations of substrate. Graphical analysis of such data will provide values for K_m and Vmax. The turnover number is defined as the number of substrate molecules converted to product per enzyme molecule in a specific period of time. K_m is not related to turnover number. It is also not dependent on the molecular weight of the enzyme. *(Stryer, pp. 187–191,199–200)*

270. **The answer is E.** Tertiary structure refers to the three-dimensional arrangement of amino acid residues in a protein. Studies of many proteins reveal that the nonpolar (hydrophobic) amino acid residues are buried in the interior of the protein structure, whereas the polar residues are on the outside in contact with the aqueous environment. The protein folds so as to shield its nonpolar groups from interaction with water molecules. These hydrophobic interactions are the driving force of protein folding. The tertiary structure is further stabilized by hydrogen bonding, polar interactions, and the formation of disulfide bonds. Peptide bonds are only involved in formation of the primary structure of a protein. *(Stryer, pp 29–34)*

271. **The answer is A.** Activation and linking of free amino acids to tRNA are catalyzed by aminoacyl-tRNA synthetases specific for each amino acid. This enzyme, like all others, can only accelerate the time in which a reaction reaches equilibrium. It cannot drive the reaction in a specific direction. During activation, amino acids are linked to AMP.

$$\text{Amino acid} + \text{ATP} \rightleftharpoons \text{aminoacyl-AMP} + \text{PP}_i$$

During transfer, the activated amino acid is linked to a specific RNA.

$$\text{Aminoacyl-AMP} + \text{tRNA} \rightleftharpoons \text{aminoacyl-tRNA} + \text{AMP}$$

Since the free energy of hydrolysis of the ester bonds formed is similar to that of the terminal phosphate of ATP, the $\Delta G°'$ of the reaction is nearly zero. The reaction is driven by the hydrolysis of pyrophosphate (PP_i).

$$\text{PP}_i + \text{H}_2\text{O} \rightarrow 2\,\text{P}_i$$

The formation of P_i by pyrophosphatase is a common cell mechanism to ensure the irreversibility of an otherwise reversible reaction. *(Stryer, pp 734–735)*

272. **The answer is B.** Most peripheral tissues, including muscle, avidly sequester glucose. The hexokinases of these tissues have a low K_m and a high affinity for glucose. Once phosphorylated, the glucose cannot leave peripheral tissues. In contrast, liver glucokinase has a very high K_m for glucose. This low-affinity enzyme will only phosphorylate glucose when blood levels are high. Phosphorylated glucose derived from glycogen stores in the liver may be released back into the blood as glucose when levels fall because of the presence of glucose 6-phosphatase in liver endoplasmic reticulum. *(Stryer, pp 187–191,352,361)*

273. **The answer is A.** Long-chain (> 10 carbon atoms) as well as medium-chain (5 to 10 carbon atoms) and short-chain (2 to 4 carbon atoms) fatty acids must be activated before β oxidation, which uses only fatty acids linked to CoA. Long-chain fatty acids are activated outside the mitochondrial matrix and then transported across the inner membrane of mitochondria as acyl carnitine complexes. In contrast, short- and medium-chain fatty acids diffuse across the inner mitochondrial membrane and are activated in the matrix. Fatty acid thiokinase (acyl-CoA synthetase) catalyzes the activation reaction in which the carboxyl group of the free fatty acid forms a thioester linkage with CoA.

$$\text{R-COO}^- + \text{ATP} + \text{HS-CoA} \rightleftharpoons \text{R-CO-S-CoA} + \text{AMP} + \text{PP}_i$$

The reaction is made irreversible by the consumption of the equivalent of two high-energy phosphate bonds and the hydrolysis of the resulting PP_i by pyrophosphatase. *(Stryer, pp 472–473)*

274. **The answer is C.** The formation of the three-carbon CoA thioester malonyl-CoA from acetyl-CoA is the regulatory step of fatty acid synthesis. Acetyl-CoA carboxylase catalyzes this reaction.

$$\text{Acetyl-CoA} + HCO_3^- + ATP \rightleftharpoons \text{malonyl-CoA} + ADP + P_i$$

Citrate, which serves as the means of transport of acetyl-CoA from the mitochondria to the cytosolic site of fatty acid synthesis, is the key allosteric regulator of acetyl-CoA carboxylase. It shifts the enzyme from an inactive protomer to an active filamentous polymer. The end product of the cytosolic fatty acid synthetase complex, palmitoyl-CoA, inhibits the carboxylase. Although acetyl-CoA carboxylase is the prime regulatory enzyme of fatty acid synthesis, it is not a part of the fatty acid synthetase complex, the site where most of the reactions of fatty acid synthesis take place. *(Stryer, pp 481–482)*

275. **The answer is A.** The first two steps of cholesterol biosynthesis lead to the formulation of 3-hydroxy-3-methylglutaryl-CoA. These are also the first two steps of ketone body synthesis. In ketogenesis, 3-hydroxy-3-methylglutaryl-CoA is cleaved to form acetoacetate and acetyl-CoA. In cholesterol biosynthesis, it is reduced to form mevalonic acid. Although these steps are common to both ketogenesis and cholesterol biosynthesis, they are separate in time and space. Cholesterol biosynthesis occurs in the cytosol of cells from excess acetyl-CoA produced from dietary surplus. In contrast, ketogenesis occurs only in the mitochondria of liver cells from acetyl-CoA derived from β oxidation of fatty acids. Ketogenesis does not occur to any great extent except in states of dietary need, such as fasting and starvation, or under abnormal circumstances, such as an excessively fat-rich diet or diabetes. *(Stryer, pp 478–479,554–559)*

276. **The answer is D.** Cholesterol is obtained from the diet as well as by de novo synthesis. Although many cells can synthesize cholesterol, the liver is the major site of its production. The rate of cholesterol production is highly responsive to feedback inhibition from both dietary cholesterol and synthesized cholesterol. Feedback regulation is mediated by changes in the activity of 3-hydroxy-3-methylglutaryl-CoA reductase. This enzyme is the first committed step in the production of cholesterol from acetyl-CoA. 3-Hydroxy-3-methylglutaryl-CoA, the substrate of the reductase, also can be synthesized into the ketone body acetoacetate by the action of 3-hydroxy-3-methylglutaryl-CoA lyase. *(Stryer, pp 560,564)*

277. **The answer is B.** Unlike phosphoglycerides, sphingomyelin lacks a glycerol backbone. Phosphoglycerides are composed of glycerol esterified to two fatty acids by an ester linkage and to a polar group by a phosphate ester linkage. Lecithin is the phospholipid phosphatidyl choline. In contrast, sphingomyelin is composed of one fatty acid esterified to the amino group of sphingosine and a polar group attached to the hydroxyl of sphingosine through a phosphate ester linkage. Choline and ethanolamine are the polar groups of sphingomyelin. All of the lipids listed in the question are important in membrane structure. *(Stryer, pp 547–553)*

278. **The answer is C.** In contrast to liver cells, adipocytes contain little or no glycerol kinase. Thus, glycerol produced from lipolysis is not used to any great extent as a source of glycerol 3-phosphate, the central substrate for esterification of fatty acids into triacylglycerols. The major source of glycerol 3-phosphate in adipocytes is dihydroxyacetone phosphate, which is derived from glycolysis of glucose. A lack of glucose, such as that that occurs in diabetes or fasting, would inhibit triacylglycerol synthesis and favor lipolysis. Ketogenesis and gluconeogenesis do not occur in adipocytes. *(Stryer, pp 471–472)*

279. **The answer is D.** In the genetic disorder known as Tay-Sachs disease, ganglioside GM_2 is not catabolized. As a consequence, the ganglioside concentration is elevated many times higher than normal. The functionally absent lysosomal enzyme is β-N-acetylhexosaminidase. The elevated GM_2 results in irreversible brain damage to infants, who usually die before the age of 3 years. Under normal conditions, this enzyme cleaves N-acetylgalactosamine from the oligosaccharide chain of this complex sphingolipid, allowing further catabolism to occur. The cause of most lipidoses (lipid storage diseases) is similar. That is, a defect in catabolism of gangliosides causes abnormal accumulation. *(Stryer, p 554)*

280. **The answer is B.** In fasting or diabetes, lipolysis predominates in adipocytes because of the inability of these cells to obtain glucose, which is normally used as a source of glycerol 3-phosphate. Glycerol 3-phosphate is necessary for the esterification of fatty acids into triacylglycerides. Circulating fatty acids become the predominant fuel source, and β oxidation in the liver becomes substantially elevated. This leads to an increased production of acetyl-CoA. Since glucose use in diabetes is reduced, gluconeogenesis is increased in the liver. This predisposes oxaloacetate and makes the citric acid cycle unavailable for heightened use of acetyl-CoA. As a consequence, acetyl-CoA is diverted to the formation of ketone bodies. *(Stryer, pp 478–480)*

281–283. The answers are 281-A, 282-C, 283-B. The curve to the left of curve Z on the reaction velocity vs. substrate concentration plot shown in the question has a lower K_m. This can be easily demonstrated since $K_m = \frac{1}{2}$ Vmax and all the curves shown have the same Vmax. Thus, curve X demonstrates higher reaction velocities at lower substrate concentrations than the other curves shown. Curve X represents a positively modulated reaction velocity of the same enzyme represented by curve Z. In contrast, curve Y represents a plot of the same enzyme shown in curve Z in the presence of a negative modulator.

In going from left to right in the figure that accompanies the question, the reaction velocity per unit substrate concentration decreases in those areas of the curves where Vmax is not being approached. The K_m of the curves to the right increases, indicating a decreased affinity for substrate. Most likely, this would be because of an increase in inhibitory modulator concentrations or a decrease in positive modulator concentrations. The Vmax is similar in all of the curves shown, and either an increase in a needed cofactor or positive cooperativity would push the curves from right to left.

Since $K_m = \frac{1}{2}$ Vmax the apparent K_m for curve Y in the question is 3 μmol/L. The Vmax of all the curves shown is 12 μmol/min. A line drawn horizontally from one-half that value on the y axis to curve Y and from that point vertically to the x axis will give the apparent K_m. *(Stryer, pp 187–195, 239–243)*

284. The answer is A. Untreated diabetes leads to high blood glucose levels (hyperglycemia) and glucosuria, as glucose exceeds the kidney threshold and spills into the urine. At the same time that blood glucose levels are high, the lack of insulin leads to a favoring of lipolysis and consequent ketogenesis by the liver. The high level of ketogenesis by the liver produces ketonemia (high blood levels of ketone bodies) and ketonuria (ketone bodies in the urine). Insulin injections help to reduce these symptoms and allow diabetic persons to live relatively normal lives. However, insulin injections when blood glucose levels are low, as well as overdoses of insulin, can cause severe hypoglycemia (low blood levels of glucose). If blood glucose levels fall below 80 mg/100 ml, insulin shock occurs. When blood levels fall below 20 mg/100 ml, convulsions and coma occur because of the deprivation of glucose to the brain. IV glucose injections can reverse insulin shock. *(Stryer, pp 641–642)*

285. The answer is A. Pro-opiocortin can give rise to five peptide hormones of the anterior pituitary. ACTH and β-lipotropin, a prohormone, are formed by cleavage of pro-opiocortin. α-Melanocyte-stimulating hormone (α-MSH) is a cleavage product of ACTH, whereas β-endorphin and γ-lipotropin are cleavage products of β-lipotropin. β-MSH is a cleavage fragment of β-endorphin. This is summarized below.

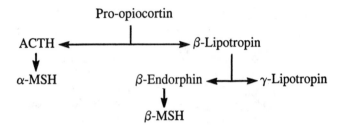

TSH is a hormone of the anterior pituitary that is not derived from pro-opiocortin. *Stryer, pp 993–994)*

286. The answer is E. Biotin serves as an intermediate carrier of CO_2 during carboxylations catalyzed by acetyl-CoA carboxylase, propionyl carboxylase, and pyruvate carboxylase. This vitamin is present in the prosthetic groups of these enzymes. Biotin is made from intestinal bacteria and is also obtained from a wide variety of foods. Avidin, a protein present in egg whites, tightly binds biotin in the gut, preventing its absorption. In individuals who consume large quantities of raw eggs, this leads to a toxic reaction due to biotin's role in carboxylation reactions. *(Stryer, pp 481–482)*

287. The answer is A. The α-amino group of many amino acids is transferred to α-ketoglutarate to form glutamate, which is then oxidatively deaminated to ammonium ion. A similar transamination reaction yields alanine from pyruvate during degradation of amino acids. The prosthetic group of all transaminases is pyridoxal phosphate (PLP), which is derived from pyridoxine. During transamination, the aldehyde group of PLP forms a Schiff's-base linkage with the α-amino group of amino acids, ultimately transferring the amino group to either a α-ketoglutarate or pyruvate. *(Stryer, pp 495–499)*

288. The answer is C. Vitamin B_1 is obtained as thiamine from pork, yeast, whole grains, and nuts. Its active form in enzymatic reactions is thiamine pyrophosphate (TPP), a form to which it is converted in the body. During decarboxylation, substrates form a hydroxyethyl-TPP intermediate, which is then oxidized to an acetyl group before being transferred off of TPP. A deficiency of thiamine leads to beriberi, a wasting disease with nervous system damage and edema. *(Stryer, pp 379–382)*

289. The answer is B. LDLs are the primary carriers of blood cholesterol. Routine plasma lipid measurements are carried out after a 12-hr fast. In this way, the major endogenous plasma lipoproteins, VLDLs, and the major exogenous plasma lipoproteins (chylomicrons) have been cleared from the blood of normal individuals. LDLs, which are the end products of VLDL delipidation, and HDLs, which are protein rich, are the only lipoproteins circulating after a 12-hr fast. LDLs are rich in cholesterol, being composed of about 45 percent cholesterol or cholesterol esters. In both dietary and familial hypercholesterolemia, circulating LDL levels are increased. *(Stryer, pp 560–561)*

290. The answer is D. A deficiency in galactose 1-phosphate uridyl transferase causes galactosemia, a disease characterized by high blood levels of galactose, defective growth, mental retardation, and in some cases death. Early diagnosis and treatment with a galactose-free diet reverse most clinical symptoms. Galactose is formed by the hydrolysis of lactose and is normally formed into glucose. First, galactose is phosphorylated to galactose 1-phosphate by galactokinase. The uridyl transferase reaction transfers UDP from UDP-glucose to the phosphorylated galactose. UDP-galactose is then converted to UDP-glucose by UDP-galactose-4-epimerase. *(Stryer, pp 357–359)*

291. The answer is B. After hydrolysis of the apoprotein of Hb in old erythrocytes in the spleen, the heme group is degraded. First, the α-methene bridge is cleaved to form biliverdin, a linear tetrapyrrole, which is green. The mono-oxegenase called heme oxygenase catalyzes the reaction, which requires molecular O_2 and the reduced form of NADPH. A methene bridge carbon is released. The enzyme biliverdin reductase catalyzes the reduction by NADPH of the central methene bridge carbon of biliverdin to form bilirubin, which is red. After these reactions, bilirubin is transported to the liver complexed to serum albumin. There, each bilirubin molecule is conjugated via UDP-glucuronate to two glucuronates to form bilirubin diglucuronide. These six-carbon, carboxylated derivatives of glucose are attached to the propionated side chains of bilirubin, making it more soluble before its excretion in the bile. Unlike bile pigments, the bile acids are conjugated to glycine or taurine. *(Stryer, pp 596–597)*

292. The answer is C. Carbohydrates attached to asparagine residues have a common inner-core structure. Such a block of oligosaccharides is built up and carried to the asparagine of proteins on a lipid carrier. That carrier is dolichol phosphate, an aliphatic chain composed of isoprene units. *N*-acetylglucosamine is the sugar residue directly bonded to dolichol phosphate and then transferred to the asparagine side chain. *(Stryer, pp 773–774)*

293. The answer is C. Except for the initial formation of malonyl-CoA by the carboxylation of acetyl-CoA, most of the reactions of fatty acid synthesis occur on the cytosolic fatty acid synthetase complex. The

intermediates are attached to the complex by the sulfhydryl group of the acyl carrier protein (ACP). When malonyl-ACP is condensed with acyl-ACP, the carbon atom derived from bicarbonate is decarboxylated as CO_2. The β-ketoacyl intermediate formed is reduced in the presence of NADPH to a β-hydroxyacyl, which then is dehydrated to form an enoyl. The enoyl is reduced by NADPH to a saturated acyl in the final step of each round of elongation. *(Stryer, pp 481–487)*

294. The answer is A. During ethanol clearance in any individual, including alcoholic persons, ethanol is first converted to acetaldehyde by the action of alcohol dehydrogenase and then to acetate by the action of acetaldehyde dehydrogenase. Both of these enzymes require the oxidized form of NAD^+ to function. During alcohol oxidation, the level of the reduced form of nicotinamide adenine dinucleotide (NADH) increases greatly in the liver, leading to an overload of the shuttle normally used to regenerate NAD^+. This causes the level of NAD^+ to be the bottleneck in the removal of alcohol from the body. The levels of alcohol dehydrogenase may be somewhat higher than normal in chronically alcoholic persons. Nevertheless, NAD^+ is still the rate-limiting factor in the oxidation of ethanol. *(Stryer, pp 362–364)*

295. The answer is C. In contrast to the glycerol 3-phosphate shuttle operating in skeletal muscle, in the heart and liver the bidirectional malate-aspartate shuttle transfers the electrons of cytoplasmic and mitochondrial NADH between the two cell compartments reversibly. The pathway is complex, with glutamate, aspartate, malate, and α-ketoglutarate serving as diffusible carriers. Mitochondrial and cytosolic oxaloacetate and NADH also serve as electron transporters. In contrast to the glycerol 3-phosphate shuttle, which yields only two ATP per pair of electrons derived from cytosolic NADH, the malate-aspartate shuttle yields three ATP per cytosolic NADH. This occurs because NADH and not the reduced form of flavin adenine dinucleotide (FADH) is the mitochondrial carrier of electrons. *(Stryer, pp 417–418)*

296. The answer is D. Except for the fact that the carrier groups for fatty acid synthesis (ACP) and β oxidation (CoA) are different, the attached intermediates are similar. In each group of reactions, the enzymatic steps result in acyl, enoyl, β-hydroxyacyl, and β-ketoacyl intermediates being formed or degraded. The enzymatic steps differ in that fatty acid synthesis is carried out in the cytosol using NADPH as a reductant. Biosynthesis is stimulated by citrate. β oxidation occurs in the mitochondrial matrix using flavin adenine dinucleotide (FAD) and NAD^+ as pyridine nucleotide acceptors of electrons. Citrate levels are low during fatty acid oxidation. *(Stryer, pp 472–488)*

297. The answer is D. Glycolysis is the only major source of ATP in erythrocytes, since they lack mitochondria. In order for glycolysis to continue uninterrupted, NADH must constantly be reoxidized to NAD$^+$ so that glyceraldehyde 3-phosphate may be oxidized. Conversion of pyruvate to lactate by lactate dehydrogenase accomplishes this. The excess lactate diffuses into the liver, where it is converted to glucose via gluconeogenesis. *(Stryer, pp 444–445)*

298. The answer is D. Increases in either hydrogen ion concentration (lowered pH), CO_2 partial pressure, or 2,3-DPG all lead to a decreased affinity of Hb for O_2. Conversely, decreases in these factors lead to an increased affinity of O_2 for Hb. A decrease in pH changes the charge on histidine residues in Hb, favoring the release of O_2. Binding of DPG to deoxyhemoglobin causes the cross-linking of the β chains, leading to a stabilization of the deoxygenated form of Hb and a lowered affinity for O_2. CO_2 binds to the un-ionized α-amino groups on the terminal ends of Hb. This results in charged carbamino derivatives, which form salt bridges. The salt bridges further reduce the affinity of Hb for O_2. *(Stryer, pp 156–157, 160–163)*

299. The answer is A. In persons with a deficiency in pyruvate kinase, glycolytic intermediates are high because the terminal step is blocked. 2,3-DPG, which is formed from the glycolytic intermediate 1,3-DPG by a mutase, accumulates in RBCs. 2,3-DPG is a regulator of O_2 transport that acts by stabilizing the structure of deoxyhemoglobin. Thus, an increase in 2,3-DPG levels leads to a low O_2 affinity in persons with pyruvate kinase deficiency. Just the opposite effect has been observed in individuals with hexokinase deficiency. Deficiencies of any of the other enzymes listed in the question would not result in accumulations of glycolytic intermediates that would lead to increases in 2,3-DPG. *(Stryer, pp 361–362, 368–370)*

300. The answer is D. The biochemical deficiency of the enzyme HGPRT results in mental retardation and compulsive self-destructive behavior. This X-linked recessive disease also results in gout because of elevated levels of urate. However, unlike gout alone, allopurinol treatment of patients with Lesch-Nyhan syndrome does not increase the rate of synthesis of purines because it does not lower the level of PRPP. In genetically normal individuals, HGPRT allows the salvage synthesis of guanosine 5′-monophosphate (GMP) or inosine 5′-monophosphate (IMP) from guanine or hypoxanthine plus PRPP. The relationship between salvage pathways of purine synthesis and de novo pathways is not yet understood. *(Stryer, pp 620–623)*

301. The answer is A. Partial defects of enzymes of the urea cycle commonly lead to hyperammonemia, since the synthesis of urea in the liver is the major route of ammonia (NH_4^+) removal. The high levels of NH_4^+ are toxic. It is thought that the increased concentration of ammonia ions depletes α-ketoglutarate levels by shifting the equilibrium of glutamate dehydrogenase toward glutamate and glutamine formation.

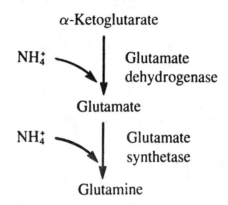

The decrease of α-ketoglutarate adversely affects the citric acid cycle, leading to a decrease in ATP levels. Development and function of brain tissue are highly vulnerable to low ATP levels. Deficiencies of urea cycle enzymes also lead to decreased amounts of urea and increases in the concentrations of certain cycle intermediates preceding the lesion. In mild forms of hyperammonemia, low-protein diets may allow clinical improvement by lowering blood NH_4^+ levels. Gout, which results from elevated levels of urate in the serum, is not related to the urea cycle. It is often caused by partial deficiencies of the enzyme HGPRT, a purine salvage pathway enzyme. *(Stryer, pp 500–502)*

302. The answer is B. The nucleotide thymine, unlike all the other nucleotides, is synthesized at the level of a deoxyribonucleoside monophosphate by the methylation of deoxyuridylate (dUMP) to deoxythymidylate (dTMP). The enzyme thymidylate synthetase catalyzes this reaction. Thus, TMP as such is not a product of the pathway of thymine synthesis. In contrast, all other nucleotides are synthesized as ribose phosphates. CTP is derived from uridine triphosphate (UTP) and is a feedback inhibitor of aspartate transcarbamoylase, the enzyme catalyzing the formation of carbamoyl aspartate, the precursor of UMP. In turn, UMP is the feedback inhibitor of the formation of carbamoyl phosphate, the precursor of carbamoyl aspartate. In purine nucleotide biosynthesis, the formation of PRPP from ribose 5-phosphate, as well as the conversion of PRPP to phosphoribosylamine, is inhibited by AMP, GMP, and IMP. The conversion of IMP to adenylosuccinate, the AMP precursor, is inhibited by AMP. The conversion of IMP to xanthylate, the G̃MP precursor, is inhibited by GMP. *(Stryer, pp 602–609,613–614)*

303. **The answer is D.** Under normal aerobic conditions, 36 net ATP are formed from the complete oxidation of glucose. Glycolysis yields 2 net ATP from substrate level phosphorylation, the citric acid cycle yields 2 ATP [as guanosine triphosphate (GTP)] from substrate level phosphorylation, and oxidative phosphorylation yields 32 ATP. In the presence of an uncoupling agent, such as dinitrophenol, substrate level phosphorylation still proceeds. Thus, 4 net ATP are produced. *(Stryer, pp 421–422)*

304. **The answer is B.** The net reaction for the complete oxidation of glucose is as follows:

$$\text{Glucose} + 36\,\text{ADP} + 36\,\text{P}_i + 36\,\text{H}^+ + 6\,\text{O}_2 \rightarrow 6\,\text{CO}_2 + 36\,\text{ATP} + 42\,\text{H}_2\text{O}$$

The phosphorus/O_2 ratio is 3, since 36 ATP are formed and 12 atoms of oxygen are consumed. Of the 36 ATP, only 4 (net) are not formed by oxidative phosphorylation. These include the 2 net ATP derived from substrate level phosphorylation in glycolysis and the 2 ATP equivalents formed as GTP from succinyl-CoA in the citric acid cycle. *(Stryer, pp 420–421)*

305. **The answer is A.** Glucose phosphate isomerase catalyzes the reversible conversion of fructose 6-phosphate to glucose 6-phosphate in both glycolysis and gluconeogenesis. In fact, most of the steps of glycolysis are simply reversed in gluconeogenesis. However, the three regulatory steps in the conversion of glucose to pyruvate are not reversible. These steps are (1) glucose → glucose 6-phosphate, which is catalyzed by hexokinase, (2) fructose 6-phosphate → fructose 1,6-diphosphate, which is catalyzed by phosphofructokinase, and (3) phosphoenolpyruvate → pyruvate, which is catalyzed by pyruvate kinase. The reversal of these steps in gluconeogenesis requires the enzymes glucose 6-phosphatase and fructose diphosphatase for the formation of glucose and fructose 6-phosphate, respectively. The formation of phosphoenolpyruvate from pyruvate is more complicated in that the four following steps are involved: (1) pyruvate carboxylase catalyzes the conversion of pyruvate to oxaloacetate, (2) oxaloacetate is reduced to malate by mitochondrial malate dehydrogenase, (3) malate is reconverted to oxaloacetate by extramitochondrial malate dehydrogenase, and (4) oxaloacetate is transformed to phosphoenolpyruvate by GTP-dependent phosphoenolpyruvate carboxykinase. *(Stryer, pp 438–440)*

306–308. **The answers are 306-B, 307-E, 308-D.** The transition state is an unstable intermediate in a reaction pathway between reactants and products.

It is usually the intermediate of highest free energy. The energy of activation (designated $\Delta G^{\ddagger}$) of any reaction is the difference in free energy between the ground state of the reactants and the transition state. There is a relationship between the rate of a reaction and its $\Delta G^{\ddagger}$: the larger the $\Delta G^{\ddagger}$, the slower the reaction. The free energy change of a reaction (ΔG) is given by the difference in free energy between the ground states of the products and reactants (i.e., $G_{prod} - G_{reac}$). A negative value for ΔG indicates that the reaction will proceed spontaneously without the input of any energy. It does not, however, indicate anything about the rate of the reaction. *(Stryer, pp 180–184)*

309–311. **The answers are 309-E, 310-D, 311-A.** The reactions of the citric acid cycle are shown in the figure below. *(Stryer, p 378)*

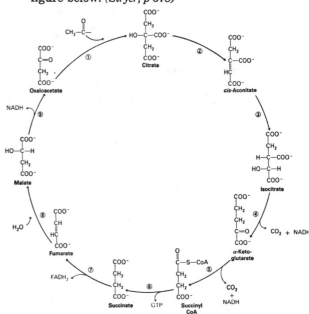

(From Biochemistry, *3rd ed, by Lubert Stryer. Copyright © 1975, 1981, 1988 by Lubert Stryer. Used by permission of W.H. Freeman and Company.)*

312–315. **The answers are 312-A, 313-D, 314-B, 315-E.** Glycogen phosphorylase catalyzes the sequential release of glucose from glycogen. The glycosidic bond between the two terminal glucose residues is split by inorganic phosphate. The reaction is

$$\text{Glycogen}_{(n)} + \text{P}_i \rightarrow \text{glucose 1-phosphate} + \text{glycogen}_{(n-1)}$$

Glucokinase catalyzes the reaction

$$\text{Glucose} + \text{ATP} \rightarrow \text{glucose 6-phosphate} + \text{ADP}$$

This enzyme in liver provides the glucose 6-phosphate necessary for glycogen synthesis. The addition of glucose units to a growing glycogen chain is catalyzed by glycogen synthase in the following reaction.

$$\text{Glycogen}_{(n)} + \text{UDP-glucose} \rightarrow \text{glycogen}_{(n+1)} + \text{UDP}$$

An activated derivative of glucose, UDP-glucose, serves as the glucosyl donor in this reaction. Glucose 6-phosphatase catalyzes the reaction.

$$\text{Glucose 6-phosphate} + H_2O \rightarrow \text{glucose} + P_i$$

The enzyme functions primarily in liver to release free glucose into the blood for uptake by other tissues, chiefly brain and muscle. Glucose 6-phosphate dehydrogenase catalyzes the conversion of glucose 6-phosphate to 6-phosphoglucono-δ-lactone. It requires NADP$^+$ as a cofactor. (Stryer, pp 361,428,451,454,456)

316–319. The answers are 316-C, 317-A, 318-D, 319-D. The carbon skeletons of glutamine, proline, arginine, and histidine enter the citric acid cycle at the level of α-ketoglutarate. All of these amino acids are converted to the common intermediate glutamate, which is oxidatively deaminated by glutamate dehydrogenase to yield α-ketoglutarate. In the formation of glycine from serine, the side chain β-carbon of serine is transferred to tetrahydrofolate to form methylenetetrahydrofolate. The reaction is catalyzed by serine transhydroxymethylase, which is a pyridoxal phosphate enzyme. This is the major source of one-carbon units for tetrahydrofolate derivatives. Transamination of oxaloacetate by glutamate results in the formation of aspartate from oxaloacetate and α-ketoglutarate from the glutamate skeleton. In turn, asparagine is produced by the amidation of aspartate with ammonium ion. During amino acid degradation, asparagine is hydrolyzed by asparaginase to aspartate. Transamination of α-ketoglutarate by aspartate forms oxaloacetate and glutamate. (Stryer, pp 503–505,578–583)

320–322. The answers are 320-E, 321-C, 322-A. Keratins contain as much as 14 percent cystine, the disulfide form of the amino acid cysteine. Hair and nails, as well as the cytoskeletal elements known as intermediate filaments, are composed of fibrous keratin proteins. Functional prothrombin contains γ-carboxylated glutamate, which results from a vitamin K-dependent posttranslational modification of nascent prothrombin. Agents that competitively block vitamin K action, such as warfarin and dicumarol, act as anticoagulants. Proline is modified to hydroxyproline by a posttranslational mechanism in collagen synthesis. The reducing agent ascorbic acid is needed for the hydroxylation reaction. Scurvy, a disease caused by dietary insufficiency of vitamin C (ascorbate), is characterized by abnormal collagen that cannot properly form fibers because of the lack of hydroxylated proline residues. Phosphorylation and dephosphorylation of serine are control mechanisms for the regulation of enzyme activity via protein kinase and phosphatase reactions that are under the control of hormonal mecha-

nisms. D-Valine is not a biologically active amino acid. Only L-amino acids are effective in mammalian systems. (Stryer, pp 250–252,261–268,459–460,938–940)

323–324. The answers are 323-A, 324-A. The variable part of nucleic acids is their sequence of bases. The base thymine, shown in **A** in the question, is found only in DNA. The base uracil, shown in **E**, replaces thymine in RNA. Uracil lacks the C-5 methyl group present in thymine. All of the other purines and pyrimidines shown in the question are common to both DNA and RNA (**B**, cytosine; **C**, adenine; **D**, guanine). Exposure to ultraviolet light, particularly in the skin, causes a cross-linking of adjacent thymine bases in DNA via bonding between each C-5 and C-6 atom. A specific repair mechanism composed of ultraviolet-specific endonuclease, DNA polymerase I (including its 5′ ⇌ 3′ exonuclease activity) and DNA ligase replace the affected area. In the autosomal recessive skin disease known as xeroderma pigmentosum, the endonuclease is functionally absent. (Stryer, pp 72,86,677–679)

325–326. The answers are 325-D, 326-C. The reduced flavin nucleotide FADH is produced at only one point in the citric acid cycle, at the conversion of succinate to fumarate. This reaction is catalyzed by succinate dehydrogenase. In contrast, NADH is formed during the two decarboxylation steps (labeled **A** and **B** on the figure that accompanies the question) and during the conversion of malate to oxaloacetate. Substrate level phosphorylation occurs during the formation of succinate from succinyl-CoA. In this step, GDP is phosphorylated to GTP using the energy of the CoA-thioester bond. (Stryer, pp 374–379)

327–328. The answers are 327-B, 328-C. Under most enzymatic conditions K_m is a measure of the affinity of the enzyme for its substrate. A low K_m value indicates tight binding of substrate to enzyme; a high value denotes weak binding. In the enzymes listed in the question, lysozyme has the lowest K_m and, thus, the greatest affinity for its substrate. k_{cat}, the catalytic rate constant, is the rate of the enzymatic reaction when the enzyme is fully saturated with substrate. In many cases, this is the turnover number of the enzyme. A high value for k_{cat} indicates that the enzyme converts its substrate to product very rapidly. The overall catalytic efficiency of an enzyme is, therefore, determined by the expression k_{cat}/K_m. The higher the value for this expression, the greater the catalytic efficiency of the enzyme. Of the enzymes listed in the problem, carbonic anhydrase has the highest value for k_{cat}/K_m and, therefore, the greatest catalytic efficiency. (Stryer, pp 190–191)

329–330. The answers are 329-C, 330-D. Most ATP is synthesized in the mitochondria via oxidative phosphorylation. A small amount of ATP, however, can be formed outside the mitochondria by phosphoryl group transfer from a high-energy compound directly to ADP. Phosphoenolpyruvate is a high-energy compound, and its phosphate group is transferred to ADP, yielding ATP and pyruvate. This reaction is catalyzed by pyruvate kinase. Under anaerobic conditions, such as pertains in muscle during vigorous exercise, pyruvate formed during glycolysis accumulates because of the inactivity of the citric acid cycle. The pyruvate is instead reduced to lactate in a reaction catalyzed by lactate dehydrogenase. This reaction requires NADH as a cofactor. *(Stryer, pp 355–357,363–364)*

331–333. The answers are 331-D, 332-C, 333-B. The first three reaction sequences are distinct parts of the glycolytic pathway. The precursor for formation of fructose 6-phosphate can be either glucose or glycogen. In the first instance, 1 mol of ATP is consumed to generate glucose 6-phosphate, which is converted to fructose 6-phosphate. In muscle, however, glycogen can be broken down via a phosphorolysis reaction involving inorganic phosphate and catalyzed by glycogen phosphorylase. The product is glucose 1-phosphate, which is converted to glucose 6-phosphate and metabolized via the glycolytic pathway. Thus, the phosphorylated sugar intermediate is generated from glycogen without expenditure of an ATP. Fructose 6-phosphate is converted to fructose 1,6-bisphosphate in a reaction that uses ATP. In the conversion of glyceraldehyde 3-phosphate to pyruvate, 2 mol of ATP are generated. Pyruvate may be used for the synthesis of glucose by gluconeogenesis. Four moles of ATP (and 2 mol of GTP) are consumed in the conversion of pyruvate to glucose via the gluconeogenic pathway. *(Stryer, pp 349–357,438–442,451–454)*

334–336. The answers are 334-B, 335-A, 336-D. Dactinomycin binds specifically to DNA and prevents its use as a template for RNA synthesis. It inhibits the growth of rapidly proliferating cells and is used for the treatment of certain cancers. Tetracycline binds to the small subunit of bacterial ribosomes and prevents the binding of aminoacyl-tRNA. It has no effect on eukaryotic ribosomes and is, therefore, a potent antibiotic. Methotrexate is an inhibitor of dihydrofolate reductase and has its major effect by blocking the synthesis of thymidylate (TMP). This, in turn, results in inhibition of DNA synthesis. It is widely used in the chemotherapy of a variety of cancers. *(Stryer, pp 614–616,715,759)*

337–339. The answers are 337-D, 338-A, 339-C. The enzymes that mediate RNA biosynthesis (transcription) are referred to as RNA polymerases. In eukaryotes, there are three different RNA polymerases that are responsible for the transcription of ribosomal RNA, messenger RNA or transfer, and 5S RNA, respectively. In contrast, a single RNA polymerase is involved in the transcription of all types of RNA in prokaryotes. The biosynthesis of all nucleic acids (both RNA and DNA) in all organisms is achieved by the sequential addition of nucleotide units to the free 3′-hydroxyl group of a growing polynucleotide chain (called a primer). Thus, transcription in both eukaryotes and prokaryotes is said to occur in a 5′ to 3′ direction. The enzyme responsible for mRNA synthesis in eukaryotes is RNA polymerase II. This enzyme is specifically inhibited by α-amanitin. RNA synthesis in all organisms begins at a specific nucleotide position. RNA polymerase binds to the DNA template at a specific sequence called a promoter. In prokaryotes, the promoter consists of two sequence elements that occur at 10 and 35 nucleotides before the transcription start site (called the −10 and −35 sequences). Similar sequences comprise eukaryotic promoters but, in general, are found 25 and between 40 and 100 nucleotides upstream of the transcription start site. *(Stryer, pp 704–710,716–718)*

340–342. The answers are 340-D, 341-A, 342-B. Cholesterol and triacylglycerides are transported in the blood by chylomicrons and VLDLs. Both of these lipoproteins are triglyceride rich. The end products of VLDL delipidation are LDLs, which are rich in cholesterol. LDLs are taken up by peripheral tissues, which recognize them through specific LDL receptors. In this manner, LDLs deliver cholesterol to peripheral tissues. HDLs are protein-rich lipoproteins synthesized by the liver and by gut epithelium. HDLs contain apolipoproteins of the A and C classes. C-II apolipoprotein is important for the activation of lipoprotein lipase, the endothelial lipase involved in delipidation of chylomicrons and VLDLs. HDLs are also important in transport of cholesterol from peripheral tissues back to the liver for excretion as bile. In Tangier disease, HDLs are deficient, leading to a buildup of excess cholesterol in peripheral tissues. Xanthomas, subcutaneous deposits resulting from abnormal cholesterol accumulation, are often observed. *(Stryer, pp 560–564)*

343–345. The answers are 343-B, 344-A, 345-C. Mitochondrial electron transport is tightly coupled to oxidative phosphorylation at three sites.

$$\underset{\text{REDUCTASE}}{\text{NADH} \rightarrow \text{NADH-Q}} \overset{1}{\rightarrow} \text{QH}_2 \overset{2}{\rightarrow} b \rightarrow c_1 \rightarrow c \rightarrow a + a_3 \overset{3}{\rightarrow} \text{O}_2$$

At each of these sites, a proton gradient is generated across the inner membrane of mitochondria and one molecule of ATP is synthesized by the flow of a pair of electrons. The oxidation of many substrates, including pyruvate, proceeds through

NADH. Rotenone specifically inhibits transfer of electrons from NADH to coenzyme Q (ubiquinone) at site 1. However, succinate oxidation donates electrons to coenzyme Q beyond the block produced by rotenone at site 1. Thus rotenone does not affect oxidation of succinate. In contrast, antimycin A inhibits electron flow specifically between cytochromes b and c_1, preventing oxidative phosphorylation at site 2. Thus antimycin A disrupts electron transport and oxidative phosphorylation dependent on succinate. Dinitrophenol dissipates the proton gradient across the inner mitochondrial membrane, thereby uncoupling oxidative phosphorylation from electron transport. It has no effect on electron transport, and the energy that normally is used to generate a proton gradient for oxidative phosphorylation is generated as heat. *(Stryer, pp 412–413,421–422)*

346–347.   The answers are 346-A, 347-C. Membranes differ greatly in their protein and lipid content. Myelin, the membrane that wraps around certain nerves as an insulator, contains only about 18 percent protein. The primary molecular species of its lipids is phosphatidyl choline. Erythrocyte plasma membrane is composed of about 50 percent protein and 50 percent lipid. Either phosphatidyl choline or sphingomyelin (or both), depending on the species of animal examined, is the major phospholipid entity. Almost 25 percent of the protein of RBC membrane is the anion channel protein. It is a glycoprotein that extends across the bilayer of the membrane, allowing the cell to be permeable to bicarbonate and chloride ions. *(Stryer, pp 284–290,301–305)*

348.   The answer is E (all). Fatty acid biosynthesis occurs in the cytoplasm. The committed step in fatty acid synthesis is the formation of malonyl-CoA, which is catalyzed by the enzyme acetyl-CoA carboxylase. Citrate stimulates the activity of acetyl-CoA carboxylase, which results in increased levels of fatty acid synthesis. The effect of citrate is counteracted by palmitoyl-CoA, which is present when fatty acid levels are high. *(Stryer, pp 481,490–491)*

349.   The answer is E (all). In the genetic disease known as sickle cell anemia, homozygous persons suffer from hemolytic anemia due to the presence of sickled erythrocytes in the venous circulation. The sickle effect is a result of the change of one amino acid at position 6 of the β chain of Hb (Glu → Val). This amino acid substitution results in aggregation of Hb S that is deoxygenated. The oxygenated form masks the stickiness caused by the valine substitution. The solubility of the deoxygenated Hb S is lower than normal, and precipitation of the aggregates causes the observed sickle shape. Substitution of the highly polar glutamate with nonpolar valine leads to a change in the electrophoretic

mobility of Hb S when compared with normal Hb. *(Stryer, pp 163–170)*

350.   The answer is B (1,3). Nerve–muscle end-plate stimulation causes the contraction of vertebrate skeletal muscle. The nervous excitation causes the release of calcium stored in the sarcoplasmic reticulum. The calcium ions interact with troponin and tropomyosin, allowing them to undergo conformational changes that permit contraction to occur. Together with actin, troponin and tropomyosin make up thin filaments of skeletal muscle. Once the conformational changes of the thin filaments occur, the myosin filaments (thick filaments) can interact with them. Contractile force is generated, and ATP is hydrolyzed until calcium is removed. During contraction, ATP is rapidly hydrolyzed. It is replaced with ATP formed from the contribution of a phosphoryl group to ADP from phosphocreatine. Creatine kinase catalyzes this reaction. Although the reverse reaction (that is, phosphate contribution to creatine from ATP) does occur to regenerate phosphocreatine stores, it can only be carried out in resting muscle when ATP levels are high. *(Stryer, pp 921–936)*

351.   The answer is C (2,4). The negative logarithm to the base 10 of the hydrogen ion concentration can be used to calculate the pH of an aqueous solution. For example, the $[H^+]$ of pure, distilled water is 1.0×10^{-7} mol/L. Thus, $pH = -\log 10^{-7} = -(-7) = 7.0$. Another way to calculate the acidity of a solution is by the Henderson-Hasselbalch equation, if the molar proportions of base and acid are known, as well as the pK of the solution. The pK of an acid is the pH at which it is half-dissociated. For a solution of acetic acid (pK of 4.8) containing 0.1 mol/L acetic acid and 0.2 mol/L acetate ion, the pH may be calculated as follows:

$$pH = 4.8 + \log \frac{2 \times 10^{-1}}{1 \times 10^{-1}} = 4.8 + \log 2 = 4.8 + 0.3 = 5.1$$

(Stryer, pp 41–42)

352.   The answer is C (2,4). UDP-glucose is an activated form of glucose. It is synthesized from glucose 1-phosphate and UTP in a reaction catalyzed by the enzyme UDP-glucose pyrophosphorylase. The addition of glucose to a growing glycogen chain is mediated by the enzyme glycogen synthase employing UDP-glucose as the glucose donor. The use of galactose by the glycolytic pathway requires its conversion to glucose 1-phosphate. This is accomplished by a series of reactions in which UDP-glucose is first used and then regenerated. *(Stryer, pp 358–359,455–456)*

353.   The answer is A (1,2,3). Albinism is a total lack of skin pigmentation because of a deficiency of tyrosine 3-monooxygenase, which allows the conversion of tyrosine to melanin in melanosome granules. Patients with alkaptonuria pass urine that turns black on standing. Affected patients lack homogentisate oxidase, an enzyme in the pathway for degradation of phenylalanine and tyrosine. Homogentisate accumulates in the urine and is oxidized and polymerized into a melaninlike substance on exposure to air. The odor of maple syrup is strong in the urine of patients with maple syrup urine disease. In these patients, the oxidative decarboxylation of the three branched-chain amino acids leucine, isoleucine, and valine is blocked. α-Keto acids derived from these amino acids accumulate and are excreted into the urine. In patients born with PKU, a phenylalanine hydroxylase is usually deficient. Phenylalanine cannot be converted to tyrosine, and it and its derivative, phenylpyruvate, accumulate in all body fluids. If infants are left untreated, severe mental retardation and a shortened life span result. Approximately 1 percent of all patients in mental institutions suffer from PKU. Screening of newborns by measuring the presence of phenylalanine in the blood allows intervention with a low-phenylalanine diet, yielding an increase in IQ compared with untreated individuals. *(Stryer, pp 510–514)*

354. The answer is B (1,3). In the pentose phosphate pathway, NADPH is generated as glucose 6-phosphate, which is oxidized to ribose 5-phosphate. This five-carbon sugar and its derivatives are precursors of ATP, CoA, NAD^+, FAD, RNA, and DNA. The first step of the pathway, conversion of glucose 6-phosphate to 6-phosphogluconolactone, is catalyzed by glucose 6-phosphate dehydrogenase, which is tightly regulated by the availability of $NADP^+$. At high levels, NADPH competes with $NADP^+$ for binding to the enzyme, inhibiting the pathway. *(Stryer, pp 427–431)*

355. The answer is A (1,2,3). In general, GTP serves as the energy source for protein synthesis on the ribosome. Binding of aminoacyl-tRNA to the ribosomal A site is mediated by formation of a ternary complex of tRNA, elongation factor EF-Tu (or EF1 in eukaryotes), and GTP. The GTP is hydrolyzed concomitant with tRNA binding to the ribosome. Similarly, binding of the specific initiator tRNA, Met-tRNA$_i$, to the ribosome involves the participation of the initiation factor IF2 (eIF2 in eukaryotes) and GTP. Hydrolysis of GTP is a necessary step for formation of productive initiation complexes on the ribosome. Polypeptide chain elongation proceeds after peptide bond formation via the process of translocation, which also is mediated by a protein factor (EF-G or EF2) and requires GTP hydrolysis. The actual formation of the peptide bond is catalyzed by the peptidyl transferase activity of the ribosome and does not require any

nonribosomal protein factors or GTP hydrolysis. *(Stryer, pp 754–758)*

356. The answer is C (2,4). During strenuous physical exertion, the rate of production of pyruvate by glycolysis exceeds the capacity of the citric acid cycle to oxidize it, and pyruvate accumulates in the blood. NADH also accumulates, since its oxidation by the respiratory chain is limited. Under these conditions glycolysis could be inhibited, since NAD^+ is needed for the continued oxidation of glyceraldehyde 3-phosphate. By converting pyruvate to lactate via lactate dehydrogenase, NAD^+ is regenerated. The levels of pyruvate and lactate increase, and these substances diffuse from muscle to the blood. The oxygen debt that continues after exercise refers to the oxidation of the high levels of lactate and pyruvate. However, while exercise continues, excess lactate and pyruvate are taken up by the liver and converted to glucose, which may then be recirculated back to muscle. *(Stryer, pp 444–445)*

357. The answer is B (1,3). Glycogen synthase is active in the dephosphorylated form. When active, it catalyzes the synthesis of glycogen by adding glucose units to a growing glycogen chain from UDP-glucose. Synthase, like all the enzymes of glycogen metabolism, is localized to glycogen particles found in the cytoplasm of cells. Activated phosphorylase kinase catalyzes the phosphorylation of glycogen phosphorylase, the enzyme controlling glycogenolysis. *(Stryer, pp 456–457,462–464)*

358. The answer is C (2,4). Actinomycin and rifamycin are antibiotic inhibitors of transcription. Actinomycin, a polypeptide-containing antibiotic obtained from *Streptomyces,* binds to double-helical DNA and prevents its acting as an effective template for RNA synthesis. Rifamycin, also obtained from *Streptomyces,* specifically inhibits initiation of RNA synthesis by interfering with the formation of the first phosphodiester bond in the RNA chain. In contrast, streptomycin and puromycin are inhibitors of protein synthesis. Streptomycin is a basic trisaccharide that inhibits initiation and causes misreading of mRNA in prokaryotes. It interferes with the binding of formylmethionyl-tRNA to ribosomes. Puromycin causes premature chain termination by acting as an analog of aminoacyl-tRNA in both prokaryotes and eukaryotes. *(Stryer, pp 714–715,759–760)*

359. The answer is D (4). Fatty acids are activated to the CoA derivatives at the outer mitochondrial membrane but are oxidized inside the mitochondria. Long-chain fatty acyl-CoA molecules do not cross the mitochondrial membrane. A special transport system involving carnitine is used for movement of the activated fatty acids into the mitochondria. The fatty acyl moiety is transferred from the

CoA to carnitine in a reaction catalyzed by carnitine acyltransferase I. Acylcarnitine thus formed is shuttled across the inner mitochondrial membrane, where the fatty acyl group is transferred back to a CoA molecule within the mitochondrial matrix. The latter reaction is catalyzed by carnitine acyltransferase II. *(Stryer, pp 473–474)*

360.   The answer is B (1,3). During β oxidation of saturated fatty acids, two-carbons in the form of acetyl-CoA are cleaved off the fatty acid during each round of oxidation. This is accomplished by subjecting a saturated acyl-CoA to the following sequence of four reactions: (1) oxidation catalyzed by FAD-linked dehydrogenase, (2) hydration catalyzed by enoyl-CoA hydratase, (3) oxidation catalyzed by NAD-linked dehydrogenase, and (4) cleavage of the acetyl-CoA by β-ketothiolase. However, when the β oxidation process reaches a double bond, two alternative enzymes can be used, depending on the position of the bond. If the double bond starts at the β position (the 3′ carbon) of the enoyl-CoA, an isomerase converts the 3′ → 4′ *cis* double bond into a 2′ → 3′ *trans* double bond. The subsequent reactions are those of regular β oxidation. Thus, the usual FAD oxidation of step 1 is replaced by the isomerase. In contrast, if the *cis* double bond starts at the α carbon (the 2′ carbon) of the enoyl-CoA, the regular hydration of step 2 above becomes the first reaction. This produces a D-3-hydroxyacyl-CoA. In order to make the hydroxyacyl available for action by the NAD-linked dehydrogenase of step 3, which does not react with the D form, an epimerase converts the D-3-hydroxyacyl-CoA to L-3-hydroxyacyl-CoA. The last two steps are those of regular β oxidation. Thus, in both cases the FAD-linked oxidation step is lost. Reductase and dehydratase enzymes are used in fatty acid synthesis but not in oxidation of fatty acids. *(Stryer, pp 477–478)*

361.   The answer is E (all). The synthesis of all steroid hormones starts with the formation of progesterone from cholesterol. An intermediate in these steps is pregnenolone, which is formed by the removal of a six-carbon unit from the side chain of cholesterol. These reactions, as well as others in the synthesis of first progesterone and then the other derivative steroid hormones, require the action of mono-oxygenases. The mono-oxygenases, which are also called mixed-function oxygenases, carry out hydroxylations of the intermediates in steroid hormone synthesis by incorporating atoms from molecular O_2 and by using the reductive potential of NADPH. This is illustrated in the following reaction sequence, in which R is the steroid nucleus.

$$RH + O_2 + NADPH + H^+ \rightarrow ROH + H_2O + NADP^+$$

(Stryer, pp 565–568)

362.   The answer is E (all). The initial step in purine nucleotide biosynthesis is the formation of phosphoribosylamine from PRPP and glutamine. This reaction is catalyzed by PRPP amidotransferase and is the committed step in purine biosynthesis. The reaction is regulated by feedback inhibition by AMP and/or GMP. Since PRPP is a substrate in this reaction, the rate of purine biosynthesis is governed by the availability of PRPP. The initial purine nucleotide product of the de novo pathway is IMP. This compound serves as a branch point in the synthesis of AMP and GMP. In one branch of the pathway, IMP is converted to AMP and requires GTP, whereas in the other branch of the pathway, IMP is converted to GMP in reactions requiring ATP. The reciprocal requirements of one purine nucleotide for the synthesis of the other serve to ensure that relatively balanced amounts of both are produced. *(Stryer, pp 602–607)*

363.   The answer is A (1,2,3). Any condition that results in elevated levels of purine nucleotides is likely to cause hyperuricemia. Glucose 6-phosphatase converts glucose 6-phosphate to free glucose. In the absence of this enzymatic activity, levels of glucose 6-phosphate increase, leading to elevated activity of the pentose phosphate pathway (in which glucose 6-phosphate is the initial substrate). This, in turn, leads to the increased production of ribose 5-phosphate, which is converted to PRPP. The latter compound is a substrate in the committed step of purine biosynthesis, and therefore, a rise in the levels of PRPP results in elevated amounts of purines. Similarly, increased activity of PRPP synthetase, which catalyzes the synthesis of PRPP from ribose 5-phosphate, will result in an overabundance of PRPP and, in turn, purines. HGPRT is a salvage pathway enzyme that catalyzes the condensation of hypoxanthine or guanine with PRPP to yield IMP or GMP. In this way, purine bases that become available in the diet or by virtue of nucleic acid degradation can be recycled into the corresponding nucleotides and used for nucleic acid biosynthesis. If this salvage is blocked, the purine bases are degraded further to uric acid. Purine nucleoside phosphorylase is a purine degradative enzyme. Its absence prevents the formation of uric acid. *(Stryer, pp 465,602–603,618–623)*

364.   The answer is A (1,2,3). Reduced glutathione is an antioxidant. It is regenerated by the transfer of electrons from NADPH to oxidized glutathione via FAD. This reaction, which transfers the electrons to a disulfide bridge of glutathione, is catalyzed by glutathione reductase. In erythrocytes, the reduced form of glutathione maintains the cysteine residues of Hb and other RBC proteins in a reduced state. It also plays a role in cell detoxification by reacting with organic peroxides and hydrogen peroxides. *(Stryer, pp 436–438)*

365. The answer is C (2,4). Arsenate replaces the P_i that normally reacts with glyceraldehyde 3-phosphate to form 1,3-DPG. Instead, an unstable intermediate, 1-arseno-3-phosphoglycerate, is produced and immediately hydrolyzes to 3-phosphoglycerate. NADH is formed as usual. Thus, glycolysis proceeds in the presence of arsenate, but the ATP normally formed in the conversion of 1,3-DPG to 3-phosphoglycerate is lost. *(Stryer, p 368)*

366. The answer is A (1,2,3). Esterification of diacylglyceride to a fatty acyl group donated by acyl-CoA is the last step in the synthesis of triacylglycerides. It is catalyzed by diacylglycerol acyltransferase. Although CDP-diacylglycerol can be the activated intermediate in the synthesis of phosphoglycerides, diacylglycerol itself can be used in salvage pathways. In salvage pathways, choline or ethanolamine is activated to form CDP-choline or CDP-ethanolamine, which then can be esterified to diacylglyceride in a one-step reaction yielding phospholipid and liberated cytidine monophosphate (CMP). Lysophosphatidic acid, which is glycerol esterified to a fatty acid at the 1' position and to phosphate at the 3' position, is an intermediate in the synthesis of diacylglyceride or an intermediate in the degradation of phosphoglycerides. *(Stryer, pp 547–550)*

367. The answer is E (all). The last step of electron transport is the transfer of a pair of electrons to molecular O_2 to form water. In this reaction, the enzyme is the cytochrome *c* oxidase complex, which includes the iron moieties of the heme groups of cytochromes *a* and a_3. Cyanide reacts with the ferric form of the heme carrier, whereas carbon monoxide reacts with the ferrous state. Electron transfer to O_2, as well as oxidative phosphorylation from generation of a proton pump at this site, is inhibited. *(Stryer, pp 412–413)*

368. The answer is C (2,4). The first step in the respiratory chain of electron transfer is the reduction of NAD^+. Electrons are collected from a variety of substrates through the action of NADH dehydrogenase. Electrons are then donated from NADH to FMN. In contrast, some respiratory substrates bypass NAD^+ and are dehydrogenated by flavin-linked dehydrogenases. These include glycerol phosphate, succinate, and fatty acyl-CoA. All of these electrons funnel into coenzyme Q and from there through cytochromes *b*, c_1, *c*, *a*, and a_3, respectively. *(Stryer, 410–413)*

369. The answer is B (1,3). The kinetic plot shown in the figure is characteristic of an allosteric enzyme. The curve in the presence of high [ATP] has a sigmoid shape (S shape) that usually means that substrate binding to the enzyme is cooperative. This indicates that the binding of one substrate molecule enhances the binding of subsequent substrate molecules to the enzyme. This behavior is distinguishable from enzymes that obey Michaelis-Menten kinetics and display kinetic plots that are hyperbolic. The substrate binding in these cases is not cooperative. Allosteric enzymes have binding sites for molecules other than the substrate. Binding of such compounds will modify the activity of the enzyme and are called allosteric effectors. In the figure, the maximum velocity ultimately is achieved at both low and high [ATP], and thus Vmax is not affected by ATP. The curve is shifted to the right, however, at high [ATP], and this means that the apparent K_m is increased. ATP is a negative effector of phosphofructokinase and inhibits the activity of the enzyme. *(Stryer, pp 193,239–243,359–361)*

370. The answer is A (1,2,3). A microsomal electron transport system for hydroxylation of a variety of organic substrates is present in the liver. NADPH-cytochrome P_{450} reductase and cytochrome P_{450} make up this system. Electrons are transferred from NADH to FAD to the iron of P_{450}. Reduced P_{450} simultaneously reduces one of the O_2 atoms of molecular O_2 to water and transfers the other to an organic substrate. In addition to hydroxylation of biologic substrates, this system also hydroxylates drugs and carcinogens. *(Stryer, p 566)*

371. The answer is B (1,3). Eukaryotic chromatin is made up of repeating units called nucleosomes. These are composed of between 160 and 240 base pairs of DNA and two molecules each of the histone proteins H2A, H2B, H3, and H4. Histones are small basic proteins that bind very tightly to DNA and the eight histone molecules form a protein core around which the DNA is wound. This arrangement is one factor that facilitates the packing of large amounts of DNA into the eukaryotic nucleus. RNA is not part of the essential nucleosome structure. The eukaryotic genome contains some nucleotide sequences that are repeated up to 1 million times. These are referred to as repetitive sequences. Some of these may serve a structural function in the chromosome; e.g., centromeres contain highly repetitive DNA sequences. *(Stryer, pp 824–829,834–836)*

372. The answer is C (2,4). An important step in the elucidation of protein structure is determination of the amino acid sequence. The initial step in this process usually is identification of the amino terminal amino acid. This can be accomplished by chemical means through the use of several possible reagents, including phenylisothiocyanate and FDNB. Both reagents react with the free α-amino group at the N-terminus of a protein to yield modified amino acids that can be identified by a variety of techniques. Ninhydrin reacts with amino acids to give a blue color and may be used for measurement of protein concentrations. Cyanogen bromide cleaves peptide bonds whose carboxyl function is donated by methionine. Treatment of a methionine-containing protein will result in its breakdown to smaller peptide fragments. *(Stryer, pp 50–57)*

373. **The answer is E (all).** Restriction endonucleases are enzymes produced by bacteria that recognize a specific base sequence in DNA and cleave the phosphodiester bonds of both DNA strands. The result is the fragmentation of DNA into smaller pieces. In bacteria, these enzymes serve the protective function of preventing transformation by the uptake of foreign DNA. The recognition sites for restriction enzymes possess a twofold axis of rotational symmetry; i.e., the sequences are palindromes. The DNA in the host cell is protected from digestion by the restriction enzyme because the recognition sequence is methylated. Restriction enzymes are widely used in the application of recombinant DNA technology. *(Stryer, pp 118–119,858–859)*

374. **The answer is A (1,2,3).** In muscle and nerve cells, cytosolic NADH produced by glycolysis must be regenerated to NAD$^+$ to permit glycolysis to proceed. This is accomplished by the glycerol phosphate shuttle. Since mitochondria are impermeable to NADH and NAD$^+$, the electrons of NADH are transferred to dihydroxyacetone phosphate, forming glycerol 3-phosphate in the cytosol. Glycerol 3-phosphate diffuses into mitochondria and is converted back to dihydroxyacetone phosphate by donating its electrons to FAD to form FADH. Dihydroxyacetone phosphate diffuses out of the mitochondria into the cytosol. Thus, glycerol 3-phosphate, and not dihydroxyacetone phosphate, is the carrier of electrons in the mitochondria and the cytosol. The electrons from FADH enter the electron transport chain at the level of coenzyme Q. Thus, only two ATP are formed from the electron pair donated by cytosolic NADH, whereas three ATP are formed from mitochondrial NADH. *(Stryer, pp 417–420)*

375. **The answer is D (4).** The net reaction of the citric acid cycle is as follows.

$$\text{Acetyl-CoA} + \text{FAD} + 3\ \text{NAD}^+ + \text{GDP} + \text{P}_i + 2\ \text{H}_2\text{O} \rightarrow \text{CoA} + \text{FADH} + 3\ \text{NADH} + \text{GTP} + 2\ \text{H}^+ + 2\ \text{CO}_2$$

Two carbon atoms in the form of acetyl-CoA enter the cycle, and two carbon atoms in the form of CO_2 leave the cycle. The two carbon atoms that are decarboxylated in the first round are different from the new ones that entered. Four pairs of electrons are transferred from intermediates to three NAD$^+$ molecules and one FAD molecule. One high-energy phosphate bond is generated when GTP is produced from the thioester linkage of succinyl CoA. The

synthesis of citrate and the hydration of fumarate consume two water molecules. *(Stryer, pp 374–379)*

376. **The answer is B (1,3).** The amino groups of amino acids are converted to urea for excretion via the urea cycle. The liver is the only organ capable of carrying this out. The human liver produces some 20 to 30 g of urea each day. Likewise, bile acid synthesis from cholesterol can only be carried out by the liver. Bile acids are synthesized or recaptured from the enterohepatic circulation and esterified to either glycine or taurine in the liver. Esterified bile acids are secreted into the gallbladder for storage between meals. Synthesis of gangliosides, which are components of all mammalian plasma membranes, can be carried out in all cells. Use of medium-chain fatty acids as an energy source occurs in most cells. Brain tissue and erythrocytes are exceptions. *(Stryer, pp 500–502,559)*

377. **The answer is C (2,4).** Tyrosine serves as a precursor for the synthesis of thyroxine, the thyroid hormone that stimulates the metabolic rate of O_2 consumption by the tissues. Tyrosine also leads to the synthesis of the adrenal hormone epinephrine in a pathway whose intermediates include levodopa, dopamine, and norepinephrine. The pigment melanin is also synthesized from tyrosine. The neurotransmitter serotonin (5-hydroxytryptamine) is derived from tryptophan, and the vasodilator histamine is formed from histidine. *(Stryer, pp 591–592,1025)*

378. **The answer is E (all).** The formation of acetyl-CoA from pyruvate is catalyzed by the enzymes of the pyruvate dehydrogenase complex.

$$\text{Pyruvate} + \text{CoA} + \text{NAD}^+ \rightarrow \text{acetyl-CoA} + \text{CO}_2 + \text{NADH}$$

As can be seen from the reaction, the stoichiometric cofactors are CoA and NAD$^+$. Pyruvate dehydrogenase requires thiamine pyrophosphate, dihydrolipoyl transacetylase requires lipoic acid as lipoamide, and dihydrolipoyl dehydrogenase requires FAD. In all, five cofactors take part in the reactions. *(Stryer, pp 379–382)*

379. **The answer is C (2,4).** Nicotinic acid is required for the synthesis of NAD$^+$. Its deficiency results in pellagra, a disease characterized by psychic disturbances, diarrhea, and dermatitis. Although it is classified as a vitamin, nicotinic acid can be synthesized from tryptophan. Thus a diet rich in either nicotinate or tryptophan will prevent pellagra. *(Stryer, pp 617–618)*

380. **The answer is C (2,4).** The binding sites for adenylate cyclase-specific hormones are located on the extracellular surface of cells. The receptor protein is distinct from the enzyme, adenylate cyclase, which ultimately synthesizes cyclic AMP from ATP. Adenylate cyclase is located on the inner surface of the plasma membrane. A guanyl nucleotide-binding protein (G protein) couples hormone receptors to adenylate cyclase after the attachment of a hormone to the receptor protein. The inactive G protein exchanges GDP for GTP and becomes activated when stimulated by a hormone–receptor complex. GTP is hydrolyzed to GDP by the G protein, and in the absence of hormone–receptor complex, it will activate itself. Activated G protein stimulates adenylate cyclase to produce cyclic AMP. *(Stryer, pp 973–983)*

381. **The answer is A (1,2,3).** Pepsin and chymotrypsin are enzymes that derive from proteolytic hydrolysis of the zymogens pepsinogen and chymotrypsinogen. The proenzyme forms of these enzymes are inactive until the covalent modulation occurs. In a like manner, phosphorylated glycogen synthase is inactive until dephosphorylation catalyzed by phosphatase occurs. In contrast, aspartate transcarbamoylase is an allosteric enzyme that is regulated by noncovalent modification. It is the first step in the pathway for CTP (cytidine triphosphate) synthesis and is inhibited by this end product. *(Stryer, pp 242–247,462–463)*

BIBLIOGRAPHY

Stryer L. *Biochemistry*. 3rd ed. San Francisco: WH Freeman and Co; 1988

Subspeciality List: Biochemistry

Question Number and Subspecialty

255. Nucleotide metabolism
256. Energy metabolism
257. Integration of metabolism
258. Blood
259. Muscle contraction
260. Thermodynamics
261. Integration of metabolism
262. pH
263. Muscle contraction
264. Carbohydrate metabolism
265. Carbohydrate metabolism
266. Carbohydrate metabolism
267. Carbohydrate metabolism
268. Nucleotide metabolism
269. Enzymes
270. Proteins
271. Molecular biology
272. Enzymes
273. Lipids
274. Lipids
275. Lipids
276. Lipids
277. Lipids
278. Lipids
279. Lipids
280. Lipids
281. Enzymes
282. Enzymes
283. Enzymes
284. Integration of metabolism
285. Hormones
286. Vitamins
287. Vitamins
288. Vitamins
289. Lipids
290. Carbohydrate metabolism
291. Small molecule metabolism
292. Proteins
293. Lipids
294. Carbohydrate metabolism
295. Energy metabolism
296. Lipids
297. Carbohydrate metabolism
298. Blood
299. Carbohydrate metabolism
300. Nucleotide metabolism
301. Amino acid metabolism
302. Nucleotide metabolism
303. Energy metabolism
304. Energy metabolism
305. Carbohydrate metabolism
306. Thermodynamics
307. Thermodynamics
308. Thermodynamics
309. Carbohydrate metabolism
310. Carbohydrate metabolism
311. Carbohydrate metabolism
312. Carbohydrate metabolism
313. Carbohydrate metabolism
314. Carbohydrate metabolism
315. Carbohydrate metabolism
316. Amino acid metabolism
317. Amino acid metabolism
318. Amino acid metabolism
319. Amino acid metabolism
320. Protein
321. Protein
322. Protein
323. Molecular biology
324. Molecular biology
325. Energy metabolism
326. Energy metabolism
327. Enzymes
328. Enzymes
329. Carbohydrate metabolism
330. Carbohydrate metabolism
331. Carbohydrate metabolism
332. Carbohydrate metabolism
333. Carbohydrate metabolism
334. Molecular biology
335. Molecular biology
336. Molecular biology
337. Molecular biology
338. Molecular biology
339. Molecular biology
340. Lipids
341. Lipids

342. Lipids
343. Energy metabolism
344. Energy metabolism
345. Energy metabolism
346. Membranes
347. Membranes
348. Lipids
349. Blood
350. Muscle contraction
351. pH
352. Carbohydrate metabolism
353. Amino acid metabolism
354. Carbohydrate metabolism
355. Molecular biology
356. Carbohydrate metabolism
357. Carbohydrate metabolism
358. Molecular biology
359. Lipids
360. Lipids
361. Lipids
362. Nucleotide metabolism
363. Nucleotide metabolism
364. Carbohydrate metabolism
365. Carbohydrate metabolism
366. Lipids
367. Energy metabolism
368. Energy metabolism
369. Enzymes
370. Energy metabolism
371. Molecular biology
372. Proteins
373. Molecular biology
374. Energy metabolism
375. Energy metabolism
376. Integration of metabolism
377. Hormones
378. Vitamins
379. Vitamins
380. Hormones
381. Proteins

Microbiology
Questions

382. Protective strategies for prevention of the septic shock syndrome could include all the following EXCEPT

    (A) anticachectin antibody
    (B) core polysaccharide-specific antibody
    (C) lipid A-specific antibody
    (D) antibody to terminal polysaccharides of O antigen
    (E) pharmacologic antileucotriene agents

383. Staphylococcal scalded skin syndrome is related to the organism's ability to produce

    (A) α-toxin
    (B) lipase
    (C) exfoliatin
    (D) hyaluronidase
    (E) coagulase

384. Of the following, the virus that is most resistant to chemical and physical agents is the one that causes

    (A) mumps
    (B) measles
    (C) influenza
    (D) serum hepatitis
    (E) polio

385. For viruses, the burst size is

    (A) the interval of time between infection and release of progeny virus
    (B) the average number of progeny viruses released per infected cell
    (C) the interval between infection and the appearance of intracellular progeny viruses
    (D) the average number of viruses that infect a cell
    (E) the number of viruses per unit volume of suspension

386. All of the following are stages of conjugation EXCEPT

    (A) effective pair formation
    (B) plasmid or chromosome mobilization
    (C) recombination
    (D) competency
    (E) transfer of a unique strand of DNA

387. Ticks are the arthropod vector of

    (A) Tsutsugamushi disease
    (B) Rocky Mountain spotted fever
    (C) murine typhus
    (D) epidemic typhus
    (E) bubonic plague

388. The plasma membrane receptor for influenza virus is

    (A) an unsubstituted protein
    (B) a glycolipid
    (C) a glycoprotein
    (D) a mucopolysaccharide
    (E) a nucleic acid

389. All of the following contribute directly to the intracellular killing of microbes by neutrophils EXCEPT

    (A) myeloperoxidase–hydrogen peroxide–halide system
    (B) oxygen metabolites
    (C) lysozyme and other hydrolytic enzymes
    (D) iron chelating proteins, such as lactoferrin
    (E) catalase

390. Which of the following statements concerning the Ouchterlony diagram below is true?

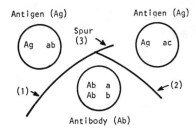

(A) line 1 will contain Ag ab and Ab b only
(B) line 2 will contain Ag ac and Ab b
(C) the spur will contain Ab a and Ag ab
(D) the spur will contain Ag ac and Ab a
(E) the spur will contain Ag ab and Ab b

391. The base pair substitution that results in the change of a purine for a pyrimidine is a

(A) transformant
(B) transition
(C) transversion
(D) transposition
(E) frame shift

392. Transformation of bacteria can be blocked by

(A) RNAse in the medium
(B) DNAse in the medium
(C) antiserum against bacteriophage
(D) bacteriophage that adsorb to sex pili
(E) preventing cell-to-cell contact between donor and recipient cultures

393. A lysogenic cell refers to a bacterial cell that

(A) is susceptible to a virulent phage
(B) is resistant to lysozyme
(C) is resistant to lysis
(D) carries a prophage
(E) excretes lysozyme

394. The antibody induced by which of the following parts of an influenza virus is most protective?

(A) envelope
(B) neuraminidase
(C) hemagglutinin
(D) nucleic acid
(E) internal protein

395. Chlamydiae and rickettsiae are correctly described as

(A) spread by the bite of an infected arthropod

(B) resistant to the usual broad-spectrum antibiotics
(C) containing either RNA or DNA but not both
(D) obligate parasites of living cells
(E) dividing solely by binary fission

396. In the following diseases, the etiologic agents are initially introduced to the host in the form of spores EXCEPT

(A) tetanus
(B) infant botulism
(C) anthrax
(D) gas gangrene
(E) diphtheria

397. A genetic test of function that depends on the interaction of the products of genes is

(A) suppression
(B) postreplication repair
(C) recombination
(D) host-induced modification
(E) complementation

398. Ultraviolet light

(A) disrupts the bacterial cell membrane
(B) removes free sulfhydryl groups
(C) is a common protein denaturant
(D) causes the formation of pyrimidine dimers
(E) acts as an alkylating agent

399. Members of the genera *Rhizobium* and *Azotobacter*

(A) are involved in nitrogen fixation
(B) grow best at a pH of 3.5 to 4.0
(C) are thermophilic
(D) contain capsules composed of D-glutamic acid
(E) adhere to human cells

400. Penicillin would be LEAST effective in treating which of the following diseases?

(A) syphilis
(B) gonorrhea
(C) pneumococcal pneumonia
(D) mycoplasmal pneumonia
(E) streptococcal pharyngitis

401. In coccidioidomycosis, which of the following is a poor prognostic sign?

(A) conversion to positive skin test
(B) positive precipitin titer
(C) decreased precipitin titer

(D) increasing complement fixation titers

(E) decreasing complement fixation titers

402. All of the following diseases are associated with herpes viruses EXCEPT

(A) central nervous system diseases

(B) congenital infections

(C) venereal diseases

(D) skin rashes

(E) scrapie

403. A rising titer of antistreptolysin O indicates a diagnosis of

(A) acute rheumatic fever

(B) glomerulonephritis

(C) a recent streptococcal infection

(D) scarlet fever

(E) erysipelas

404. Secretory IgA consists of IgA dimer, secretory component (SC), plus

(A) paraprotein

(B) J chain

(C) SC epitope

(D) γ chain

(E) ε chain

405. The antiphagocytosis property of group A streptococci is associated with

(A) M protein

(B) hyaluronidase

(C) streptolysin O

(D) streptolysin S

(E) DNAse

406. The mutagen 5-bromouracil (5-BU) preferentially causes

(A) frame shift mutations

(B) transitions

(C) transversions

(D) deletions

(E) recombinations

407. Antigens can best be processed for presentation by

(A) macrophages

(B) Kupffer cells

(C) B cells

(D) young erythrocytes

(E) suppressor T cells

408. All of the following substances affect lymphocytes EXCEPT

(A) migration inhibitory factor (MIF)

(B) interleukin 1

(C) transfer factor

(D) interleukin 2

(E) blastogenic factor

409. One of the first events that occurs after poliovirus infects a cell is

(A) hydrolysis of viral DNA

(B) synthesis of viral DNA

(C) hydrolysis of viral protein

(D) hydrolysis of host DNA

(E) cessation of host cell macromolecular biosynthesis

410. Damage to DNA caused by bifunctional alkylating agents that damage both strands of DNA is repaired by

(A) photoreactivation

(B) excision repair

(C) direct repair

(D) recombination of postreplication repair

(E) microinsertion

411. Patients with X-linked infantile agammaglobulinemia are known to

(A) exhibit profound deficiencies of cell-mediated immunity

(B) have very low quantities of immunoglobulin in their serum

(C) have normal numbers of B lymphocytes

(D) have a depletion of lymphocytes in the paracortical areas of lymph nodes

(E) be particularly susceptible to viral and fungal infections

412. During a routine pelvic examination, a woman is found to have a tender, open lesion on the vagina. The patient states that she had similar lesions 12 months previously. The causative agent is most likely to be

(A) echovirus

(B) coxsackievirus

(C) rubella virus

(D) herpes simplex virus

(E) measles virus

413. Antibodies against acetylcholine neural receptors are thought to be involved in the pathogenesis of

(A) myasthenia gravis
(B) multiple sclerosis
(C) acute idiopathic polyneuritis
(D) Guillain-Barré syndrome
(E) postpericardiotomy syndrome

414. A 7-month-old child is hospitalized for a yeast infection that does not respond to therapy. The patient has a history of acute pyogenic infections. Physical examination reveals that the spleen and lymph nodes are not palpable. A differential WBC count shows 95 percent neutrophils, 1 percent lymphocytes, and 4 percent monocytes. A bone marrow specimen contains no plasma cells or lymphocytes. X-ray reveals absence of a thymic shadow. Tonsils are absent. These findings are most compatible with

(A) multiple myeloma
(B) severe combined immunodeficiency disease
(C) X-linked agammaglobulinemia
(D) Wiskott-Aldrich syndrome
(E) chronic granulomatous disease

415. The figure below represents the

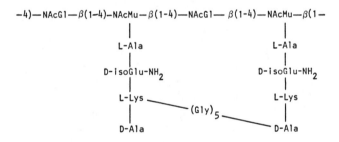

(A) O antigen of *Salmonella typhimurium*
(B) peptidoglycan of *Staphylococcus aureus*
(C) C substance of *Streptococcus pneumoniae*
(D) peptidoglycan of *Mycoplasma pneumoniae*
(E) H antigen of *S. typhimurium*

416. A stage of competence of recipient cells is necessary for

(A) complementation
(B) transduction
(C) transformation
(D) conjugation
(E) transposition

417. Enteroviruses are the causative agents of all of the following diseases EXCEPT

(A) aseptic meningitis

(B) gastrointestinal infections
(C) myocarditis
(D) pleurodynia
(E) shingles

418. A rabbit is repeatedly injected with a hapten. Two weeks later, its serum is subjected to a gel diffusion assay with the hapten and a carrier protein. It would be expected that

(A) no precipitin line will be present
(B) a line of identity between the serum and carrier protein will be detected
(C) a line of identity between serum and both the carrier and the hapten will be present
(D) a line of partial identity between serum, carrier, and hapten will be detected
(E) a line of nonidentity between serum, carrier, and hapten will be detected

419. All of the following are components of R plasmids EXCEPT

(A) R determinant
(B) the pilus
(C) RTF component
(D) insertion sequences
(E) antibiotic resistance genes

420. Skeletal muscle, cardiac, and central nervous system involvement occurs with which of the following

(A) *Wuchereria bancrofti*
(B) *Onchocerca volvulus*
(C) *Enterobius vermicularis*
(D) *Trichinella spiralis*
(E) *Necator americanus*

421. The infectiveness of *Chlamydia trachomatis* has been related to its

(A) elementary body (EB)
(B) capsule
(C) cell wall
(D) reticulate body (RB)
(E) phagosome

422. All of the following viruses have hemagglutinin in their viral envelope EXCEPT

(A) rubeola virus
(B) influenza B virus
(C) Parainfluenza virus 3
(D) rubella virus
(E) human papovavirus

423. The Vi or virulence antigen of *Salmonella* serotype *typhi* is

(A) the polysaccharide capsule
(B) the core polysaccharide of the lipopolysaccharide molecule
(C) the flagellar antigen
(D) a plasmid encoded exotoxin
(E) the lipid A portion of the LPS molecule

424. Muscle pains, eosinophilia, facial edema, and gastrointestinal upsets are classic symptoms of clinical

(A) hookworm infection
(B) trichinosis
(C) toxoplasmosis
(D) onchocerciasis
(E) pediculosis

425. High-molecular-weight substances that possess both immunogenicity and specificity are termed

(A) simple haptens
(B) determinant groups
(C) adjuvants
(D) antigens
(E) complex haptens

426. A laboratory test used to identify *Staphylococcus aureus* is based on the clotting of plasma. The microbial product that is responsible for this activity is

(A) coagulase-reactive factor
(B) coagulase
(C) prothrombin
(D) thrombin
(E) thromboplastin

427. The Weil-Felix reaction is correctly described as

(A) useful in the diagnosis of rickettsial diseases
(B) based on the agglutination of species of *Salmonella* by the patient's convalescent serum
(C) a test to detect antiviral antibodies
(D) based on scrotal swelling in a male guinea pig infected with the organism
(E) positive for Q fever when *Proteus* OXK is agglutinated

428. The most common cause of meningitis in children in the age range of 6 months to 5 years is

(A) *Haemophilus influenzae* type B
(B) pneumococcus
(C) meningococcus

(D) *Escherichia coli*
(E) *Streptococcus agalactiae*

429. The most common medium used for cultivation of fungi is

(A) tellurite medium
(B) SS agar
(C) Lowenstein-Jensen medium
(D) selenite F medium
(E) Sabouraud's glucose agar

430. Congenital rubella syndrome is most prominent in an infant when a pregnant woman becomes infected

(A) during the first trimester of pregnancy
(B) one week before full-term delivery
(C) one month before a full-term delivery
(D) hours before childbirth
(E) during the third trimester of pregnancy

431. The causative agents for the following infections are dimorphic fungi EXCEPT

(A) sporotrichosis
(B) candidiasis
(C) cryptococcosis
(D) histoplasmosis
(E) blastomycosis

432. A burn patient developed a wound infection, and a bacteriologic culture of the site indicates a gram-negative rod that was oxidase positive and produced a bluish green pigment. The organism was relatively resistant to antibiotics but susceptible to ticarcillin, gentamicin, and tobramycin. The organism is likely to be identified as

(A) *Escherichia coli*
(B) *Klebsiella pneumoniae*
(C) *Proteus mirabilis*
(D) *Serratia marcescens*
(E) *Pseudomonas aeruginosa*

433. Acute glomerulonephritis is a sequela of a previous infection by

(A) any M type of group A streptococci
(B) a few M types of group A streptococci
(C) only lysogenic group A streptococci
(D) all of the Lancefield groups of streptococci
(E) only encapsulated strains of *Streptococcus pneumoniae*

434. *Cryptococcus neoformans* differs from other pathogenic fungi in that it

(A) has a capsule
(B) is an intracellular parasite
(C) has septate hyphae
(D) reproduces by binary fission
(E) is dematiacious

435. *Diphyllobothrium latum* causes anemia by

(A) its blood-sucking activities
(B) the production of a toxin that affects hematopoiesis
(C) competition with the host for vitamin B_{12}
(D) occlusion of the common bile duct
(E) inhibition of the absorption of iron

436. Which of the following zoonotic diseases is usually transmitted to humans by the bite of an arthropod vector?

(A) anthrax
(B) brucellosis
(C) salmonellosis
(D) plague
(E) leptospirosis

437. The greatest amount of chromosomal DNA can be transferred by

(A) Hfr $\times$ F$^-$ mating
(B) F$'$ $\times$ F$^-$ mating
(C) plasmid transfer
(D) transportation of transposable elements
(E) specialized transduction

438. The specific biochemical reaction that describes the mechanism of action of diphtheria toxin is the

(A) inhibition of acetylcholine release
(B) glycosylation of mRNA
(C) inhibition of oxidative phosphorylation
(D) ADP-ribosylation of elongation factor 2 (EF-2)
(E) activation of adenylcyclase

439. All of the following are true statements about *Streptococcus pneumoniae* EXCEPT

(A) colonies form readily on blood agar
(B) colonies are beta hemolytic
(C) organisms may be isolated in small numbers from normal human throat cultures
(D) colonies are inhibited by optochin
(E) organisms are bile soluble

440. The substance responsible for the adherence of *Streptococcus mutans* to smooth surfaces is

(A) peptidoglycan
(B) lipoteichoic acid
(C) glucose
(D) fructan
(E) dextran

441. The best method for assessing the total number of B lymphocytes is

(A) quantitative immunoglobulin levels
(B) Fc receptor assay
(C) E rosette assay
(D) surface immunoglobulin (sIg) assay
(E) phytohemagglutinin A (PHA) mitogenicity

442. Functional assessment of T lymphocytes includes

(A) E rosette assay
(B) surface immunoglobulin (sIg) evaluation
(C) transformation of lymphocytes by phytohemagglutinin A (PHA)
(D) serum immunoglobulin determination
(E) enumeration of θ-bearing cells

443. Lyme disease

(A) is transmitted by mites
(B) is caused by *Leptospira interrogans*
(C) is a disease in which the serum levels of IgM correlate with disease activity
(D) has not been associated with arthritis
(E) does not respond to tetracycline treatment early in the acute illness

444. A gram-negative bacterium is isolated from a patient's cerebrospinal fluid (CSF). It grows on enriched chocolate agar but does not grow on blood agar except adjacent to a streak of staphylococci. The organism most probably is

(A) *Neisseria meningitidis*
(B) *Neisseria gonorrhoeae*
(C) *Haemophilus influenzae*
(D) *Streptococcus pneumoniae*
(E) *Listeria monocytogenes*

445. A common cause of pneumonia in children that is becoming increasingly common in adults with chronic obstructive pulmonary disease is

(A) *Streptococcus pneumoniae*
(B) *Streptococcus pyogenes*
(C) *Klebsiella pneumoniae*

(D) *Haemophilus influenzae*

(E) *Staphylococcus aureus*

446. The most common cause of bacterial meningitis in newborns is

(A) *Staphylococcus aureus*

(B) *Escherichia coli*

(C) *Streptococcus pyogenes*

(D) *Neisseria meningitidis*

(E) *Streptococcus pneumoniae*

DIRECTIONS (Questions 447 through 459): Each group of items in this section consists of lettered headings followed by a set of numbered words or phrases. For each numbered word or phrase, select the <u>ONE</u> lettered heading that is most closely associated with it. <u>Each lettered heading may be selected once, more than once, or not at all.</u>

Questions 447 and 448

For each parasitic organism listed below, choose the mode by which it is usually transmitted to humans.

(A) ingestion of infective egg

(B) ingestion of cyst stage

(C) ingestion of animal tissue that contains the larva

(D) penetration of skin by infective larva

(E) ingestion of adult form

447. *Entamoeba histolytica*

448. *Schistosoma mansoni*

Questions 449 through 451

For each of the components described below, choose the letter on the diagram that represents the portion of the immunoglobulin molecule with which it is associated.

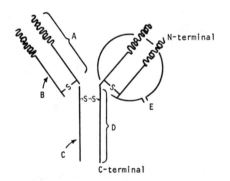

449. Fab fragment

450. Complement-binding area

451. Constant region of the light chain

Questions 452 through 454

For each descriptive term below, choose the letter on the figure that represents the corresponding phase of antigen clearance in vivo.

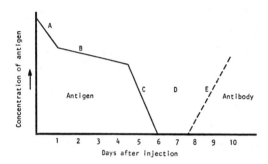

452. Immune elimination

453. Metabolic clearance

454. Equilibration phase

Questions 455 and 456

(A) pili

(B) endotoxin

(C) calcium dipicolinate

(D) heat-stable protein (HPr)

(E) H antigen

455. Participation in bacterial conjugation

456. Spore component

Questions 457 through 459

Two triple auxotrophic strains of *Escherichia coli*, Trp⁻ Lys⁻ His⁻ Pro⁺ Pan⁺ Bio⁺ and Trp⁺ Lys⁺ His⁺ Pro⁻ Pan⁻ Bio⁻, are allowed to conjugate in liquid medium for 30 min. After dilution of the broth, the bacteria are plated onto a complete medium. After 24 hr of growth, six replicas are made, each into a plate containing minimal medium and additional nutrient or nutrients as indicated in the figure below. For each of the following genotypes of the colony, choose the mutant strain with which it is associated.

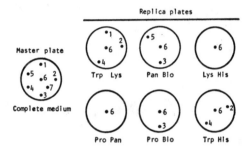

(A) Trp⁻
(B) Trp⁻ Lys⁻
(C) Bio⁻
(D) Pan⁻ Bio⁻
(E) Trp⁻ Lys⁻ Bio⁻

457. The genotype of colony 1

458. The genotype of colony 4

459. The genotype of colony 5

DIRECTIONS (Questions 460 through 465): Each group of items in this section consists of lettered headings followed by a set of numbered words or phrases. For each numbered word or phrase, select

A if the item is associated with (A) <u>only</u>,
B if the item is associated with (B) <u>only</u>,
C if the item is associated with <u>both (A) and (B)</u>,
D if the item is associated with <u>neither (A) nor (B)</u>.

Questions 460 and 461

(A) amantadine hydrochloride
(B) *N*-methylsatin-β-thiosemicarbazone
(C) both
(D) neither

460. Effective antiviral agent that prevents virus capsid protein synthesis

461. Must be administered daily to block infection by influenza A virus

Questions 462 and 463

(A) *Bacillus*
(B) *Clostridium*
(C) both
(D) neither

462. Gram-positive, sporeforming, rod-shaped bacteria

463. Contain(s) no superoxide dismutase

Questions 464 and 465

(A) human immunodeficiency virus (HIV)
(B) lymphadenopathy virus (LAV)
(C) both
(D) neither

464. Reduction of the CD-4⁺ lymphocytes

465. Bar-shaped nucleoid

DIRECTIONS (Questions 466 through 508): For each of the items in this section, <u>ONE</u> or <u>MORE</u> of the numbered options is correct. Choose the answer

A if only <u>1, 2 and 3</u> are correct,
B if only <u>1 and 3</u> are correct,
C if only <u>2 and 4</u> are correct,
D if only <u>4</u> is correct,
E if <u>all</u> are correct.

466. Pili of *Neisseria gonorrhoeae* are known to
    (1) be responsible for the absence of secretory IgA in urethral exudates
    (2) impart resistance to intracellular killing on piliated strains
    (3) have endotoxic properties
    (4) be organelles of attachment

467. Which of the following agents may cause clinical disease in an immunosuppressed patient?
    (1) *Pneumocystis carinii*
    (2) varicella virus
    (3) *Toxoplasma gondii*
    (4) *Streptococcus pneumoniae*

468. Isolated routinely from renal transplant recipients
    (1) rotavirus
    (2) cytomegalovirus (CMV)
    (3) Creuztfeld-Jakob prion
    (4) human papovavirus, BK

469. The pharmacologically active mediators of anaphylaxis include

(1) histamine and slow reacting substance of anaphylaxis (SRS-A)

(2) bradykinin and platelet-activating factor

(3) eosinophil chemotactic factor and serotonin

(4) IgE

470. Human T cell leukemia (lymphoma) virus is correctly described as

(1) a retrovirus

(2) horizontally transmitted

(3) associated with several cases of acquired immunodeficiency syndrome (AIDS)

(4) similar antigenically to other mammalian retroviruses

471. The bacterial phosphotransferase system is known to

(1) concentrate transported substances

(2) produce a phosphorylated product

(3) include two proteins, enzyme I and HPr, which are common to several phosphotransferase systems

(4) be used by bacteria to transport amino acids

472. Q fever is an acute infectious disease of worldwide occurrence that

(1) is caused by *Rickettsia akari*

(2) stimulates the production of *Proteus* agglutinins

(3) involves a rash that spreads from the trunk to the extremities

(4) is acquired by inhaling dust containing infected animal excreta

473. Rotaviruses are a group of wheel-shaped, double-stranded RNA viruses that

(1) cause gastroenteritis

(2) are antigenically related to the Norwalk agents

(3) produce electrolyte imbalance and malabsorption

(4) are a common cause of traveler's diarrhea

474. Laboratory diagnosis of a viral respiratory tract infection can be made using the following

(1) demonstration of a fourfold rise in antibody titer to a particular virus

(2) isolation of virus from throat swabbings, nasal secretions, or sputum specimens

(3) lack of evidence of a bacterial infection

(4) visualization of inclusion bodies in stained smears of infected cells

475. A viral cause has been linked to which of the following forms of neoplasia?

(1) nasopharyngeal carcinoma

(2) hepatocellular carcinoma

(3) Burkitt's lymphoma

(4) molluscum contagiosum

476. Virulence factors of *Salmonella typhi* include

(1) endotoxin

(2) enterotoxin

(3) Vi antigen

(4) V-W antigen

477. A 46-yr-old cattle rancher develops a low-grade fever 5 days after his 20th high school reunion, which included a rabbit hunt. Standard febrile agglutinin titrations reveal low levels of antibodies to the following organisms: *Francisella tularensis, Brucella abortus, Salmonella typhi,* and *Proteus* OX-19. The differential diagnosis should include

(1) tularemia

(2) brucellosis

(3) typhoid fever

(4) Rocky Mountain spotted fever

478. *Clostridium perfringens* is accurately described as

(1) involved in most cases of gas gangrene

(2) producing a lecithinase

(3) growing well in a reduced environment

(4) able to cause food poisoning

479. Plasmid encoded genes specify

(1) multiple drug resistance

(2) enterotoxins of *Escherichia coli*

(3) bacteriocins

(4) exotoxin production

480. The Arthus reaction has been associated with

(1) agglutinins

(2) leukotrienes

(3) mainly IgM

(4) complement C3a and C5a

481. Transposons are nucleotide sequences that

(1) often contain inverted DNA repeats

(2) require no significant DNA homology for integration

(3) require plasmids for transfer to other hosts

(4) can integrate within other transposons

482. In tuberculosis control, chemoprophylaxis is designed primarily

   (1) to prevent tuberculous infection from becoming disease
   (2) for persons with active infection
   (3) for individuals whose purified protein derivative (PPD) skin test recently converted from negative to positive
   (4) for persons who are not able to receive BCG vaccination

483. A positive purified protein derivative (PPD) skin test may indicate that the individual tested has

   (1) inactive tuberculosis
   (2) has been exposed to *Mycobacterium tuberculosis*
   (3) received BCG vaccine
   (4) active tuberculosis

484. Substances that are mitogenic for T lymphocytes include

   (1) phytohemagglutinin (PHA)
   (2) specific antigen
   (3) concanavalin A
   (4) endotoxin

485. Immunologic suppression for transplantation may occur by

   (1) lymphoid irradiation
   (2) antilymphocyte globulin
   (3) cyclosporine
   (4) steroids

486. Rheumatoid factor is correctly described as

   (1) detected via latex agglutination test
   (2) consisting mainly of IgM antibody
   (3) accompanying certain autoimmune diseases
   (4) consisting of anti-DNA antibody

487. Epstein-Barr virus is associated with which of the following conditions?

   (1) nasopharyngeal carcinoma
   (2) infectious mononucleosis
   (3) Burkitt's lymphoma
   (4) systemic lupus erythematosus

488. Immune complexes appear to be involved in the pathogenesis of

   (1) poststreptococcal glomerulonephritis
   (2) the Arthus reaction
   (3) glomerulonephritis of systemic lupus erythematosus
   (4) serum sickness

489. Individuals with tuberculoid leprosy are correctly described as

   (1) having lesions containing very few *Mycobacterium leprae*
   (2) a health hazard to contacts
   (3) usually having a positive lepromin skin test response
   (4) showing suppressed cell-mediated immunity

490. The polymyxins are a group of cyclic polypeptides that

   (1) attach to cell membranes lacking sterols
   (2) attach to both eukaryotic and prokaryotic cell membranes
   (3) are used against septicemias caused by gram-negative bacteria
   (4) are drugs of choice for fungal infections

491. The superoxide anion generated by phagocytizing neutrophils is rapidly converted (via superoxide dismutase) to

   (1) hydrogen peroxide
   (2) hydroxyl radicals
   (3) oxygen
   (4) singlet oxygen

492. Cytomegalovirus is known to

   (1) induce an antibody response in most persons by the age of 35 yr
   (2) result in heterophil antibody production in infected persons
   (3) cause a generalized infection in infants
   (4) grow readily in human epithelial cells in vitro

493. Desirable properties of a vector plasmid for use in molecular cloning include

   (1) high copy number
   (2) selectable phenotype
   (3) autonomous replication
   (4) single sites for restriction enzymes

494. Functions of flora that normally reside in the body include

(1) production of bacteriocins effective against pathogens

(2) synthesis of potent neurotoxins

(3) continuous antigenic stimulation of the immune response

(4) inhibition of phagocytosis

495. An acutely ill child is brought to the emergency room. The presence of petechiae and a stiff neck suggests meningococcal meningitis. If the diagnosis is correct, the examination of spinal fluid should reveal an increased

(1) number of neutrophils

(2) opening pressure

(3) protein content

(4) glucose content

496. Toxins produced by *Staphylococcus aureus* include

(1) exfoliative toxin

(2) verotoxin

(3) enterotoxin

(4) erythrogenic toxin

497. Which of the following statements may correctly describe the mumps virus?

(1) live vaccine is recommended in childhood to prevent clinical infection

(2) aseptic meningitis may result from infection

(3) the wild-type virus may cause inapparent infection

(4) orchitis can be prevented by vasectomy

498. Mechanisms of viral cytocidal effects include

(1) shutdown of cellular macromolecular synthesis

(2) release of lysosomal enzymes

(3) toxic effects of viral proteins

(4) complement activation by the alternate pathway

499. The molecular action of streptomycin on bacteria includes

(1) misreading of the UUU codon in RNA

(2) prevention of aminoacyl-tRNA binding to the 50S ribosome

(3) prevention of initiation of protein synthesis

(4) terminating protein synthesis

500. Characteristics of strains of *Neisseria gonorrhoeae* that may assist in its hematogenous dissemination include

(1) Arg⁻Ura⁻Hyx⁻ phenotype

(2) tendency to cause asymptomatic urethritis

(3) resistance to the complement-mediated killing of normal human serum

(4) opaque colony type

501. Rickettsia

(1) couple the conversion of ADP to ATP with the oxidation of glutamic acid

(2) are generally resistant to tetracycline and chloramphenicol

(3) multiply in the endothelial cells of small blood vessels

(4) possess highly impermeable cytoplasmic membranes

502. Bacterial resistance to aminoglycosides encountered in clinical isolates is usually attributable to

(1) an adenyltransferase

(2) a phosphoryltransferase

(3) an acetyltransferase

(4) decreased permeability

503. *Legionella pneumophila*

(1) can survive for months in tap water at 25°C

(2) is the major cause of legionellosis in humans

(3) is not usually demonstrable in gram stains of clinical specimens

(4) has been found in air-conditoning systems

504. A patient is complaining of a sore throat. Physical examination of the throat indicates a severe redness and an exudate; lymphadenopathy is also evident. This triggers key thoughts of

(1) throat culture

(2) bacitracin discs

(3) blood agar

(4) penicillin

505. Serodiagnosis of autoimmune disease usually involves the detection of which of the following in a person's serum?

(1) elevated levels of γ-globulin

(2) depressed levels of complement

(3) immune complexes

(4) excess autoantigen

SUMMARY OF DIRECTIONS				
A	**B**	**C**	**D**	**E**
1, 2, 3 **only**	**1, 3** **only**	**2, 4** **only**	**4** **only**	**All are** **correct**

506. Poliovirus vaccine is correctly described by which of the following statements?

(1) the Sabin vaccine is a live attenuated virus cell-culture preparation

(2) the Salk vaccine contains formalin-inactivated cell-culture prepared virus

(3) it is a polyvalent preparation

(4) active virus is excreted in the feces of Sabin vaccine-immunized individuals

507. The Venereal Diseases Research Laboratories (VDRL) and the Rapid Plasma Reagin (RPR) tests

(1) detect antibodies directed against *Treponema pallidum*

(2) are used to follow response to treatment in people with syphilis

(3) remain positive for life in most people after treatment of primary or secondary syphilis

(4) detect IgM and IgG antibodies directed against a cardiolipin antigen

508. Bacteria differ from animal cells in that bacterial cells lack

(1) a nuclear membrane

(2) a well-defined mitotic apparatus

(3) histones

(4) polyribosomes

Answers and Explanations

382. **The answer is D.** Multiplication of a given gram-negative bacterium within the blood stream leads to release of its specific endotoxin that produces the septic shock syndrome. The endotoxin is composed of three regions. Region I contains the nonspecific, nontoxic, O antigen. Thus, administration of antibodies to the terminal polysaccharide of the O antigen, that already are present in the blood stream is not likely to constitute an effective protective strategy for prevention of the septic shock syndrome. Region II of the endotoxin contains the core polysaccharide that is linked to the region III, or lipid, moiety of the endotoxin. The toxicity of the endotoxin resides mostly in the lipid A moiety. Therefore, administration of specific antibody to lipid A and its associated core-linked polysaccharide should assist in prevention of the septic shock syndrome. Cachectin plays a pivotal role in the pathophysiology of sepsis and by itself can produce the septic shock syndrome in experimental animals. Conversely, animals that have been previously immunized against cachectin will survive an otherwise lethal dose of endotoxin. A well-known effect of endotoxin is that it induces vasodilatation, hypotension, and increased permeability. This action is prolonged by leucotrienes. Thus, administration of anti-leucotriene agents should be indicated in septic shock syndrome. *(Joklik et al, pp 70–72,461; Roitt, p 9)*

383. **The answer is C.** Staphylococcal scalded skin syndrome is an intoxication in which exfoliatin, produced by phage group II organisms growing somewhere in the body (usually the gut), obtain access to the blood stream. The resultant toxemia is evidenced by changes in the integrity of the integument: The skin separates at the stratum granulosum because of the effect of the toxin on the desmosomes located there. This causes the skin to appear to float. It has no resilience and will stay wrinkled if pushed in one direction (Nikolsky's sign). *(Joklik et al, pp 350–352)*

384. **The answer is D.** Hepatitis B virus is practically indestructible; hence the need for the use of disposable syringes, needles, and other equipment that may carry the pathogen. This agent has taken on particular significance in the dental profession, where cold sterilization with disinfectant solutions is commonly practiced. The virus is not inactivated by most of the agents used. It is now recommended that dentists be vaccinated against hepatitis B. The increased use of self-injected drugs by a segment of our society has greatly increased the occurrence of hepatitis B in the population and, thus, has also increased the danger of transmission by any procedures that involve skin puncture or bleeding. *(Jawetz et al, p 452)*

385. **The answer is B.** The term burst size is defined as the average number of progeny viruses released per infected cell. *(Joklik et al, pp 667–674)*

386. **The answer is D.** The stages of conjugation are as follows: (1) specific pair formation, in which the donor and recipient make contact through the F pili, (2) effective pair formation with cell-to-cell contact, (3) chromosome mobilization, (4) transfer of a unique strand of DNA to the recipient cell, which leads to (5) formation of partial diploids, or merozygotes (entire recipient chromosome and partial chromosome from the donor), and (6) genetic recombination, in which the donor chromosome replaces segments of the recipient chromosome. Competency is a condition that is necessary for transformation of cells and is *not* a stage of conjugation. *(Joklik et al, pp 114–117)*

387. **The answer is B.** Rocky Mountain spotted fever is spread from its reservoir in nature (e.g., rodents, dogs) to humans by the bite of infected ticks, primarily the wood tick (*Dermacentor andersoni*) in the western USA and the dog tick (*Dermacentor variabilis*) in the eastern areas. Tsutsugamushi disease is spread by mites, epidemic typhus is spread by human body lice, and endemic (murine) typhus and bubonic plague are transmitted by rat fleas. There is no vector in Q fever, which is acquired by inhalation of infectious particles. *(Joklik et al, pp 596–598,602–603)*

388. **The answer is C.** Viral infection is initiated with the attachment of the viral hemagglutinin to a specific host cell membrane glycoprotein (mucopeptide) receptor. The viral particles then fuse with the membrane, and the nucleocapsid enters the cell to begin the replicative cycle. The virus enters the eclipse phase, during which no viral material can be detected in the cell by conventional procedures. During this time viral proteins and nucleic acids are being produced. The next phase is assembly, when mature virus is manufactured. Release follows, and the cycle is repeated in a new cell. *(Joklik et al, p 696)*

389. **The answer is E.** The increased metabolic activity associated with the phagocytosis of microbes by neutrophils results in the formation of such oxygen metabolites as the superoxide radical O^-_2, H_2O_2 which may be lethal for many microorganisms. H_2O_2 in the presence of cofactors, such as myeloperoxidase, and the halides chlorine, iodine, or bromine result also in microbial death. Nonoxidative mechanisms, such as the action of lactoferrin, lysozyme, and other hydrolytic phagocytic enzymes, may be directly lethal for various microorganisms. Catalase is an enzyme that degrades H_2O_2 to O_2 and H_2O. Thus, since it destroys an antimicrobial agent, it cannot contribute to the intracellular killing of microbes by neutrophils. *(Joklik et al, pp 281–282)*

390. **The answer is E.** In the Ouchterlony diagram that accompanies the question, each antibody will react with its homologous determinant group on the antigen molecule. Thus, both antibodies a and b will react with antigen ab, but only antibody a will react with antigen ac. Antibody b will diffuse through the line of precipitate formed by antibody a and antigen ac to precipitate with antigen ab, forming the spur at position 3. Line 1 will contain both antibodies. The spur (3) will contain antibody b, not antibody a. Line 2 will contain antigen ac and antibody a only. *(Joklik et al, p 198)*

391. **The answer is C.** A transformant is a recipient cell that is transformed by naked DNA and gains new properties in the process of transformation. A transition refers to a base pair substitution that results in the substitution of a purine for a purine or a pyrimidine for a pyrimidine. A transversion is a base pair substitution that results in the substitution of pyrimidines for purine and vice versa (AT → CG). Transposition is the process in which a transposon is translocated from one position to another in a replicon or is transferred to a different replicon. A frame shift mutation generates shifts in the reading frame of the transcribed DNA by insertion or deletion of a single nucleotide. On translation of the transcribed DNA (containing the insertion or deletion), the reading frame is shifted, and a

nonfunctional protein is produced. *(Joklik et al, pp 106–109)*

392. **The answer is B.** Transformation is the transfer of genetic information from one bacterial cell to another by the introduction of naked DNA into a bacterial cell. Transformation is not affected by RNAse in the medium, since DNA is resistant to RNAse. However, DNAse in the medium destroys the transforming material (DNA), and hence transformation of bacteria can be blocked by DNAse. Antiserum against bacteriophage is not effective in blocking transformation because bacteriophage are not involved in transformation. Antiserum to bacteriophage will block transfer of genetic information by transduction. In contrast to transformation, transfer of genetic information by conjugation requires effective pair formation or cell-to-cell contact. In some bacteria, the sex pili are involved in cell-to-cell contact, and bacteriophage that bind to the tips of the pili block effective pair formation. Therefore, bacteriophage that adsorb to sex pili block conjugation but do not affect transformation. As already stated, transformation does not require cell-to-cell contact, and prevention of cell-to-cell contact between donor and recipient cultures does not hinder transformation. *(Joklik et al, pp 113–117)*

393. **The answer is D.** When a temperate bacteriophage infects a susceptible bacterium, the phage may enter either the lytic cycle or the lysogenic cycle of replication. If the phage enters the lytic cycle, the phage replicates, the cell is lysed, and viable progeny phage are released. With the lysogenic cycle, the bacteriophage DNA integrates into the host chromosome, where it is maintained until the lytic cycle is induced. The integrated viral DNA is referred to as a prophage, and the bacterial cell carrying the prophage is referred to as a lysogenic bacterium, or a lysogen. *(Joklik et al, pp 768–769)*

394. **The answer is C.** The attachment of influenza virus to host cells occurs through a reaction of the hemagglutinin with a receptor on the membrane. Thus, antibody that blocks this reaction will prevent the disease. Antineuraminidase antibodies reduce viral spread and can diminish the severity of the disease. *(Joklik et al, p 696)*

395. **The answer is D.** Chlamydiae and rickettsiae are the largest of the obligate intracellular parasites. They are bacteria-like in that they have a cell wall, contain both DNA and RNA, and are susceptible to certain antibiotics (e.g., tetracyclines and chloramphenicol). Most rickettsiae are spread by arthropod vectors; chlamydiae are spread by direct contact or by the respiratory route. In addition, chlamydiae divide by binary fission and by an unequal divisional process involving elementary and reticulate body formation. *(Joklik et al, pp 592–596)*

396. The answer is E. The causative agents of tetanus, botulism, gas gangrene, anthrax, and diphtheria are *Clostridium tetani, Clostridium botulinum, Clostridium perfringens, Bacillus anthacis,* and *Corynebacterium diphtheriae,* respectively. Spore formation is a property that is found in bacteria belonging to the genus *Clostridium* and genus *Bacillus. (Joklik et al, pp 23,414–417,519–520,537–551)*

397. The answer is E. Genetic complementation is a genetic tool that is employed to determine whether two mutants lacking the same functions have mutations in the same location on the genes. If the genetic information from one of the mutants is introduced into the other mutants and the resulting diploid organism regains the ability to synthesize the proper end product, one may conclude that the two mutations are located in regions of distinct genetic function. The two types of genetic complementation are intragenic (within the same gene) and intergenic (within different genes) complementation. Intragenic complementation requires an end product that is an oligomeric polypeptide with two or more identical subunits. For example, one mutant may have a mutation that causes a conformational change in the subunit that makes the enzyme inactive. On association with another mutationally altered subunit due to a mutation in the same gene at a different location, the restraints may cancel out to produce an active enzyme. In this case, the peptide subunits coded for by two genes from two mutants can complement each other and produce an active protein. With intergenic complementation, two nonidentical gene products from two mutants complement each other. For example, introduction of a P⁻ Lys⁺ phage (unable to replicate) into a bacterium containing a P⁺ Lys⁻ phage (unable to produce lysozyme) will result in release of viable progeny from the bacterium. Suppression is a method in which a second mutation corrects the damage done by the first mutation. The remainder of the choices listed in the question are not genetic tests of function. *(Joklik et al, 103–123)*

398. The answer is D. The germane mode of action of ultraviolet light on microorganisms is related to its absorption by the DNA. This absorption leads to the formation of covalent bonds between adjacent pyrimidine bases. These pyrimidine diamers alter the form of the DNA and thus interfere with normal base pairing during the synthesis of DNA. Disruption of the bacterial cell membrane, removal of free sulfhydryl groups, protein denaturation, and addition of alkyl groups to cellular components are induced by detergents, heavy metals, heat or alcoholic compounds, and ethylene oxide or formaldehyde, respectively. *(Joklik et al, pp 163–170)*

399. The answer is A. Members of the genera *Rhizobium* and *Azotobacter* produce nitrogenase, which converts atmospheric N_2 to NH_4^+. The reduction of N_2 to HN_4^+ by nitrogenase permits the assimilation of NH_4^+ into amino acids and other cellular components. Members of the genera *Rhizobium and Azotobacter* grow best at a pH close to 7.0 and will not grow at temperatures of 50 to 60°C, at which thermophilic bacteria thrive. Capsules may be present in *Rhizobium* and *Azotobacter,* but they do not contain D-glutamic acid, which is the key component of the *Bacillus anthracis* capsule. Attachment to human cells of members of the genera *Rhizobium* and *Azotobacter* is not known to occur. *(Joklik et al, pp 44–45,121)*

400. The answer is D. Mycoplasma organisms do not have a cell wall and are therefore resistant to penicillin. Other forms of bacteria that lack a cell wall are spheroplasts and protoplasts, which are formed from gram-negative and gram-positive bacteria, respectively, through the action of penicillin or by other procedures that remove the cell wall or interfere with its formation. The remaining organisms listed in the question are all susceptible to the action of penicillin, although certain strains of the gonococcus have acquired a β-lactamase-producing plasmid. Tetracyclines, erythromycin, and the aminoglycosides are effective antibiotics for the treatment of mycoplasmal infections. *(Davis et al, p 786)*

401. The answer is D. Complement-fixing antibodies tend to appear relatively late in coccidioidomycosis. With chemotherapeutic treatment they will persist longer than the precipitins detected in the serum of affected patients. In disseminated disease the titers may increase dramatically, which is a poor prognostic sign. Conversion to skin test negativity would also be a poor prognostic sign, as it can signal the terminal anergy that may occur when the system is overloaded with antigen. Precipitins normally decrease with time, so decreased precipitin titers would have no particular prognostic significance. *(Davis et al, p 840)*

402. The answer is E. A severe form of encephalitis may be produced by herpesvirus type, and is thought to be the result of a lesion in the temporal lobe. Herpesvirus type 2 may be transmitted to the newborn during passage through an infected birth canal. Severely infected infants who survive may have permanent brain damage. Genital herpes caused by herpesvirus type 2 is characterized by vesiculoulcerative lesions of the penis, cervix, vulva, vagina, or perineum and may be transmitted venereally. Vesicles and skin rashes are also caused by the varicella-zoster virus (herpesvirus type 3). Scrapie is a degenerative central nervous disease of sheep. The causative agent has been associated with a proteinaceous material devoid of detectable amounts of nucleic acid, and it is called prion instead of virus. (Jawetz, pp 464,504)

403.   The answer is C. All of the conditions listed in the question are of streptococcal etiology; therefore, a rise in antistreptolysin O would occur in all of these. The only valid diagnostic conclusion regarding patients with a rising antistreptolysin O titer is that a recent streptococcal infection has occurred. Two of the diseases listed, scarlet fever and erysipelas, are distinguished on the basis of clinical signs. The former is a generalized, febrile disease with an associated sore throat and scarlatinal rash, whereas the latter is a local cellulitis that occurs in the subcutaneous tissues and may radiate locally, involving draining lymphatics. Rheumatic fever and glomerulonephritis are postinfection sequelae of group A streptococcal infections. The organisms cannot be isolated from the patient at the time the disease is developing. As the diseases involve different organs, the symptoms will be correspondingly diverse. (Davis et al, pp 617–620)

404.   The answer is B. Polymeric forms of IgM and IgA are held together by a 15,000-dalton polypeptide chain called the J chain. It does not share antigenic determinants or amino acid sequences with H or L chains. The J chain is S-S bonded to the heavy chains in the polymeric forms of these immunoglobulins. (Davis et al, pp 350–351)

405.   The answer is A. Group A streptococci produce two antiphagocytic surface components, hyaluronic acid and M protein, which interfere with ingestion. The streptolysins and DNAse are able to kill phagocytic cells by membrane disruption (streptolysin O) or by leukotoxicity exhibited only after phagocytosis. Other streptococcal extracellular products that may have a deleterious effect on leukocytes include DNAse, proteinase, and RNAse. Hyaluronidase and streptokinase are virulence factors that may play a role in the organism's spread through the body. (Davis et al, pp 613,617)

406.   The answer is B. The base analog 5-BU causes transitions or subtransitions of AT for GC (or vice versa) to occur in the DNA of cells or viruses. 5-BU is a thymine analog, and on DNA replication, the 5-BU can be incorporated into the new DNA in place of the normal thymine base. Once incorporated, the 5-BU may undergo transient internal rearrangement (tautomerization) from the keto state to the enol state, in which it pairs with guanine instead of adenine. In subsequent replications, the cytosine will be paired with the guanine and the AT will be replaced by a GC. Transversions, which are caused by mutagens, such as the alkylating agent ethylethane sulfonate, result in the substitution of a pyrimidine for a purine and vice versa (AT $\rightarrow$ GC). Frame shift mutations are induced by acridine de-

rivatives. The acridines shift the reading frame by intercalating between successive base pairs of DNA. The shift of the reading frame produces a nonfunctional protein. Deletions in DNA are induced by agents such as introus acid, bifunctional alkylating agents, and irradiation. These agents cause cross-links between complementary DNA strands, and on DNA replication the DNA around the cross-links is not replicated, while the segments on each side replicate and join together. Finally, recombinations are not considered a type of mutation. (Joklik et al, pp 106–108)

407.   The answer is A. There is evidence that antigens must be metabolically processed by macrophages before they can be recognized by the T helper cells. For example, T helper cells from F_1 hybrids between two inbred strains ($P_1 \times P_2$) that have been sensitized on antigen-pulsed macrophages from one parent (P_1) will proliferate in response to a second challenge of the antigen only if F_1 macrophages or macrophages from P_1 are present. Kupffer cells, young erythrocytes, or suppressor T cells from P_1 are not considered as inducers of T helper cell proliferation. B cells may be involved in antigen processing but are not the best antigen processors. (Joklik et al, pp 158,216–217)

408.   The answer is A. Mediators affecting lymphocytes include the following: interleukin 1 (IL-1), which potentiates mitogenic responses of T cells and thymocytes, interleukin 2 (IL-2), which promotes and maintains the proliferation of T lymphocytes, transfer factor, which prepares nonsensitive lymphocytes to respond to specific antigens and to the transfer of delayed hypersensitivity, and the blastogenic factor, which is involved in lymphocytes proliferation. The MIF does not affect lymphocytes, but it inhibits the migration of macrophages from an antigen reaction site. (Roitt, pp 110–112)

409.   The answer is E. One of the early steps in viral infections is the cessation of host cell synthesis of macromolecules. Cellular nucleic acids are not degraded, but chromosomal breaks may occur. Polyribosomes are disaggregated, favoring a shift to viral synthetic processes. The virus first directs the synthesis of new proteins (which may require a brief burst of mRNA synthesis), then viral nucleic acids are synthesized, and assembly and release occur. In poliovirus, the viral nucleic acid is tRNA, which thus serves as its own messenger. (Joklik et al, pp 670–671)

410.   The answer is D. Excision repair follows damage by bifunctional alkylating agents or ultraviolet (UV) irradiation. With excision repair, a specific endonuclease makes a nick adjacent to the damaged base or dimers. Next, the altered bases are excised from the DNA, DNA polymerase I fills the gap, and the two strands are ligated. Bifunctional alkylating agents [e.g., mechlorethamine (nitrogen mustard) and mitomycin] cause cross-links between the complementary strands of DNA. These cross-links are removed by two steps. First the altered base on one strand is removed, and then the altered base on the opposite strand is removed. Photoreactivation is a method of repairing DNA that has been damaged by UV light. Exposure of bacterial cells to UV light results in the formation of pyrimidine dimers in the DNA. Subsequent exposure to light in the visible region of the spectrum induces an enzyme that cleaves the dimers and restores the original pyrimidine bases. Direct repair is synonymous for photoreactivation. Postreplication repair or recombination repair may occur in bacteria that are incapable of excision repair or photoreactivation. In this type of repair, replication of the DNA occurs, and the new strands contain gaps corresponding to areas of pyrimidine dimers. Multiple crossovers between the daughter strands restore the intact molecule. Since bifunctional alkylating agents cross-link DNA, DNA damaged by this method cannot replicate. Therefore, this is not an acceptable method for repair. *(Joklik et al, pp 107–113)*

411. The answer is B. Bruton's hypogammaglobulinemia is a B cell immunodeficiency disorder. Affected patients are deficient in B cells in the peripheral blood and in B-dependent areas of lymph nodes and spleen. Most of the serum immunoglobulins are absent, and the IgG level is <200 mg/L. Recurrent pyogenic infections usually begin to occur at 5 to 6 months of age, when maternal IgG has been depleted. *(Joklik et al, pp 230–232)*

412. The answer is D. Recurrent vesiculating lesions in the genital region suggest herpesvirus type II, although type I is seen in some cases. The remaining organisms listed in the question either are not recurring or do not produce vesicular lesions. Rubella and measles are associated with maculopapular rashes that do not progress to vesicles. Coxsackievirus and echovirus produce a wide variety of diseases, including meningitis, encephalitis, upper respiratory tract infections, and enteritis. A macular rash may accompany some of these conditions, but its presence has no particular diagnostic significance. *(Joklik et al, p 792)*

413. The answer is A. Antiacetylcholine receptor antibodies are found in more than 90 percent of myasthenia gravis patients. If the clinical symptoms are suggestive of myasthenia gravis, this finding alone is often considered diagnostic. Multiple sclerosis patients tend to have high levels of measles virus antibodies in their spinal fluid. However, the role of this agent in the disease is undetermined.

Guillain-Barré syndrome (also called acute idiopathic polyneuritis) is a demyelinating disease of peripheral nerves. It commonly occurs after a viral infection or an injection, such as influenza immunization. The disease seems to be caused by a T cell response to nervous tissue. *(Joklik et al, pp 273,551)*

414. The answer is B. The patient described in the question has a profound deficiency of both the B cell and T cell components of the immune response (i.e., severe combined immunodeficiency disease). The dramatic absence of lymphocytes and lymphoid tissue would not be found in any of the other conditions listed. Patients with acquired immunodeficiency syndrome (AIDS) may have a similar immune function deficit (absence of effective B and T cell responses); however, they will have adequate lymphoid tissues. The cells are present, perhaps in diminished numbers, but are not mature and functional. *(Joklik et al, pp 234–236)*

415. The answer is B. The figure that accompanies the question represents the peptidoglycan of *S. aureus*. Although the general features of this structure are essentially the same in all bacteria possessing a cell wall (the mycoplasmas lack a cell wall), species-specific variations are present. Variations in the cell walls of other species may occur in the amino acids of the tetrapeptide attached to *N*-acetylmuramic acid or in the cross-linking peptide bridge. Both the C substance from *S. pneumoniae* and the O antigen from *S. typhimurium* are carbohydrates and do not contain peptides. The H antigen of *S. typhimurium* is composed of a small basic protein of approximately 20,000 daltons. *(Joklik et al, pp 20,63–74)*

416. The answer is C. Competent cells are necessary for the uptake of naked DNA. Therefore, recipient cells need to be in a state of competency for transformation to occur. A protein called competence factor is produced by bacterial cultures during a brief period of the growth cycle. This protein increases competency of noncompetent bacterial cells when added to the cell culture. Additionally, one can artificially induce competence in a cell culture by making the cell envelope more permeable to DNA by exposure to calcium chloride. Transduction, conjugation, and transposition do not require competent cells for exchange of genetic information from a donor (F⁺, Hfr) to a recipient cell (F⁻). Transduction requires infection of a cell by a phage that is carrying chromosomal genes. Transposition is the translocation of genetic information from a plasmid to a chromosome (or vice versa) by a transposon. Complementation involves the interaction of gene products (proteins) and does not require competent cells. *(Joklik et al, pp 113–114)*

417. The answer is E. The enterovirus group includes such RNA-containing viruses as the polomyelitis virus, the coxsackieviruses, which cause pleurodynia, aseptic meningitis, myocarditis, or diarrhea in neonates, and the echoviruses types 4,6,9,11,14, 16,18, and others, which have been associated with aseptic meningitis. Shingles is caused by the DNA-containing herpesvirus type 3. *(Jawetz et al, pp 432–440,506–507)*

418. The answer is A. By definition, a hapten is a substance of low molecular weight that by itself does not elicit the formation of antibodies. However, when attached to a carrier protein, antibody production becomes feasible. The hapten–carrier approach has been employed to produce antibodies against penicillin, steroids, nucleotides, lipids, and even 2,4-dinitrophenol. Since the rabbits have been repeatedly injected with the hapten only, their serum cannot be expected to have antibodies against the hapten. Thus, when the rabbit serum is subjected to the gel diffusion assay with the hapten and a carrier protein that was not used to complex the hapten during immunization, no antigen–antibody precipitin lines of either identity, partial identity, or nonidentity can be expected. *(Joklik et al, pp 181,198)*

419. The answer is B. R plasmids are large plasmids composed of two functionally distinct parts: (1) the RTF and (2) the resistance determinant (R determinant). The RTF constitutes the major part of the R plasmid and contains the genes for autonomous replication and conjugation. The R determinant contains the genes for antibiotic resistance. The RTF and R determinant usually exist together in the cell as one unit. However, the IS elements at the boundaries of these two parts promote crossover and allow the R determinant and the RTF to dissociate. When the R determinant and the RTF are in the same cell, they may associate and dissociate, and the R determinant may be exchanged with a different RTF. The pilus is not a component of the R plasmid but is an appendage of the bacterial cell. *(Joklik et al, pp 122–124)*

420. The answer is D. *T. spiralis* can damage many tissues, such as skeletal muscle, cardiac muscle, or nervous tissue. Myositis is the most prominent feature of trichinosis. However, myocarditis with congestive heart failure and neurologic symptoms also is often encountered. *W. bancrofti* attacks the lymphoid system, leading to what is known as filariasis, lymphangitis, hydrocele, or elephantiasis. *O. volvulus* is responsible for dermatologic nodules and rashes, and ocular onchocerciasis frequently results in visual impairment or blindness. *E. vermicularis* causes anal itching (pruritis) and occasional abdominal discomfort in children, and it is thought to be the most commonly encountered hel-

minth parasite in the United States. *N. americanus* attacks the lungs, producing hemorrhages and pneumonitis. *(Joklik et al, pp 972–973,978–979,983–987)*

421. The answer is A. *C. trachomatis* can be found in two forms, a small spherical body 0.2 to 0.4 μm, the EB, which is the infective form, and a large 0.6 to 1.0 μm circular-oval structure, the RB. The EB is responsible for binding and entrance of *C. trachomatis* to the host cells. The EB has a cell wall, but no known capsule, that allows it to survive for brief periods in the extracellular environment. *(Joklik et al, p 609)*

422. The answer is E. The viral envelopes of rubeola, influenza B, parainfluenza, and rubella viruses all possess hemagglutinins on their viral envelopes. The human papovavirus is not known to have hemagglutinins. Hemagglutinins are glycoproteins occurring as spikes on viral envelopes and serve as points of attachment to host cells. Five major hemagglutinin types for influenza virus have been identified, H swine, HO, H1, H2, and H3. Influenza virus mutates its hemagglutinin types (antigenic drift), and this accounts for the loss of immunity to influenza virus that has led to influenza virus epidemics. *(Joklik et al, pp 645–646,822)*

423. The answer is A. The Vi antigen of *Salmonella* serotype *typhi* is believed to act as a capsule, composed of polysaccharide, that prevents phagocytosis, or the intracellular destruction of *S. typhi* by the phagocytes. For example, studies with human volunteers have shown that *S. typhi* mutants lacking Vi antigen are less virulent than those that contain Vi antigen. *(Joklik et al, pp 461–462,476)*

424. The answer is B. Trichinosis is acquired by ingestion of *Trichinella spiralis* larvae in undercooked meat (usually pork). The larvae quickly excyst and invade the mucosal epithelium, where they mature into adult worms by the second day of infection. Mating ensues, and the fertilized eggs develop into minute larvae. By the sixth day of infection, the larvae migrate into the intestinal lymphatics or mesenteric venules and are disseminated throughout the body. The pathologic changes associated with this disease occur in the gastrointestinal tract (associated with the presence of the adult worms), lungs, skeletal muscles, heart, CNS, eyes, and other organs where the larvae take up residence and become encysted. The severity of symptoms is related to the number of worms, the size, age, and immunologic status of the host, and the tissues invaded. The primary symptoms of hookworm are mainly intestinal. Anemia may occur as a consequence of severe infection. *Toxoplasma* infections usually are asymptomatic in adults but may produce serious CNS disease in the developing fetus. *Onchocerca* larvae develop into adult worms in subcutaneous tissue and cause tumorlike nodules. Microfiliarial forms may migrate through the eyes and cause blindness. Pediculosis is an infestation with the human body louse, *Pediculus humanus. (Joklik et al, pp 983–984)*

425. **The answer is D.** Antigens have the ability to induce an immune response (immunogenicity) and also react specifically with the products of that response, either humoral antibodies or specifically sensitized lymphocytes. Determinant groups are the portions of the antigen molecule that determine its specificity. Haptens are partial, or incomplete, antigens. They have specific reactivity but are not immunogenic by themselves. Adjuvants are substances that have the ability to enhance the immune response to antigens without necessarily being antigenic themselves. For example, *Bordetella pertussis* will cause the host to produce large amounts of IgE antibodies to antigens that normally would not induce the production of this antibody at all. Similarly, mycobacterial presence in a vaccine will encourage the development of cell-mediated immunity to other antigens in the vaccine. *(Joklik et al, pp 180–184)*

426. **The answer is B.** In a laboratory test used to identify *S. aureus*, coagulase reacts with a prothrombin-like compound in plasma to produce an active enzyme (a complex of thrombin and coagulase) that converts fibrinogen to fibrin. This activity of the staphylococcal organism has a very high correlation with the organism's virulence, although coagulase-negative organisms may also cause disease, which are usually less severe. The necessity for a relatively accurate test to predict virulence stems from the presence of nonpathogenic staphylococci as indigenous flora of many areas of the human body. Another test that is used to identify a pathogenic isolate is the production of DNAse. This assay is somewhat more easily performed than is the coagulase test. Consequently, many laboratories have switched to the DNAse agar plate test. *(Joklik et al, p 348)*

427. **The answer is A.** The Weil-Felix reaction, which is based on the agglutination of differing strains of *Proteus vulgaris* by serum from patients with rickettsial diseases, is a useful diagnostic test. Another test, rarely used in diagnosis of rickettsial diseases today, is the Neill-Mooser reaction, in which viable murine typhus organisms are injected into laboratory animals. Scrotal swelling is the end point of this test. Q fever does not induce the production of *Proteus* agglutinins. OXK agglutination suggests a diagnosis of scrub typhus. *(Joklik et al, pp 595–604)*

428. **The answer is A.** *H. influenzae* type B is responsible for 70 percent of the bacterial meningitides in children between the ages of 2 months and 5 years. The pneumococcus causes meningitis in debilitated adults. Meningococcal meningitis occurs sporadically in all age groups and takes on epidemic proportions in military populations. *E. coli* and *S. agalactiae* cause meningitis in neonates, who acquire the infection during passage through the birth canal. *(Jawetz et al, p 262)*

429. **The answer is E.** Cultivation of fungi requires a medium that is adjusted to the optimal pH of growth for fungi, that is, a pH of 4.0 to 5.0. Such a medium is the one developed by Sabouraud. The SS medium is a medium used to isolate bacterial species belonging to the genus *Salmonella* or *Shigella*. Selenite medium is employed to enrich the number of *Salmonella* species that may be present in small numbers in fecal or other clinical specimens. Tellurite medium is used for the selective isolation of *Corynebacterium diphtheriae*, which is not as sensitive to the concentration of tellurite incorporated into the medium as the other bacteria that may be encountered in specimens submitted for the microbiologic diagnosis of diphtheria. Lowenstein-Jensen medium is used for the cultivation of *Mycobacterium tuberculosis* and other mycobacteria. *(Jawetz et al, pp 242,285,322; Joklik et al, 415)*

430. **The answer is A.** The route of infection of rubella virus is the respiratory tract, with spread to lymphatic tissue and then to the blood (viremia). Maternal viremia is followed by infection of the placenta, which leads to congenital rubella. Many organs of the fetus support the multiplication of the virus, which does not seem to destroy the cells but reduces the rate of growth of the infected cells. This leads to fewer than normal numbers of cells in the organs at birth. Therefore, the earlier in pregnancy infection occurs, the greater the chance for the development of abnormalities in the infected fetus. A vast percentage of maternal infections that occur during the first trimester of pregnancy result in such fetal defects as pulmonary stenosis, ventricular septal defect, cataracts, glaucoma, deafness, mental retardation, and other maladies. *(Joklik et al, pp 839–841)*

431. **The answer is C.** A common feature of the cytology of the fungi is their ability to exist in a yeastlike form as well as filaments, or hyphae, depending on the temperature (25°C or 37°C) or environment in which they are grown. This ability to exist in either the yeastlike or hyphae form is known as dimorphism. Cryptococcosis is meningitis caused by *Cryptococcus neoformans*, which when cultured on Sabouraud's agar at either 25°C or 37°C appears as a budding yeast with a large capsule. Sporotrichosis, candidiasis, histoplasmosis, and blastomycosis are all caused by dimorphic fungi. *(Jawetz et al, pp 332–333)*

432.   The answer is E. *P. aeruginosa* is a gram-negative, oxidase-positive, aerobic rod that produces a green-blue pigment called pyrocyanin. This microorganism has been associated frequently with wound infections in burn patients, and it is considered as the second leading cause of burn infections after *Staphylococcus aureus*. *P. aeruginosa* tends to develop resistance to various antibiotics. However, it may respond to ticarcillin, gentamicin, tobramycin, piperacillin, or azlocillin. *E. coli, K. pneumoniae, P. mirabilis,* and *S. marcescens* may cause urinary or pulmonary tract infections but are not considered leading causes of burn infections. Furthermore, these bacteria are oxidase negative and do not produce blue-green pigments. *(Jawetz et al, pp 146,233–249; Joklik et al, pp 488–490)*

433.   The answer is B. There are two nonsuppurative sequelae of group A streptococcal disease, rheumatic fever and acute glomerulonephritis. Although rheumatic fever can follow pharyngeal infection with practically any group A streptococcal organism, the majority of nephritogenic strains belong to only six or seven M types. Types 1, 4, 12, 25, and 49 are the most commonly associated with acute glomerulonephritis. The preceding streptococcal infection need not be restricted to the upper respiratory tract to trigger this condition, and streptococcal erysipelas is a frequent cause. *(Joklik et al, pp 362–363)*

434.   The answer is A. *C. neoformans* is the only encapsulated yeast that is pathogenic for humans. Visualization of a capsule around yeast cells in an India ink preparation of spinal fluid is diagnostic for cryptococcal disease, although soluble capsular antigen could also be detected by countercurrent immunoelectrophoresis or latex agglutination. This organism is considered to be an opportunistic pathogen, as over 80 percent of the individuals who become clinically ill are immunosuppressed in some way or have compromised respiratory functions. The organism is abundant in pigeon excreta-contaminated soil, which is most probably the source of human infections. *(Joklik et al, p 937–939)*

435.   The answer is C. *D. latum,* also known as the fish or broad tapeworm, is the biggest worm and can reach 10 m in size. Humans acquire the infection by eating raw fish containing the larvae of the tapeworm. The worm attaches to the small intestine and causes abdominal discomfort. Nausea, diarrhea, weight loss, and pernicious anemia can result. The anemia is induced by the tapeworm's tendency to compete with humans for vitamin B_{12}, which it

easily accumulates from the intestinal contents. *(Joklik et al, pp 987–989)*

436.   The answer is D. Plague, a zoonotic disease caused by the bacillus *Yersinia pestis,* is transmitted to humans from its animal reservoir (rats in urban plague; squirrels and other wild animals in sylvatic plague) by fleas (e.g., *Xenopsylla cheopis,* the rat flea). Anthrax is an industrial disease, usually acquired by wool and leather workers. The spores contaminate the hides and raw wool and are inhaled by the workers during processing. Brucellosis and salmonellosis are acquired by ingestion of contaminated foods. Humans may develop leptospirosis if they come in contact with groundwater that has been contaminated with the urine from rodents who are harboring the agent in their normal flora or in a subclinical infection. This disease occurs usually in campers and hunters. Veterinarians are particularly prone to develop zoonotic infections because of their constant contact with infected animals. *(Joklik et al, p 495)*

437.   The answer is A. Hfr × F⁻ mating results in the transfer of the greatest amount of chromosomal DNA as compared to F′ × F⁻ mating, specialized transduction, or transposition. Incorporation of the F plasmid into the chromosome produces an Hfr or high frequency of recombination bacterium. When the Hfr bacterium encounters an F⁻ recipient bacterium, the donor bacterial chromosome is mobilized and is transferred to the F⁻ cell. Theoretically, given enough time, the entire donor bacterial chromosome and the F factor can be transferred to the F⁻ recipient. Hfr cells can revert to F⁺ cells by excision of the F plasmid from the bacterial chromosome. Occasionally, the excision is imprecise, and the F plasmid carries a segment of chromosomal DNA adjacent to the integration site of the F plasmid. The resulting F′ hybrid plasmid can then introduce the chromosomal DNA into F⁻ cells with high efficiency. The amount of chromosomal DNA that is transferred by this procedure can vary but is usually not as much as that transferred by Hfr × F⁻ mating. Specialized transduction is the transfer of chromosomal DNA adjacent to the site of integration of a temperate phage in the bacterial chromosome. A very limited amount of DNA is transferred by specialized transduction because of the limited size of the phage capsid. Plasmid transfer is not a common method of transfer of chromosomal DNA, since plasmids other than the F factor rarely integrate into the bacterial chromosome. Plasmid transfer of chromosomal markers occurs only if a transposon transfers chromosomal DNA to the plasmid. Transposons can transfer chromosomal DNA, but the amount of chromosomal DNA transferred is limited to the DNA adjacent to IS elements of the transposon. *(Joklik et al, pp 115–117)*

438. The answer is D. There are two portions of the diphtheria toxin molecule; the B fragment is responsible for bringing the molecule into proximity of a mammalian cell, whereas the A fragment is the proenzyme that, when activated by mild proteolysis, will catalyze the ADP-ribosylation of EF-2, thus blocking protein synthesis. Certain strains of pseudomonads also have a toxin with similar biologic activity. Botulinum toxin inhibits acetylcholine release in the peripheral nervous system. Choleragen and the enterotoxin from certain strains of *Escherichia coli* activate adenylcyclase. *(Joklik et al, pp 416–417)*

439. The answer is B. *S. pneumoniae* is a gram-positive lancet-shaped diplococcus that may be present in small numbers in the human throat. This microorganism is lysed by 10 percent bile salts, such as desoxycholate at pH 7.0, and it is inhibited by optochin (ethyl hydrocuprein hydrochloride). When it is grown on blood agar, it converts the hemoglobin of the red blood cells to methemoglobin, so that there is a green coloration around the colonies of *S. pneumoniae,* which is called alpha hemolysis. Beta hemolysis refers to the complete breakdown of the hemoglobin of the red blood cells around the colonies of *Streptococcus pyogenes* but not of *S. pneumoniae. (Joklik et al, pp 358,368–369)*

440. The answer is E. High-sucrose diets are cariogenic because the *S. mutans* organisms use sucrose as a substrate for the synthesis of dextran, which causes the organisms to adhere to the teeth in the form of plaques of microbial colonies. This is the first step in the development of caries and also is an important component in the initiation of peridontal disease. *(Joklik et al, pp 580–582)*

441. The answer is D. Quantitative immunoglobulin levels reflect the secretory activity of B lymphocytes and could be misleading as to the actual number of such cells; for example, in multiple myeloma or other B cell malignancies, one would expect to find a marked hypergammaglobulinemia. B cells are not the only cells that have receptors for the Fc fragment of immunoglobulin. Phagocytic cells also have such receptors and thus could be included in an Fc receptor assay. E rosetting is a property of T lymphocytes, as is PHA mitogenic response; hence neither of these assays would be appropriate for the enumeration of B lymphocytes. *(Joklik et al, pp 215–217)*

442. The answer is C. The E rosette assay measures the number of T lymphocytes and does not indicate their functional status. Enumeration of θ-bearing cells also would not give any information of their functional status. Both sIg and serum immunoglobulin determinations would measure B cell functions. PHA induces mitosis in thymus-derived lymphocytes (T cells). The mitosis is detected in the assay by measuring the amount of radioactive thymidine that is incorporated into the T cells during a 24-hr period of incubation with this nucleotide. *(Joklik et al, pp 215–217)*

443. The answer is C. Lyme disease is a recently discovered illness caused by *Borrelia burgdorferi,* which is transmitted to humans by tick bites. The disease produces a unique annular skin lesion called erythema chromicum migrans (ECM). Certain patients develop neurologic and cardiovascular symptoms and arthritis. Diagnosis of the disease may be assisted by correlating the serum levels of IgM with Lyme disease activity because these patients develop IgM antibodies to *B. burgdorferi* 3 to 6 weeks after infection. *(Jawetz et al, pp 297–298)*

444. The answer is C. The organisms of the genus *Haemophilus* are small, gram-negative, nonmotile, nonsporeforming bacilli with complex growth requirements. *H. influenzae* requires a heat-stable factor found in blood (X factor), which can be replaced by hematin, and nicotinamide adenine dinucleotide (V factor), which can be added to the medium as a supplement or, can be supplied by other microorganisms, such as staphylococci (satellite phenomenon). *(Joklik et al, pp 394–395)*

445. The answer is C. *K. pneumoniae* is present in 5 to 10 percent of healthy adults and frequently occurs as a secondary pathogen in the lungs of patients with chronic pulmonary disease. It causes about 3 percent of all acute bacterial pneumonias, primarily acting as an opportunistic pathogen in individuals whose respiratory system is in some way compromised. It is an important pathogen because of its resistance to many of the antibiotics commonly employed in the treatment of pneumonia, and it usually develops into a pulmonary abscess as a complication of the pneumonic process. The major virulence factor of this pathogen is an antiphagocytic capsule. The organism is gram negative and has a lipopolysaccharide endotoxin that also contributes to its virulence. Other diseases caused by *K. pneumoniae* include bronchitis, bronchiectasis, and urinary tract infections. *(Jawetz et al, pp 239–240)*

446. The answer is B. *E. coli* is the most frequent cause of meningitis in neonates, who acquire the organism during birth. Group B streptococci also are an important cause of this disease in this age group. The remaining organisms listed in the question cause meningitis in all age groups on a relatively sporadic basis, with the exception of *N. meningitidis,* which can become epidemic in closed populations such as army training camps. *(Hoeprich, pp 1035–1036)*

447–448.   The answers are 447-B, 448-D. A few parasitic diseases are acquired by ingestion of the eggs of organisms, such as *Enterobius vermicularis, Ascaris lumbricoides, Toxocara canis,* and *Trichuris trichiura.* Cysts are the infective form of *Entamoeba, Toxoplasma,* and *Giardia.* Ingestion of larvae is the source of *Trichinella* and *Taenia* infestations. Larval penetration of skin is the mode of transmission for hookworms, *Strongyloides,* and *Schistosoma.* Larval inoculation by vector insects occurs in onchocercal and wuchererial infections. Although both organisms have an intestinal phase in their life cycle in humans, major pathology involves tissues other than the gut. In addition to the primary abscesses affecting the large intestine of patients with *E. histolytica* infection, secondary abscess formation may occur in the liver or, rarely, in other organs. *S. mansoni* (and *Schistosoma japonicum* as well) causes granulomatous reactions in the host to the eggs deposited in intestinal venules or to those trapped in the liver or other organs. *(Joklik et al, pp 951–952,992–995)*

449–451.   The answers are 449-E, 450-C, 451-B. The antibody molecule is composed of two identical light chains and two identical heavy chains. The light chains are either κ or λ chains and have two domains, a constant domain (represented by the straight line in the figure that accompanies the question) and a variable domain (represented by the wavy line). The heavy chains carry the determinant group responsible for the immunoglobulin class of the molecule and are either α, γ, μ, δ, or ε chains. They have either four or five domains, only one of which is variable (represented by the wavy line). The portion of the molecule marked **A** is called the Fd fragment; this is the heavy-chain portion of the fragment antigen binding (Fab) fragment, which results from mild proteolysis of the molecule. Another fragment of the pepsin digestion of the molecule is the fragment crystallizable (Fc) fragment, marked by the **D** in the diagram. It is in this area of the molecule where most of the carbohydrate is located. Various biologic properties are controlled by this area as well. For example, complement is bound in this portion, and the ability of the IgE molecule to fix to mast cells is controlled here. *(Joklik et al, pp 186–187)*

452–454.   The answers are 452-C, 453-B, 454-A. When an antigen is injected into an animal, it first undergoes an equilibration (choice A in the question) in which the concentration in the intravascular compartment is equalized with that outside this compartment (if the material can readily escape through the vascular endothelium), and any aggregated material is rapidly removed by the reticuloendothelial system. The next phase (**B**) is the phase of normal metabolic decay that reflects the molecule's half-life intravascularly. This will vary in slope depending on the half-life of the molecule in question. If the substance is antigenic, the host will respond immunologically to it and a phase of immune elimination, or clearance (**C**), will ensue. It is during this period of rapid removal of the antigen in the form of antigen-antibody complexes that tissue damage can occur (such as that seen in serum sickness). If the host has been exposed to the antigen before, the metabolic clearance (or decay) phase will be very short, since there either are already circulating antibodies present to opsonize the antigen, or the anamnestic response will occur, in which event new antibodies will be produced very rapidly. *(Joklik et al, pp 211–213)*

455–456.   The answers are 455-A, 456-C. Pili are hairlike proteinaceous appendages found on some bacteria. Pili are of two kinds. The thin, abundant, short ones (ordinary pili) are responsible for the adherence of bacteria to host cells. The few, long pili, known as sex pili, play a role in the transfer of genetic information from one bacterial cell to the other during the process of bacterial conjugation. The sex pili appear to be responsible for the attachment of DNA donor and recipient cells in bacterial conjugation. Members of the genus *Bacillus* and *Clostridium* produce spores. These are considered resting cells that are resistant to dryness, heat, and chemical agents. When spores are returned to an appropriate growth environment, they germinate to produce a vegetative cell. Part of their heat resistance has been attributed to a unique chemical known as calcium dipicolinate. *(Jawetz et al, pp 24–27)*

457–459.   The answers are 457-B, 458-A, 459-D. Conjugation is the contact-dependent transfer of DNA from one bacterial cell to another. Auxotrophic mutants are those that differ from the wild-type organism in having one or more additional nutritional requirements. In the case presented in the question, one organism requires exogenous tryptophan, lysine, and histidine (Try⁻ Lys⁻ His⁻) and is able to synthesize its own proline, pantothenic acid, and biotin (Pro⁺ Pan⁺ Bio⁺). The second organism in the pair has the opposite genetic capabilities (i.e., it is Try⁺ Lys⁺ His⁺ Pro⁻ Pan⁻ Bio⁻). Conjugation that resulted in complete restitution of biosynthetic capabilities would produce an organism (Try⁺ Lys⁺ His⁺ Pro⁺ Pan⁺ Bio⁺) that could grow on minimal medium devoid of any of these nutrients. Colony 6 in the question is such an organism. Colony 1 still needs tryptophan and lysine for growth, as it was only able to grow on a plate supplemented with these two amino acids; its genotype then is Try⁻ Lys⁻. Colonies 2 and 4 both need tryptophan only; they are Try⁻. Colony 3 is Bio⁻, 5 is Pan⁻ Bio⁻, and colony 7 needs something in the complete medium that has not been added to the plates used in this experiment. *(Joklik et al, pp 115–117)*

460–461. The answers are 460-B, 461-A. The number of antiviral agents available today is quite limited. Among the ones currently employed for the treatment of certain viral diseases are amantadine hydrochloride, which when given for 3 days before and 7 days after influenza A viral infection may reduce the occurrence and intensity of the disease. Amantadine hydrochloride is believed to block the entrance of the influenza A virus into susceptible cells. *N*-methylsatin-β-thiosemicarbazone appears to inhibit the multiplication of the poxviruses and vaccinia virus by interfering with the synthesis of the viral capsid proteins. Data indicate that proper administration to contacts of smallpox cases 1 to 2 days after exposure yields significant protection against smallpox. *(Jawetz et al, pp 157–158)*

462–463. The answers are 462-C, 463-B. Both the genus *Bacillus* and the genus *Clostridium* contain bacteria that are gram-positive, sporeforming, rod-shaped microorganisms. However, members of the genus *Bacillus* are aerobic bacteria and, therefore, possess the enzyme superoxide dismutase, as well as catalase. Superoxide dismutase converts the toxic superoxide radical $\bar{O}_2^-$ to H_2O_2, which is then degraded to water and oxygen by catalase. Members of the genus *Clostridium* lack superoxide dismutase, and this may provide a partial explanation as to why clostridia cannot be grown in the presence of oxygen, which during biologic oxidations is converted to the superoxide radical $\bar{O}_2$. *(Joklik et al, pp 46,519–520,537–538)*

464–465. The answers are 464-C, 465-C. The HIV is also known as the LAV. An early clue to HIV, or LAV, infection is a decrease of the CD-4+ helper T lymphocytes in which HIV multiplies. This multiplication leads to the reduction of CD-4+ T lymphocytes. Another useful diagnostic feature of the HIV is that it has a bar-shaped nucleoid. *(Joklik et al, pp 862–867)*

466. The answer is D (4). The pili of *N. gonorrhoeae* confer on the cells an enhanced ability to adhere to each other and to host cells. This has been demonstrated in vitro, where piliated organisms of colony types 1 and 2 adhere to cultured human cells better than do nonpiliated organisms of colony type 4. The pili are composed of proteins; therefore, they do not have endotoxin activity. Secretory IgA can be detected early in the urethral secretions of infected males. Thus, pili do not inhibit IgA secretion. Although the piliated strains are relatively resistant to phagocytosis, inside the phagocytic cell they are as readily destroyed as nonpiliated cells. *(Joklik et al, pp 19,385–386)*

467. The answer is E (all). Immunosuppression, whether it is genetically acquired (as in the case of Bruton's agammaglobulinemia) or is caused by such diseases as cancer or autoimmunity or is the result of some of the therapeutic modalities employed today, will definitely predispose an individual to infections by all manner of microbes. Indigenous flora will become opportunistic pathogens. Latent infections, such as those caused by the Herpesviridae, will exacerbate, and infections that would be mild or even subclinical in a normal individual will become life threatening. The majority of adult humans carry the agents listed in the question either as a latent infection or as normally occurring flora. *(Joklik et al, pp 233–234,341,967–968)*

468. The answer is C (2,4). CMV is an enveloped DNA virus belonging to the human herpesvirus group. CMV virus has been associated with congenital cytomegalic inclusion disease, mononucleosis in children, and posttransplantation infection. Primary and reactivation CMV illness appears to involve almost all renal transplant recipients and approximately 50 percent of bone marrow transplant recipients. The BK virus (BKV) is a member of the human papovaviruses that has been isolated from an immunosuppressed individual who received a kidney and a ureter transplant. The prevailing thought is that most BKV infections are the result of viral reactivation induced by immunosuppression. Immunosuppression is commonly used to minimize transplant rejection. Rotavirus is involved in gastrointestinal tract infections occurring primarily in infants and young children. The Creutzfeldt-Jacob disease is a degenerative central nervous system illness that occurs in middle life. The causative agent does not seem to be a usual virus, and pathogenicity appears to be correlated with a macromolecule containing protein but free from any detectable levels of nucleic acid. This agent has been called prion. *(Jawetz et al, p 464; Joklik et al, pp 797,808,815–816)*

469. The answer is A (1,2,3). Pharmacologically active mediators of anaphylaxis released from mast cells and basophils include histamine, SRS-A, bradykinin, platelet-activating factor, eosinophil chemotactic factor, and serotonin. IgE is a trigger for the release of the mediators; that is, when adsorbed onto a mast cell, it will induce that cell to release mediators when it reacts with its homologous allergen. *(Joklik et al, pp 311–316)*

470. The answer is A (1,2,3). Human T cell leukemia virus is a retrovirus that can be transmitted both horizontally and vertically. It is antigenically unique among this group of viruses. There are two, or possibly three, antigenic subgroups of these viruses that are distinguishable from other retroviruses by nucleic acid hybridization, immunologic analysis of structural proteins, and reverse transcriptase studies. These viruses have been isolated from patients suffering from T cell malignancies, as well as from individuals with AIDS and from clinically healthy humans. *(Joklik et al, pp 299,719, 749,773,862)*

471. **The answer is A (1,2,3).** The phosphotransferase system is a mechanism for the uptake of sugars in which the transported sugars are converted to their 6-phosphate derivative as they cross the membrane. Enzyme I transfers a phosphate group from phosphoenolpyruvate to a low-molecular-weight membrane protein (HPr) with histidine at the active site, which in turn transfers it to an enzyme III that is specific for the sugar to be transported. The enzyme III, along with membrane-bound enzyme II complex, also sugar specific, transfers the phosphate to the specific substrate and transports it across the membrane. Enzyme I and HPr are common to several systems, whereas enzyme III and the enzyme II complex are substrate specific. *(Joklik et al, p 48)*

472. **The answer is D (4).** Q (query) fever is a zoonosis caused by *Coxiella burnetii*. It is a respiratory disease that may be severe enough to develop into interstitial pneumonia. The microorganism is a natural parasite of cattle and sheep, and humans are incidental hosts, being infected by inhalation of infected excreta or contact with animal tissues. *C. burnetii* is spread from animal to animal by ticks and remains as an inapparent infection in the mammalian host until parturition. The organisms multiply readily in the placenta and other birth tissues and also are found in the urine and stool. These wastes contaminate the soil and serve as the source of infection for humans. *(Joklik et al, pp 815–817)*

473. **The answer is B (1,3).** The human rotavirus causes sporadic acute enteritis with electrolyte imbalance and malabsorption in infants and young children. Severe diarrhea and fever, sometimes accompanied by vomiting, are common symptoms. The rotaviruses are antigenically distinct from the Norwalk agents, which cause an epidemic form of acute gastroenteritis. Traveler's diarrhea is caused by enteropathogenic strains of *E. coli*.

474. **The answer is E (all).**

475. **The answer is E (all).** Epstein-Barr virus has been associated with three diseases—infectious mononucleosis, Burkitt's lymphoma, and nasopharyngeal carcinoma. It has been proposed that hepatitis B virus is causally related to liver cancer, based on the evidence of geographic correlation in the occurrence of the two diseases as well as the high frequency of HBsAg in the serum of patients with hepatocarcinoma. Moluscum contagiosum is a benign neoplasm of humans that is caused by a poxvirus, the molluscum contagiosum virus. It is

not a life-threatening infection but can be very disfiguring, causing wartlike lesions on any portion of the body. *(Joklik et al, pp 649,735–736,788)*

476. **The answer is B (1,3).** *S. typhi* does not produce any exotoxins. It contains the classic lipopolysaccharide endotoxin in its cell wall, and some strains will have a polysaccharide capsule (Vi), which acts as a phagocytosis barrier. *Escherichia coli* and *Vibrio cholerae* are classic enterotoxic agents. The V-W antigen, a cell wall component of *Yersinia pestis,* has antiphagocytic activities. *(Joklik et al, pp 461–462,476)*

477. **The answer is E (all).** The history of the patient described in the question would require careful consideration of all of the diseases listed, and the serology would not serve to rule out any. In the acute phase of the illness, an elevation of antibodies specific for the causative agent might not occur. Usually the rise in antibody levels does not occur until the second or third week of the infection, thus the significance of paired (acute and convalescent) serum samples, which allow the observation of an increase in the antibody specific for the causative agent of the infection. Identifying the cause of most bacterial infections is ideally accomplished by culture of the organism. Serology is used to confirm these identifications and is used also when the agent is slow growing or very expensive to culture or when the agent cannot be grown at all (as in the case of syphilis). *(Joklik et al, pp 478,504–505,516–517,598)*

478. **The answer is E (all).** The anaerobic, gram-positive, sporeforming rod known as *C. perfringens* can cause a variety of diseases in humans. Histotoxic infections include gas gangrene, cellulitis, bacteremia, and intrauterine disease. In addition, it is the second most common cause of food poisoning, after *Staphylococcus aureus*. One of its major virulence factors is a lecithinase, or α-toxin, which splits lecithin in cell membranes, making this a molecule with broad toxicity. *(Joklik et al, pp 537–542)*

479. **The answer is E (all).** Plasmid encoded genes specify a variety of functions that include multiple drug resistance, resistance to heavy metals, and sex pilus formation (F plasmids). Bacteriocinogens are a group of plasmids that specify the production of the bactericidal proteins known as bacteriocins. The heat-labile and heat-stable enterotoxins of *E. coli* are plasmid encoded. The gene for exfoliative toxin, an exotoxin responsible for the staphylococcal scalded skin syndrome, is also located on a plasmid. Plasmids also contain genes responsible for the production of proteases (of *Streptococcus lactis*), resistance to phages (*E. coli*), metabolism of sugars and hydrocarbons, exotoxin of *Clostridium bot-*

ulinum, and tumorigenesis in plants. *(Joklik et al, pp 121–124)*

480. The answer is C (2,4). The Arthus reaction is a type III hypersensitivity. It has been associated with significant levels of precipitation of IgG. The C3a and C5a complement moieties induce mast cell degranulation and release of leukotrienes and histamine. *(Roitt, pp 205,210,213)*

481. The answer is E (all). Transposons are nucleotide sequences that can transfer from one replicon to another replicon or from one position to another within a replicon. The insertion of the transposon occurs by a *recA*-independent mechanism and requires little sequence homology. Because of this mechanism, the transposon is able to transfer genetic information back and forth between the cell chromosome and plasmids. Transposons cannot replicate autonomously, and therefore they must depend on plasmids or conjugation methods to be transferred from one host to another. All transposons are flanked by identical nucleotide sequences, 80 to 1700 base pairs long, which are in either the direct or inverted orientation. Transposons with inverted terminal repeats take on a lollipop configuration after denaturation and reannealing have occurred. Some transposons are flanked by a class of transposons known as IS elements. This indicates that transposons may insert within transposons. *(Joklik et al, pp 117–118)*

482. The answer is B (1,3). Chemoprophylaxis in tuberculosis control is used for individuals who have been recently exposed or whose skin test has converted to positive. Treatment involves administration of INH for 1 yr. Chemotherapy consists of combined treatment with two or more drugs because drug-resistant mutants commonly occur in tuberculosis. The probability that a mutant would be resistant to both antibiotics is extremely small—it would require a double mutation. Combinations used include INH together with rifampin or ethambutol. Other useful drugs include streptomycin, para-aminosalicylate, cycloserine, and kanamycin. *(Joklik et al, p 434)*

483. The answer is E (all). A positive PPD skin test indicates that the individual has experienced mycobacterial infection at some time. It does not necessarily indicate current disease or give any information on the health status of the individual. Conversion to negative does not occur naturally and, if it occurs, has grave significance. Conversions occur in the terminal stages of tuberculosis and in certain immunodeficiency states (e.g., AIDS). *(Joklik et al, pp 432–434)*

484. The answer is A (1,2,3). Endotoxin is a mitogen for B lymphocytes. PHA, specific antigen, and con-

canavalin A would all induce blastogenesis in T lymphocytes. The two plant lectins, PHA and concanavalin A, induce mitosis by interaction with lectin receptors in the membranes of T lymphocytes. Although specific antigen should induce mitosis in all immunologically committed cells of the lymphocytic series (both B and T cell components), it is only when the numbers of such committed cells are relatively large that the blastogenic effect would be detected. Thus, specific antigen is considered to be a T cell mitogen when the individual has a cell-mediated immunity to that antigen (as in the case of tuberculosis, when the patient's T lymphocytes should undergo blastogenesis when exposed to PPD). *(Joklik et al, pp 70,213,215–216,229,307,310,335–336)*

485. The answer is E (all). The immunologic basis of graft rejection was proved by the classic experiments, which showed that accelerated destruction of second grafts from the original donor could be reproduced by infusion of B and T cells from a graft recipient into a naive animal before transplantation. It is logical, then, to expect that destruction of the effector B and T cells would suppress graft rejection. Irradiation, antilymphocyte globulin, and steroids all have been shown to cause lymphoid cell destruction when they were administered in appropriate doses. Cyclosporine is thought to inhibit interleukin 2, which drives antigen-activated cells into proliferation. *(Roitt, pp 215–221)*

486. The answer is A (1,2,3). Rheumatoid factor is one of the antibodies produced in autoimmune diseases. It is usually of the IgM class and has specificity for a region on the Fc portion of IgG. If IgG is coated onto latex particles, they will agglutinate in the presence of rheumatoid factor. Although anti-DNA antibodies may be found in the serum of patients with rheumatoid arthritis, they are more common in the serum of patients with systemic lupus erythematosus. *(Joklik et al, p 273)*

487. The answer is A (1,2,3). One of the most important oncogenic herpesviruses is the Epstein-Barr virus, which is associated with all of the diseases listed in the question except systemic lupus erythematosus. The latter disease, which is autoimmune in nature, does not seem to have a viral cause, although viral particles have been observed in tissues from affected individuals. *(Joklik et al, pp 735–736)*

488. The answer is E (all). Immune complexes are involved in the pathogenesis of all of the diseases listed in the question. They contribute to tissue damage by activating complement and attracting neutrophils that, through a process of exocytosis, release lysosomal enzymes into the microenvironment. Poststreptococcal nephritis is a nonsuppurative sequela of infection by a few M types of group streptococci. The Arthus reaction is a laboratory phenomenon that is usually evoked in the skin of an immune rabbit by the intradermal injection of antigen. Lupus glomerulonephritis is one of the most significant complications of this autoimmune disease and occurs as a result of DNA/antiDNA antibody complexes (and others) being deposited on the glomerular basement membrane. Serum sickness occurs in humans after the injection of foreign materials. Any foreign substance against which the host can produce antibody can cause this disease, although horse serum historically was the culprit. The immune complexes in serum sickness may localize in the vascular bed, producing vasculitis, or may cause arthritis or glomerulonephritis. *(Davis et al, pp 484–491)*

489. **The answer is B (1,3).** People with tuberculoid leprosy usually have a favorable prognosis and will not have many organisms in their lesions. Their cell-mediated immune response to lepromin will be intact. Lepromatous leprosy patients, on the other hand, have lesions teeming with mycobacteria. They are a health hazard. They often are immunologically anergic and will most probably have a negative lepromin skin test response. *(Joklik et al, pp 442–445)*

490. **The answer is B (1,3).** The polymyxins cause membrane damage by a detergentlike action, resulting in leakage of cell contents. Their activity both in vivo and in vitro is restricted to gram-negative organisms. They have been clinically useful against infections with *Pseudomonas aeruginosa*. The polymyxin antibiotics are effective against bacteria that contain large amounts of phosphatidyl ethanolamine in their membranes. Mammalian and fungal membranes contain sterols in place of this bacterial component and are, therefore, not susceptible to the action of the polymyxins. *(Joklik et al, pp 138–139)*

491. **The answer is B (1,3).** The superoxide anion $(O_2{}^-)$ generated by phagocytizing neutrophils is destroyed by superoxide dismutase and changed to hydrogen peroxide (H_2O_2) and oxygen. Hydroxyl radicals $(OH\cdot)$ and singlet oxygen (O_2^-) are other bactericidal oxygen intermediates that are generated during phagocytosis. These antimicrobial compounds are by-products of the hexose monophosphate shunt, which is activated during phagocytosis. *(Davis et al, p 564)*

492. **The answer is B (1,3).** Cytomegalovirus is a ubiquitous member of the family Herpesviridae. It is a significant cause of infant morbidity. In vitro cultivation is difficult, so diagnosis usually is accomplished by microscopic observation of large, cytomegalic cells, either by means of conventional stains or with the aid of immunofluorescence. In contrast to another Herpesviridae—the Epstein-Barr virus, which causes infectious mononucleosis—this agent does not induce the production of the sheep erythrocyte heterophilic hemagglutinins detected in the Paul-Bunnell test. *(Joklik et al, pp 796–798)*

493. **The answer is E (all).** To be useful as a cloning vector, a plasmid should possess several properties. It should code for one or more selectable markers (such as antibiotic resistance) to allow identification of transformants and to allow maintenance of the plasmid in a bacterial population. Also, it should contain single sites for restriction enzymes in regions of the plasmid that are not essential for replication. Single sites for restriction enzymes allow for insertion of foreign DNA molecules that have been cleaved with the restriction enzymes. Autonomous replication is necessary and allows a high copy number of plasmids to be obtained. With high copy numbers, large amounts of a specific segment of foreign DNA can be obtained readily in pure form. *(Joklik et al, pp 121–124)*

494. **The answer is B (1,3).** Flora that normally reside in the body stimulate the immune system and are responsible for the wide array of antibodies found in normal serum. These indigenous flora do not produce potent neurotoxins or inhibit phagocytosis. Bacteriocins are protein products of certain bacteria possessing plasmids called bacteriocinogens. They exert a lethal effect on other bacteria in the area. (Bacteriocins are somewhat like antibiotics but are larger molecules and have a more narrow range of activity.) Their bactericidal activity allows bacteriocins to operate in the exclusion of potential pathogens by bacteriocinogenic flora. *(Joklik et al, pp 337–342)*

495. **The answer is A (1,2,3).** The glucose content in the spinal fluid usually shows a decrease in persons suffering from meningococcal meningitis. The increased metabolic activity due to the inflammatory process will cause this change. The other observations listed in the question are consistent with bacterial meningitis. If lymphocytes predominate, the diagnostic possibilities shift to viruses and perhaps fungi as causes of the illness. *(Hoeprich, pp 137,1041–1043)*

496. **The answer is B (1,3).** Most *S. aureus* strains isolated from clinical specimens produce various types of enterotoxins, known as A, B, C, C_2, D, and E, which are responsible for food poisoning. Staphylococcal food poisoning is the most common form of microbial food intoxication. It is caused by the ingestion of food that contains preformed enterotoxin. The symptoms include abdominal pain, nausea, vomiting, and diarrhea and appear 2 to 6 hr after the ingestion of food containing enterotoxin. Another toxin produced by *S. aureus* is exfoliative toxin, also known as epidermolytic toxin. This toxin induces the staphylococcal scalded skin syndrome that afflicts usually neonates and children less than 4 yr old. Erythrogenic toxin is produced by *Streptococcus pyogenes* and is responsible for the development of scarlet fever. Verotoxins are produced by some strains of *Escherichia coli*. *(Joklik et al, pp 350–353,465–466)*

497.   The answer is A (1,2,3). Mumps vaccine is a live, attenuated agent. Its use in children induces persistent immunity similar to that that follows the natural disease. The wild-type virus may cause a subclinical infection, may involve local respiratory organ glandular tissues only (mumps), or may be disseminated throughout the body to produce orchitis or meningitis. The route of spread is hematogenous; hence the presence or absence of an intact vas deferens has nothing to do with the occurrence of orchitis. *(Jolik et al, pp 727,833)*

498.   The answer is A (1,2,3). Of the mechanisms of viral cytocidal effects listed in the question, only complement activation by the alternate pathway is not a method of virally induced cellular damage. In fact, viruses do not activate the alternate pathway. Factors that contribute to cytopathic effects include depression of cellular macromolecule synthesis, increase in lysosomal permeability, alteration in membrane composition (usually by inserting virally coded glycoproteins into the cell membrane), and toxic effects of high concentrations of viral particles or subunits, such as capsid proteins. *(Joklik et al, pp 773–778)*

499.   The answer is B (1,3). Streptomycin added to in vitro protein-synthesizing systems has two major effects—inhibition of protein synthesis and misreading of messenger. It inhibits protein synthesis by preventing initiation. Streptomycin binds irreversibly to the 30S ribosomal subunit, producing a conformational change in the aminoacyl-tRNA binding site. The streptomycin–ribosome complex forms a blocked initiation complex that is unstable. The complex is released from mRNA, but the bound ribosome recycles onto mRNA, forming another blocked initiation complex. Streptomycin also causes misreading of messenger, resulting in the incorporation of incorrect amino acids. *Joklik et al, p 254)*

500.   The answer is A (1,2,3). It is interesting that most strains of *N. gonorrhoeae* that have been cultured from disseminated gonococcal infection require ar-

ginine, uracil, and hypoxanthine for growth (Arg⁻Ura⁻Hyp⁻). These strains contain a low molecular weight outer membrane protein known as PI. A correlation has been found between *N. gonorrhoeae* strains with a low molecular weight PI and their ability to induce disseminated gonococcal infection. Furthermore, *N. gonorrhoeae* with low molecular weight PI tend to be resistant to the complement-mediated killing of normal human serum. Finally, hematogenous dissemination of *N. gonorrhoeae* from foci of infection in the urogenital tract may occur because many cases of gonococcal urethritis in females remain asymptomatic. *N. gonorrhoeae* produces four types of colonies: T_1, T_2, T_3, and T_4. T_1 and T_2 are formed by virulent piliated organisms, whereas colony types T_3 and T_4 are formed by nonpiliated, nonvirulent organisms. However, colonies of both virulent and nonvirulent *N. gonorrhoeae* show variation in the opacity of their colonies. *(Joklik et al, pp 384–386)*

501.   The answer is B (1,3). Rickettsia cannot catabolize glucose. They satisfy their energy needs by coupling the conversion to ADP to ATP with the oxidation of glutamic acid, which is used readily as an energy source. The nature of their obligate intracellular parasitism is not entirely understood. However, it may be related to the provision by the host cell's cytoplasm of various metabolites that appear to leak from the rickettsial cell. Therefore, the rickettsial cytoplasmic membrane is thought to be quite permeable. The determinants of rickettsial pathogenicity remain uncertain, although multiplication of rickettsia within the endothelial cells of the small blood vessels leads to perivascular infiltration and thrombosis. Rickettsial infections generally respond to proper chloramphenicol and tetracycline treatment. *(Joklik et al, pp 594–604)*

502.   The answer is A (1,2,3). Resistance of gram-negative organisms to the aminoglycoside antibiotics occurs because of the production of enzymes that modify the antibiotic so that it is no longer able to interact with its target. Nine inactivating enzymes have been identified; four enzymes phosphorylate hydroxyl groups on the antibiotics, three enzymes acetylate amino groups, and two adenylate hydroxyl groups. *(Joklik et al, pp 157–158)*

503.   The answer is E (all). Legionellosis, or legionnaire's disease, was first detected in 1976 when an outbreak of deadly pneumonia occurred in over 200 persons attending an American Legion convention. Epidemiologic investigations showed that the disease was caused by a gram-negative rod that was named *L. pneumophila*. The organism was spread from water reservoirs, contaminated air-conditioning units, nebulizers filled with water, or evaporative condensers. The organism can survive for over a year in tap water at room temperature (23 to 25°C). *L. pneumophila* is difficult to stain with the gram stain or other common bacterial stains. It will stain faintly gram-negative when the safranin is left on for an extended period. The organism can be demonstrated by the direct fluorescent antibody procedure or by the silver impregnation method. *(Joklik et al, pp 588–590)*

504.   The answer is E (all). The physical examination supports a provisional diagnosis of streptococcal pharyngitis. This is a common infection caused by Group A, beta hemolytic streptococci, which are usually susceptible to penicillin and bacitracin. Laboratory diagnosis of Group A streptococcal pharyngitis is based on blood agar cultures, bacitracin sensitivity tests, and various serologic assays. *(Joklik et al, pp 358–362)*

505.   The answer is A (1,2,3). Serodiagnosis of autoimmune disease usually involves the detection of elevated levels of γ-globulin composed of autoantibodies against self-components. These antibodies may be present free in the serum, or they may be complexed with the autoantigens involved. Another consequence of the presence of these complexes is the depression in the complement level, since these serum components are consumed in the complexes that are found either in the serum or in the tissues. There is no serum elevation of autoantigen in autoimmune disease. In fact, the amount of autoantigen in the serum usually is very low, and any that is present would be in the form of immune complexes. *(Joklik et al, pp 275–276)*

506.   The answer is E (all). Salk developed the first poliovaccine, which consisted of attenuated, formalin-killed viruses. Later, through further attenuation, Sabin was able to use live viruses for vaccination. The immunity imparted by the latter is more long-lasting, as the agent actually multiplies in the intestine of the host and maximally stimulates the immune system. The virus is excreted from Sabin vaccine-immunized individuals, thus serving to boost immunity in the family and community because of its ready spread via the fecal–oral route. There are three antigenic types of poliovirus—types I, II, and III. All three must be present in either vaccine. By careful attention to the proportions of each type in the vaccine, it has been possible to have all three antigenic components administered at the same time, thus greatly increasing the efficacy of the vaccines and minimizing the number of visits to the physician. *(Joklik et al, pp 813–814)*

507.   The answer is C (2,4). The VDRL and RPR tests are both the standard nontreponemal tests employed routinely for the initial diagnosis of syphilis. The tests are conducted by using the patient's serum as the source of antibody in the VDRL test or the patient's plasma as the source of antibody in the RPR test. Both tests employ beef heart cardiolipin as an antigen and are called nontreponemal. Treponemal tests, such as the fluorescent treponemal antibody absorption test (FTA-ABS), or the treponemal immobilization test (TPI) employ the treponemas of *T. pallidum* as antigens. Thus, they are called treponemal tests for syphilis and are used primarily for confirmatory purposes. The VDRL and the RPR tests will detect IgM and IgG antibodies directed against the cardiolipin antigen. These antibodies will remain in the patient's blood as long as there is active infection to destroy human tissue, release sequestered cardiolipin into the circulation, and stimulate the immune system to produce anticardiolipin antibodies. Once the spirochetes have been killed by antibiotics, the anticardiolipins will decrease. For this reason, VDRL or RPR antibody titers are used to follow response to treatment in syphilitic patients. On the other hand, once the syphilitic patient develops antibodies to *T. pallidum*, these antibodies remain high for many years and thus cannot be used to follow response to antibiotic treatment. *(Joklik et al, pp 560–562; Jawetz, et al, pp 294–295)*

508.   The answer is A (1,2,3). Bacteria are prokaryotic cells, whereas animal cells are eukaryotic cells. Prokaryotes, by definition, do not have a nuclear membrane and lack mitotic processes, and their DNA does not contain detectable amounts of histones. Prokaryotes can readily synthesize proteins, which requires polyribosomes. Therefore, bacteria must have polyribosomes. *(Jawetz et al, pp 1–10)*

BIBLIOGRAPHY

Braude AI, Davis CE, Fieber J. *Infectious and Medical Microbiology*. 2nd ed. Philadelphia, Penn.: W.B. Saunders Company; 1986.

Boyd RF, Hoerl BG. *Basic Medical Microbiology*. 3rd ed. Boston, Mass.: Little, Brown and Company; 1986.

Darnell J, Lodish H, Baltimore D. *Molecular Cell Biology*. New York, N.Y.: W.H. Freeman and Company; 1986.

Davis BD, Dulbecco R, Eisen NH, et al. *Microbiology*. 3rd ed. New York, N.Y.: Harper & Row; 1980.

Finegold SM, Sutter VL. *Anaerobic Infections*. 5th ed. Kalamazoo, Mich.: Scope Publications, Upjohn Company; 1983.

Hoeprich PD (ed). *Infectious Diseases.* 3rd ed. New York: Harper & Row; 1983.

Jawetz E, Melnick JL, Adelberg EA, et al. *Review of Medical Microbiology.* 17th ed. Norwalk, Conn.: Appleton & Lange; 1987.

Joklik WK, Willett HP, Amos DB, Wilfert CM. *Zinsser Microbiology.* 19th ed. Norwalk, Conn.: Appleton & Lange; 1988.

Roitt IM, Brostoff J, Male DK. *Immunology.* St. Louis, Mo.: C.V. Mosby Company; 1985.

Subspecialty List: Microbiology

Question Number and Subspecialty

382. Antigen-antibody reaction
383. Pathogenic bacteriology
384. Virology
385. Virology
386. Microbial genetics
387. Pathogenic bacteriology
388. Virology
389. Cellular immunology
390. Antigen-antibody reactions
391. Microbial genetics
392. Microbial genetics
393. Microbial genetics
394. Virology
395. Pathogenic bacteriology
396. Pathogenic bacteriology
397. Microbial genetics
398. Physiology
399. Physiology
400. Physiology
401. Mycology
402. Virology
403. Pathogenic bacteriology
404. Antibody structure
405. Pathogenic bacteriology
406. Microbial genetics
407. Cellular immunology
408. Cellular immunology
409. Virology
410. Microbial genetics
411. Immune deficiency disease
412. Virology
413. Autoimmune disease
414. Immune deficiency disease
415. Microbial physiology
416. Microbial genetics
417. Virology
418. Antigen-antibody reaction
419. Microbial genetics
420. Parasitology
421. Pathogenic bacteriology
422. Virology
423. Antigen-antibody reaction
424. Parasitology
425. Antigenicity
426. Pathogenic bacteriology
427. Serology
428. Pathogenic bacteriology
429. Mycology
430. Virology
431. Mycology
432. Pathogenic bacteriology
433. Pathogenic bacteriology
434. Mycology
435. Parasitology
436. Pathogenic bacteriology
437. Microbial genetics
438. Pathogenic bacteriology
439. Pathogenic bacteriology
440. Pathogenic bacteriology; Oral microbiology
441. Cellular immunity
442. Cellular immunity
443. Pathogenic bacteriology
444. Pathogenic bacteriology
445. Pathogenic bacteriology
446. Pathogenic bacteriology
447. Parasitology
448. Parasitology
449. Antibody structure
450. Antibody structure
451. Antibody structure
452. Immune response
453. Immune response
454. Immune response
455. Physiology
456. Physiology
457. Genetics
458. Genetics
459. Genetics
460. Virology
461. Virology
462. Pathogenic bacteriology
463. Pathogenic bacteriology
464. Virology
465. Virology
466. Physiology
467. Acquired immunity
468. Virology

469. Allergy
470. Oncogenic viruses
471. Physiology
472. Pathogenic bacteriology
473. Virology
474. Virology
475. Virology
476. Pathogenic bacteriology
477. Pathogenic bacteriology
478. Pathogenic bacteriology
479. Microbial genetics
480. Allergy
481. Microbial genetics
482. Pathogenic bacteriology
483. Pathogenic bacteriology
484. Cellular immunity
485. Cellular immunology
486. Autoimmune diseases
487. Virology
488. Autoimmune disease

489. Pathogenic bacteriology
490. Physiology
491. Innate immunity
492. Virology
493. Microbial genetics
494. Pathogenic bacteriology
495. Pathogenic bacteriology
496. Pathogenic bacteriology
497. Virology
498. Virology
499. Microbial genetics
500. Pathogenic bacteriology
501. Pathogenic bacteriology
502. Physiology
503. Pathogenic bacteriology
504. Immune response
505. Autoimmunity
506. Virology
507. Pathogenic bacteriology
508. Physiology

Pathology
Questions

509. Which of the following chronic pulmonary conditions is associated with α_1-antitrypsin deficiency?

    (A) Goodpasture's syndrome
    (B) panlobular emphysema
    (C) bronchiectasis
    (D) Hamman-Rich syndrome
    (E) bronchitis

510. The major pathologic change found in the hearts of persons with hypertensive heart disease is

    (A) right ventricular dilatation
    (B) right ventricular hyperplasia
    (C) right ventricular hypertrophy
    (D) left ventricular dilatation
    (E) left ventricular hypertrophy

511. "Bronze diabetes" is a term used to describe

    (A) melanoma
    (B) hemosiderosis
    (C) diabetes mellitus
    (D) kwashiorkor
    (E) hemochromatosis

512. The inflammatory process depicted in the illustration below shows a preponderance of which of the following cell types?

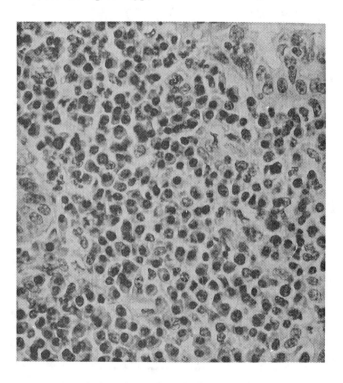

    (A) polymorphonuclear leukocytes
    (B) plasma cells
    (C) eosinophil leukocytes
    (D) macrophages
    (E) giant cells

513. Which of the following is the most common cause of spontaneous subarachnoid hemorrhage?

(A) primary brain tumors
(B) blood dyscrasias
(C) arteriovenous malformations
(D) intracranial congenital aneurysms
(E) tumors metastatic to the brain

514. Which of the five major classes of immunoglobulins has the highest mean serum concentration in humans?

(A) IgA
(B) IgD
(C) IgE
(D) IgG
(E) IgM

515. All of the following statements are true about gout EXCEPT that

(A) it is caused by elevated uric acid levels
(B) affected patients suffer transient attacks of acute arthritis
(C) multiple joints are typically affected
(D) tophi are the characteristic lesions
(E) precipitated urate crystals damage lysosomal membranes

516. Metaplasia is defined as

(A) an increase in the size of cells
(B) an increase in the number of cells
(C) irregular, atypical proliferative changes in epithelial or mesenchymal cells
(D) replacement of one type of adult cell by another type of adult cell
(E) loss of cell substance producing shrinkage of cell size

517. Niacin deficiency is associated with

(A) night blindness
(B) a bleeding diathesis
(C) altered formation of connective tissues
(D) neuromuscular and cardiac problems and edema
(E) dermatitis, diarrhea, and dementia

518. Adult polycystic disease of the kidneys is characterized by the following EXCEPT

(A) autosomal dominant inheritance
(B) autosomal recessive inheritance
(C) associated with polycystic change in the liver in some cases
(D) associated with polycystic change in the pancreas in some cases

(E) associated with berry aneurysm of the circle of Willis in some cases

519. Which statement is false about vitamin C?

(A) water-soluble vitamin
(B) necessary for synthesis of clotting factors
(C) lack causes bleeding in joints and gums
(D) deficiency state is termed scurvy
(E) necessary for synthesis of normal collagen

520. An elevation in the serum of which substance would be an unexpected finding in chronic liver disease?

(A) alanine aminotransferase
(B) aspartate aminotransferase
(C) albumin
(D) gamma globulin
(E) lactate dehydrogenase

521. The type of inflammatory change depicted in the illustration below is seen characteristically in all of the following EXCEPT

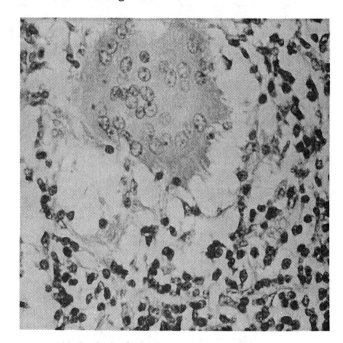

(A) Crohn's disease
(B) sarcoidosis
(C) ulcerative colitis
(D) temporal arteritis
(E) tuberculosis

522. Patients with Sjögren's syndrome show an increased risk for the development of

(A) pleomorphic adenoma
(B) melanoma
(C) lymphoma

(D) esophageal carcinoma

(E) leukemia

523. The human embryo or fetus is most susceptible to malformation caused by environmental factors during

(A) days 1 to 15

(B) days 15 to 60

(C) the second trimester

(D) the third trimester

(E) delivery

524. Which of the following disorders is considered to be caused by the human immunodeficiency (HIV) group of viruses?

(A) DiGeorge's syndrome

(B) acquired immunodeficiency syndrome (AIDS)

(C) thymic aplasia

(D) hypocomplementemia

(E) agammaglobulinemia

525. The constellation of abnormalities seen in Di-George's syndrome includes

(A) an immune defect that improves with age

(B) a deficiency of B lymphocytes

(C) a decrease in serum immunoglobulin levels

(D) developmental failure of the second and third pharyngeal pouches

(E) an autosomal recessive genetic defect

526. Diverticulosis occurs most frequently in the

(A) cecum

(B) ascending colon

(C) transverse colon

(D) descending colon

(E) sigmoid colon

527. Which of the following disease states characteristically produces the nephrotic syndrome?

(A) interstitial nephritis

(B) membranous glomerulonephritis

(C) unilateral hydronephrosis

(D) acute crescentic glomerulonephritis

(E) polycystic disease of the kidneys

528. Which condition would not occur as a tumorous lesion in the duodenum?

(A) ulcer

(B) celiac sprue

(C) ectopic pancreas

(D) Brunner gland adenoma or hamartoma

(E) leiomyoma

529. The histologic changes seen in the connective tissue from the joint space of the great toe shown in the photomicrograph below are pathognomonic for

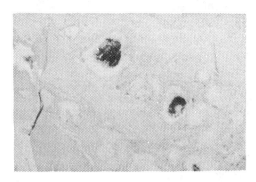

(A) rheumatoid arthritis

(B) suppurative arthritis

(C) gout

(D) osteoarthritis

(E) ankylosing spondylitis

530. Which of the following statements is LEAST appropriate regarding the lesion depicted in the photomicrograph below?

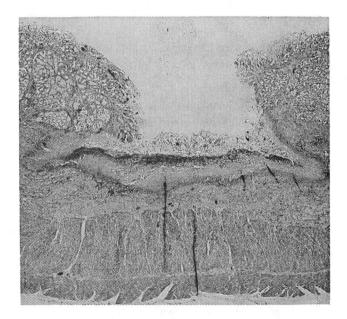

(A) focal loss of epithelial continuity

(B) associated with increased acid and pepsin secretion

(C) may be complicated by hemorrhage

(D) a malignant neoplasm

(E) may be complicated by perforation of the organ

531. A focus of normal cells or tissue identified in an abnormal location is known as

(A) a hamartoma

(B) a chloroma

(C) a choristoma

(D) an adenoma

(E) a polyp

532. Which of the following tumors is LEAST characteristically seen in early childhood?

(A) neuroblastoma

(B) retinoblastoma

(C) medulloblastoma

(D) astrocytoma

(E) meningioma

533. All of the following are characteristic of neuroblastoma EXCEPT that it

(A) is rare in childhood

(B) may arise in the adrenal medulla

(C) may arise in the posterior mediastinum

(D) secretes catecholamines

(E) shows a rosette pattern

534. Which of the following neoplasms is benign?

(A) adenocarcinoma

(B) cystadenoma

(C) fibrosarcoma

(D) lymphocytic leukemia

(E) melanoma

535. Which characteristic best determines the genotype of an organism?

(A) number of microvilli

(B) DNA structure

(C) pinocytosis

(D) lysosomal content

(E) rate of metabolism

536. All of the following statements are true about the relationship of leukocytes to the sequence of events occurring in acute inflammation EXCEPT that

(A) in response to the inflammation, neutrophils tend to marginate or pavement along the blood vessel walls

(B) endothelial cell contractions allow neutrophils to emigrate from the blood vessels through intercellular gaps

(C) WBCs may stick to endothelial cells by undergoing surface changes and by the formation of pseudopods

(D) neutrophils arrive at the site of the inflammation in response to bacterial chemotactic products

(E) C3 and C5 complement compounds are important factors in the chemotaxis of neutrophils

537. The characteristic inflammatory cell seen in the tissues in response to infection by *Salmonella typhi* is the

(A) polymorphonuclear leukocyte

(B) eosinophil leukocyte

(C) monocyte

(D) multinucleate giant cell

(E) plasma cell

538. All of the following are true about a fibrinous exudate EXCEPT that it

(A) induces connective tissue organization

(B) is associated with pneumococcal pneumonia

(C) has a low protein content

(D) is seen in bread-and-butter pericarditis

(E) has fibrin precipitates

539. Renal cell carcinoma is characterized by all of the following EXCEPT

(A) it may reach a large size before hematuria occurs

(B) it is usually seen in infants or in early childhood

(C) it invades the renal capsule and perirenal fat

(D) it invades the renal vein frequently

(E) frequent metastases include those to bone and lung

540. Identify the false statement about breast cancer

(A) incidence in United States is higher than in Japan

(B) increased incidence with early menarche

(C) increased incidence with family history of breast cancer

(D) increased incidence with high fat diet or late menopause

(E) decreased incidence with atypical mammary hyperplasia

541. A rectal biopsy is the usual approach to the morphologic documentation of Hirschsprung's disease. Which of the following findings is considered diagnostic of Hirschsprung's disease on histologic examination of the rectal biopsy specimen?

(A) hypertrophy of the muscle coat of the wall of the rectum

(B) atrophy of the mucosal lining of the wall of the rectum

(C) absence of the nerve fibers that innervate the wall of the rectum

(D) absence of parasympathetic ganglion cells in the submucosal and myenteric plexus

(E) presence of multiple small polyps along the mucosal surface of the rectal wall

542. The most common cause of neonatal cholestasis is

(A) intrahepatic biliary atresia

(B) extraheptic biliary atresia (EBA)

(C) choledochal cyst

(D) primary biliary cirrhosis

(E) Budd-Chiari syndrome

543. Adult respiratory distress syndrome is characterized by all of the following EXCEPT

(A) hyaline membrane formation

(B) proliferation of type I pneumonocytes

(C) intra-alveolar fibrosis

(D) heavy, meaty lungs

(E) unresponsiveness to oxygen therapy

544. Red hepatization is a pathologic term characterizing

(A) fibroblast proliferation

(B) WBCs, RBCs, and fibrin filling the alveolar spaces

(C) hyaline membrane formation

(D) congestion of the hepatic sinusoids

(E) hemorrhage and abscess formation

545. Chronic granulomatous disease includes all of the following EXCEPT that

(A) there is poor bacterial killing by neutrophils

(B) it usually afflicts males

(C) there are symptoms of pneumonia, lymphadenitis, or splenomegaly

(D) it is usually manifest in the first 2 yrs of life

(E) there is increased nitroblue tetrazolium (NBT) reduction

546. Which of the following is NOT a characteristic feature or complication of syphilis and its effects on the heart and great vessels?

(A) endarteritis obliterans and perivascular plasma cell infiltration of the vasa vasorum of the aortic arch

(B) dissecting aneurysm of the aorta

(C) stellate fibrosis and loss of elastic tissue in the media

(D) saccular aneurysm of the ascending thoracic aorta

(E) narrowing of the coronary ostia

547. The vegetation characteristically seen in acute rheumatic carditis most commonly occurs in

(A) the aortic sinuses of Valsalva

(B) the line of closure (free margins) of mitral valve

(C) the insertion of the chordae tendinae

(D) the mitral valve annulus

(E) just lateral to the coronary artery ostia

548. Edema is caused by all of the following mechanisms EXCEPT

(A) increased vascular permeability

(B) obstruction to lymphatic flow

(C) sodium retention

(D) increased plasma proteins

(E) increased capillary blood pressure

549. All of the following statements are true about radiation-induced carcinogenesis EXCEPT that

(A) the amount of damage is related to the dose of radiation

(B) RNA is the major cell target for radiation injury

(C) cells can repair radiation-induced cell damage

(D) past history of therapeutic radiation has been implicated in carcinogenesis

(E) occupational exposure to radiation is a well-documented cause of cancer

550. The teratogenic effect of high-dose radiation to the fetus in utero may produce all of the following abnormalities EXCEPT

(A) microcephaly

(B) mental retardation

(C) skeletal malformation

(D) mutation in fetal germ cells

(E) masculinization of the female fetus

551. All of the following statements concerning skin melanocytes and the response of skin melanocytes to ultraviolet (UV) light are true EXCEPT that

(A) in whites, an increase in the size and functional activity of melanocytes can be seen after a single exposure to UV light

(B) in whites, repeated UV light exposure produces an increase in the concentration of melanocytes

(C) melanocytes may undergo mitosis when exposed repeatedly to UV light

(D) blacks have a higher concentration of melanocytes for any given area of skin than do whites

(E) the skin of blacks has larger melanocytes with more dendritic processes than does the skin of whites

552. All of the following statements concerning Duchenne muscular dystrophy are true EXCEPT that

(A) pseudohypertrophy of the calf is the result of regeneration of the muscle

(B) it is the most common type of muscular dystrophy

(C) it occurs as symmetrical involvement of the pelvic girdle muscles

(D) Becker's muscular dystrophy is a more benign form of the disease

(E) elevated serum creatine phosphokinase (CPK) levels may be helpful in detecting the carrier state

553. Prenatal exposure to diethylstilbestrol (DES) has been linked to the development of

(A) granulosa cell tumor of the ovary

(B) squamous cell carcinoma of the endometrium

(C) clear cell carcinoma of the vagina

(D) carcinoma in situ of the cervix

(E) adenomatous hyperplasia of the endometrium

554. The bone marrow biopsy specimen shown below is diagnostic of

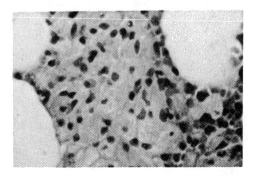

(A) amyloidosis

(B) acute myelocytic leukemia

(C) chondrosarcoma

(D) Gaucher's disease

(E) Pompe's disease

555. Which of the following is the most correct statement concerning acquired immunodeficiency syndrome (AIDS)?

(A) the disease is most prevalent in the United States in homosexual males

(B) the disease is most frequent in Central Africa in homosexual males

(C) the disease is most frequent in Central Africa in intravenous drug users

(D) the disease is most frequent in Scandinavia in prostitutes

(E) the disease is most frequent in the United States in hemophiliacs

556. Which of the following statements concerning carcinoma of the uterine cervix is FALSE?

(A) the majority of tumors are squamous cell in type

(B) the 5-yr survival in treated stage I is 90 percent

(C) the 5-yr survival in stage IV is 10 percent

(D) the disease is rare in black Africans

(E) there is often a recognizable preinvasive stage

557. Which of the following statements concerning *Schistosoma mansoni* infestation is FALSE?

(A) the eggs are usually shed in the feces

(B) liver fibrosis may be a long-term complication

(C) one of the phases in the life cycle includes the fresh water snail

(D) the initial phase of infection in humans is from water contact with the skin

(E) it is a frequent cause of hematuria

558. An expected finding in an anaphylactic reaction, or type I immunologic response, would be

(A) reaction to an antigen on first exposure to the antigen

(B) an interaction of antibody with the eosinophilic leukocyte

(C) release of vasoactive amines

(D) IgA antibody as the mediator of response

(E) tuberculin type giant cells

559. Malignant neoplasms differ from benign neoplasms by showing all of the following features EXCEPT

(A) metastases to distant viscera

(B) encapsulation

(C) blood vessel invasion

(D) rapid, erratic growth

(E) disorganized cell architecture

560. Hyponatremia secondary to the inappropriate secretion of ADH is seen most often in association with which type of lung tumor?

(A) squamous cell carcinoma

(B) adenocarcinoma

(C) large cell carcinoma

(D) oat cell carcinoma

(E) bronchioloalveolar carcinoma

561. The major scavenger cell involved in the inflammatory response is the

(A) neutrophil

(B) lymphocyte

(C) plasma cell

(D) eosinophil

(E) macrophage

562. Liquefaction necrosis is the characteristic result of infarcts in the

(A) brain

(B) heart

(C) kidney

(D) spleen

(E) small intestine

563. Which is least likely to produce an intravascular thrombus?

(A) damage to endothelium

(B) hypercoagulable states

(C) warfarin therapy

(D) stasis of blood

(E) hyperviscosity syndromes

564. A child has a vesicular skin rash. His immunization history is not available. The Tzanck test smear shown in the photomicrograph below supports the preliminary diagnosis of

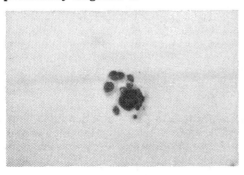

(A) measles

(B) Rocky Mountain spotted fever

(C) German measles

(D) chickenpox

(E) none of the above

Questions 565 and 566

A 60-yr-old man is suffering from the nephrotic syndrome and microscopic hematuria. A renal biopsy is performed.

565. The electron micrograph (EM) of the glomerular lesions, shown below, demonstrates

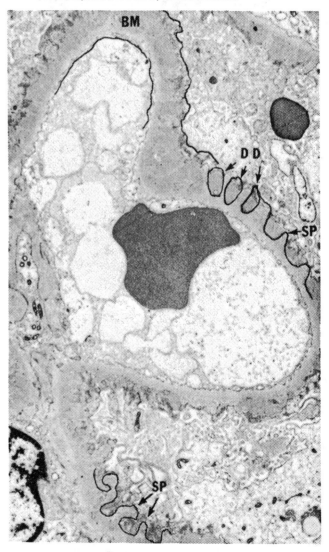

(A) acute or postinfection glomerulonephritis (AGN)

(B) membrane glomerulonephritis (MGN)

(C) minimal change disease (MCD)

(D) membranoproliferative glomerulonephritis (MPGN)

(E) focal glomerulonephritis (FGN)

566. Immunofluorescence (IF) studies performed on the biopsy specimen reveal granular staining with IgG and complement antibodies. This patient's renal disease is most likely

(A) postinfectious glomerulonephritis
(B) secondary to diabetes mellitus
(C) idiopathic
(D) IgA nephropathy (Berger's disease)
(E) a manifestation of Goodpasture's syndrome

567. A photomicrograph of immunohistochemical stain of a lesion in the region of the pituitary gland of a 50-yr-old woman with Cushing's syndrome is shown below. The lesion is most likely

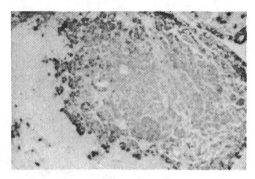

(A) a pituitary granuloma
(B) a parapituitary glioma
(C) a craniopharyngioma
(D) an adrenocortical carcinoma
(E) a pituitary adenoma

568. Auer rods are most characteristic of

(A) chronic lymphocytic leukemia (CLL)
(B) acute lymphoblastic leukemia(ALL)
(C) chronic myelocytic leukemia (CML)
(D) acute myeloblastic leukemia (AML)
(E) erythroleukemia (DiGuglielmo's syndrome)

569. A neoplastic disease of T cell lymphocytes is

(A) multiple myeloma
(B) macroglobulinemia
(C) chronic myelocytic leukemia (CML)
(D) acute myeloblastic leukemia (AML)
(E) mycosis fungoides

570. All of the following statements characterize chronic lymphocytic leukemia (CLL) EXCEPT that

(A) it is a malignancy of elderly persons
(B) patients may be asymptomatic at diagnosis
(C) patients may exhibit hepatosplenomegaly
(D) patients often have a history of fever
(E) the peripheral blood smear alone may be diagnostic

571. Hypochromic microcytic anemia is classically caused by

(A) recent blood loss
(B) vitamin B_{12} deficiency
(C) iron deficiency
(D) folic acid deficiency
(E) accelerated erythropoiesis

572. The lactate dehydrogenase (LDH) isoenzyme pattern shown below is diagnostic of

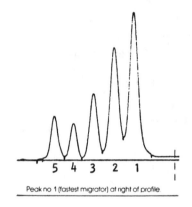

Peak no 1 (fastest migrator) at right of profile

(A) pulmonary embolism
(B) hepatitis
(C) meningitis
(D) myocardial infarction
(E) skeletal muscle trauma

DIRECTIONS (Questions 573 through 584): Each group of items in this section consists of lettered headings followed by a set of numbered words or phrases. For each numbered word or phrase, select the ONE lettered heading that is most closely associated with it. Each lettered heading may be selected once, more than once, or not at all.

Questions 573 through 575

For each description below, choose the compound with which it is usually associated.

(A) histamine
(B) bradykinin
(C) C567
(D) prostaglandin E
(E) neutral proteases

573. Vasodilatory product of Hageman factor with no chemotactic action

574. Important in early increases in vascular permeability

575. Lysosomal product important in extracellular degradation

Questions 576 through 578

    (A) Klinefelter's syndrome
    (B) Turner's syndrome
    (C) Down's syndrome
    (D) Edwards' syndrome
    (E) normal male karyotype

576. 47,XXY

577. 46,XY

578. 45,XO

Questions 579 through 581

For each infectious agent listed below, select the disease for which it is responsible.

    (A) tularemia
    (B) lymphogranuloma venereum
    (C) pertussis
    (D) plague
    (E) Rocky Mountain spotted fever

579. *Rickettsia rickettsi*

580. *Chlamydia trachomatis*

581. *Yersinia pestis*

Questions 582 through 584

For each organism listed below, select the microscopic or anatomic finding with which it is associated.

    (A) relatively intact colonic mucosa
    (B) ulceration of esophageal mucosa
    (C) necrotizing interstitial pneumonia
    (D) ulceration of colonic mucosa
    (E) diffuse reticuloendothelial hyperplasia

582. *Salmonella* species

583. *Shigella* species

584. *Vibrio cholerae*

DIRECTIONS (Questions 585 through 598): Each group of items in this section consists of lettered headings followed by a set of numbered words or phrases. For each numbered word or phrase, select

    A if the item is associated with (A) <u>only</u>,
    B if the item is associated with (B) <u>only</u>,
    C if the item is associated with <u>both</u> (A) <u>and</u> (B),
    D if the item is associated with <u>neither</u> (A) <u>nor</u> (B).

Questions 585 through 587

    (A) Graves' disease
    (B) Hashimoto's disease
    (C) both
    (D) neither

585. Autoimmune thyroid disease

586. Primarily a disease of young men

587. Characterized by Hürthle or Askanazy cells

Questions 588 through 590

    (A) cervical cancer
    (B) endometrial cancer
    (C) both
    (D) neither

588. High incidence in prostitutes and multiparous women

589. High incidence in postmenopausal women

590. High incidence in women with a history of diethylstilbestrol (DES) exposure

Questions 591 and 592

    (A) hydatidiform mole
    (B) choriocarcinoma
    (C) both
    (D) neither

591. Proliferation of trophoblasts

592. Hydropic villi

Questions 593 through 595

    (A) left-to-right shunt

    (B) right-to-left shunt

    (C) both

    (D) neither

593. Ventricular septal defect

594. Patent ductus arteriosus

595. Tetralogy of Fallot

Questions 596 through 598

    (A) asbestos

    (B) beryllium

    (C) both

    (D) neither

596. Carcinoma

597. Diffuse fibrosis

598. Allergy

DIRECTIONS (Questions 599 through 635): For each of the items in this section, <u>ONE</u> or <u>MORE</u> of the numbered options is correct. Choose the answer

    A if only <u>1, 2, and 3</u> are correct,
    B if only <u>1 and 3</u> are correct,
    C if only <u>2 and 4</u> are correct,
    D if only <u>4</u> is correct,
    E if <u>all</u> are correct.

599. Goodpasture's syndrome is characterized by

    (1) its predominance in elderly females

    (2) its rapid progression to glomerulonephritis

    (3) being immune complex mediated

    (4) necrotizing hemorrhagic interstitial pneumonia

600. Acute rheumatic fever (ARF) is characterized by

    (1) endocarditis

    (2) myocarditis

    (3) polyarthritis

    (4) hepatitis

601. Carcinoma in situ (CIS) has the potential to

    (1) regress and disappear

    (2) persist unchanged

    (3) progress without histologic change

    (4) progress to carcinoma

602. True statements about islet cell tumors of the pancreas include

    (1) they may be hormonally functional or nonfunctional

    (2) they may be single or multiple

    (3) they may produce insulin or gastrin

    (4) they only produce symptoms after widespread metastases

603. MEN IIa (Sipple syndrome) can include

    (1) medullary carcinoma of the thyroid

    (2) pheochromocytoma

    (3) adrenocortical hyperplasia or cortical adenoma

    (4) medulloblastoma

604. The lesion pictured below almost exclusively affects the

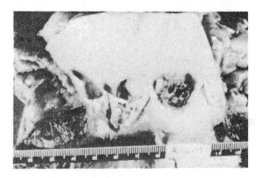

    (1) aortic valve

    (2) pulmonary valve

    (3) mitral valve

    (4) tricuspid valve

605. Diseases with autosomal dominant inheritance include

    (1) achondroplasia

    (2) Huntington's chorea

    (3) Milroy's disease (hereditary lymphedema)

    (4) albinism

606. Persons suffering from diabetes mellitus may show such pathologic changes of the kidneys as

    (1) diffuse basement membrane thickening

    (2) pyelonephritis with papillary necrosis

    (3) glycogen accumulation in tubular cells

    (4) hyalinized mesangial nodules

607. Populations at high risk for acquired immunodeficiency syndrome (AIDS) include

(1) homosexual males with multiple partners
(2) intravenous drug users
(3) recipients of multiple blood transfusions
(4) infants born to mothers with AIDS

608. Which of the following statements may correctly describe sarcoidosis?

(1) more than 80 percent of cases resolve spontaneously
(2) absence of thoracic disease on x-ray reflects a poor prognosis
(3) it may mimic a variety of disease processes
(4) bilateral hilar adenopathy is pathognomonic for sarcoidosis

609. Expected findings in pernicious anemia include

(1) leukocytosis
(2) megaloblastic anemia
(3) thrombocytosis
(4) autoantibodies to intrinsic factor or parietal cells

610. Infection by the fungus *Cryptococcus neoformans* produces

(1) little tissue damage or necrosis in affected sites
(2) skin lesions in about 10 percent of infected individuals
(3) asymptomatic or very mild pulmonary disease
(4) specific antibody that directly kills the fungus

611. The Stein-Leventhal syndrome is characterized by

(1) polycystic ovaries
(2) primary amenorrhea
(3) sterility
(4) large breasts

612. Hemolytic disease of newborn infants due to Rh blood group incompatibility is known to

(1) be preventable by the use of Rh hyperimmune globulin
(2) often result in severe congenital deformities
(3) usually be more severe that ABO blood group incompatibility
(4) results when maternal IgM antibodies cross the placenta and gain access to fetal RBCs

613. Phagocytosis is an activity of certain types of cells that involves

(1) the toxic products superoxide and hydrogen peroxide
(2) recognition of opsonin-coated particles
(3) pseudopod engulfment of foreign particles
(4) leakage of hydrolytic enzymes into the external environment

614. The differential diagnosis of the pathologic changes in the liver biopsy specimen shown below includes

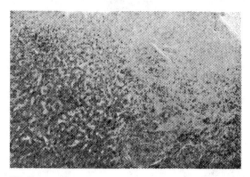

(1) hepatoma
(2) sarcoidosis
(3) metastatic adenocarcinoma of the colon
(4) primary biliary cirrhosis

615. Primary pulmonary tuberculosis is characterized by

(1) a Ghon complex
(2) caseating granulomas with Langhans' giant cells
(3) airborne transmission
(4) bilateral lung involvement

616. Amyloid is an abnormal protein compound that is

(1) composed of antiparallel β-pleated sheets
(2) apple-green birefringent on Congo red staining
(3) produced by dysplastic plasma cells
(4) seen in patients with chronic tuberculosis

617. Follicular adenomas of the thyroid characteristically are

(1) single, firm, nodular tumors
(2) composed of variable-sized follicles
(3) completely encapsulated by fibrous tissue
(4) tumors of high malignant potential

618. During thrombus formation, blood platelets cause

(1) activation of plasmin
(2) release of ADP
(3) megakaryocyte replication
(4) adherence to collagen

SUMMARY OF DIRECTIONS				
A	**B**	**C**	**D**	**E**
1, 2, 3 only	1, 3 only	2, 4 only	4 only	All are correct

619. Connective tissue repair of inflammation is correctly described as

(1) first occurring 7 to 10 days after injury
(2) showing fibroblast proliferation
(3) showing constricted large arteries
(4) granulation tissue

620. Chronic inflammation is characterized by

(1) mononuclear cell infiltration
(2) neovascularization
(3) fibroblast proliferation
(4) abscess formation

621. Carcinoma of the prostate is correctly described as

(1) usually arising centrally in the prostate gland
(2) showing the pattern of an adenocarcinoma
(3) responsive to androgen therapy
(4) commonly affecting elderly men

622. Carbon monoxide poisoning is associated with

(1) systemic asphyxiation
(2) bronchopneumonia
(3) cherry-red blood
(4) bacterial infections

623. Immunoperoxidase stains of a malignant pleural tumor reveal the following pattern of reactivity: cytokeratin positive, leukocyte common antigen negative, S100 negative. Possible diagnostic choices include

(1) lymphoma
(2) metastatic adenocarcinoma
(3) metastatic melanoma
(4) mesothelioma

624. The carcinoid syndrome is associated with

(1) tricuspid valve fibrosis
(2) transitional cell carcinoma of the bladder
(3) diarrhea, cramps, and nausea
(4) glioblastoma multiforme

625. The agent responsible for the histologic changes seen in the mucosa of the biopsy specimen of the gastroesophageal junction shown below is known to be

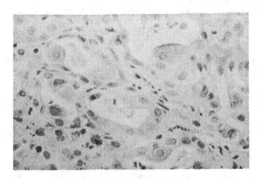

(1) a cause of an infectious mononucleosis-like syndrome
(2) transmitted by intimate sexual contact
(3) a member of the TORCH group of diseases
(4) sensitive to a number of antibiotics

626. The extent to which a substance acts as an antigen depends on

(1) its molecular size
(2) its chemical composition
(3) the dose and route of introduction
(4) the genetically determined host response

627. Which are true statements about cystic fibrosis?

(1) it is a disease of infants, children, and young adults
(2) it has a genetic basis
(3) it has repeated pulmonary infections
(4) bronchiectasis is common

628. Vitamin A deficiency is associated with

(1) xerophthalmia
(2) night blindness
(3) follicular hyperkeratosis
(4) rickets

629. Premature infants whose eyes are exposed to high concentrations of oxygen may develop

(1) retinal dysplasia
(2) retinal detachment
(3) intraocular melanoma
(4) retrolental fibroplasia

630. Exstrophy of the bladder describes

(1) communication between the bladder and rectum

(2) a condition that is incompatible with life

(3) diverticular disease of the bladder

(4) abnormal formation of the abdomen and bladder

631. Temporal arteritis is characterized by

(1) female predilection

(2) cranial artery predilection

(3) granulomatous reaction

(4) steroid responsiveness

632. Wilson's disease is characterized by

(1) abnormal copper metabolism

(2) Kayser-Fleischer rings

(3) hepatitis and cirrhosis

(4) absent α_1-antitrypsin activity

633. Fluid homeostasis between tissue and plasma is maintained by

(1) plasma osmotic pressure

(2) interstitial osmotic pressure

(3) capillary fluid pressure

(4) intracellular fluid pressure

634. Significant microscopic features of Alzheimer's disease would include

(1) senile plaques

(2) granulovacuolar degeneration

(3) neurofibrillary tangles

(4) Negri bodies

635. Which tumors can be testicular neoplasms?

(1) seminoma

(2) choriocarcinoma

(3) embryonal carcinoma

(4) teratoma

Answers and Explanations

509. The answer is B. Panlobular emphysema is a diffuse loss of alveolar septa throughout the lung, extending from the hilum to the periphery. In 1963, an association was shown between patients with a hereditary deficiency of α_1-antitrypsin and patients with severe panlobular emphysema. These patients have bilateral emphysema, primarily basilar, which occurs in both sexes and at an earlier age than do other forms of chronic obstructive pulmonary diseases. This disease has an autosomal recessive inheritance pattern. Heterozygous individuals with the α_1-antitrypsin deficiency gene also may show an increased risk of developing emphysematous changes in their lungs, especially with environmental and smoking insults. Homozygous patients with α_1-antitrypsin deficiency account for fewer than 10 percent of all patients with emphysema. *(Robbins et al, pp 717–723)*

510. The answer is E. Hypertensive heart disease is a common form of heart disease in the elderly population, affecting men more often than women and blacks more often than whites. The majority of cases are of idiopathic origin, but some cases are secondary to renal, cerebral, endocrine, or cardiovascular disease. Because of the increased resistance to blood flow, the most significant pathologic change is left ventricular hypertrophy with increasing size of the myocardial cells. There is no actual increase in cell number (hyperplasia). There is thickening of the left ventricular muscle wall concentrically, with narrowing of the chamber size. Endocardial fibrous thickening also may occur. The left ventricular wall thickness is increased as much as 2 cm, and the heart weight may be doubled. With long-standing hypertrophic heart disease, there is gradual dilatation and hypertrophy of the right ventricle and dilatation of the right and left atria. Enlargement of the myocardial cells, an increased number of nuclei per cell (boxcar nuclei), degenerative changes, and fibrosis may be seen microscopically. *(Kissane, pp 639–643)*

511. The answer is E. Hemochromatosis, or bronze diabetes, is an inherited disease characterized by cirrhosis, diabetes, and increased skin pigmentation. Affected persons are usually middle-aged or elderly, often male, and have elevated serum iron levels, high saturation of total iron-binding capacity, elevated serum ferritin levels, and increased urinary iron excretion. Sufferers are thought to have a defect in mucosal iron absorption in the gastrointestinal tract, resulting in increased iron absorption with iron overload. The excess iron accumulated is stored in parenchymal organs, especially in the liver, pancreas, endocrine glands, myocardium, and skin. Iron is not stored to any great extent in the reticuloendothelial system, as is the case of hemosiderosis with iron overload secondary to increased intake or release. In patients with hemochromatosis, the excess iron deposits in organs cause parenchymal destruction and fibrosis. This is manifested as cirrhosis and hepatic failure and diabetes due to islet cell destruction in the pancreas. Sufferers also have an increased risk of developing hepatomas. Hyperpigmentation results from increased melanin production in the epidermis and not from increased iron pigment in the dermis, as was previously thought. Affected patients have diabetes, hepatomegaly, and endocrine abnormalities, such as impotence or adrenal dysfunction. Treatment is aimed at reducing the iron load by phlebotomy or the use of iron chelators. *(Robbins et al, pp 924–928)*

512. The answer is B. The photomicrograph shows tissue in which there are sheets of plasma cells with eccentric nuclei and ample cytoplasm, typical of these cells. The recognition of plasma cells implies either that the disorder is one in which there may have been a transient acute inflammatory change that has now subsided or the disease has not yet gone into a more long-term, or chronic, phase. It is of some interest that plasma cells, although associated with such subacute inflammations, are not always seen and sometimes can be seen characteristically in certain settings. Plasma cells, for instance, are seen very frequently in these large numbers, being the predominant cell in the primary chancre of syphilis and maybe, as in the illustration, the predominant cell in chronic salpingitis. It is still not entirely clear why plasma cells that secrete immunoglobulin should be in the tissues in such large numbers in certain types of inflammation. *(Kissane, pp 45–47)*

513. The answer is D. The most common cause of spontaneous subarachnoid hemorrhage is a ruptured intracranial aneurysm. Intracranial congenital aneurysms (berry aneurysms) account for 85 percent of spontaneous subarachnoid hemorrhages. Such aneurysms are seen in 4 percent of adults at autopsy; in 20 percent of these cases, they are multiple. The cause is thought to be related to a combination of congenital and acquired factors. A defect in the media of the artery wall is believed to be the major congenital defect and is particularly significant at arterial bifurcation sites. Atherosclerosis and hypertension appear to be the most significant acquired factors causing fragmentation of the elastic lamina. The cerebrovascular lesion most commonly responsible for death in young adults is the intracranial aneurysm. Other causes of spontaneous subarachnoid hemorrhage include arteriovenous malformations (10 percent of cases), tumors, blood dyscrasias, and mycotic aneurysms (5 percent of cases combined). *(Wirz)*

514. The answer is D. Five major classes of immunoglobulins are identified in humans on the basis of the characteristics of their heavy-chain constituents. Of the five, IgG is the major immunoglobulin in humans. It has the highest mean immunoglobulin serum concentration, 1200 mg/100 ml, and accounts for approximately 75 percent of the body's total γ-globulin pool. The remaining four major immunoglobulin classes have mean serum concentrations as follows: IgA, 250 mg/100 ml; IgM, 120 mg/100 ml; IgD, 3 mg/100 ml; and IgE, 0.03 mg/100 ml. *(Kissane, p 457)*

515. The answer is C. Gout is a disease caused by elevated uric acid levels. It may be idiopathic or secondary to enzyme defects causing overproduction of uric acid. Patients with secondary gout may also have hyperuricemia due to increased production from cell breakdown or decreased excretion. The uric acid tends to build up in joint fluids and precipitate out. Initially, affected patients suffer transient attacks of acute arthritis because of an acute inflammatory reaction to the precipitated urate crystals. One or two joints are typically affected, most commonly the great toe and ankle joints. The precipitated urate crystals are taken up by macrophages and neutrophils in phagosomes. These crystals then damage the lysosomal membranes, causing release of the inflammatory mediators, enzymes, and cell debris, which stimulate the arthritis. The tophus is the characteristic lesion of gout and is caused by the inflammatory reaction. It is a

urate deposit composed of chronic inflammatory cells, macrophages, and foreign body giant cells. These tophi are found in the external ear, around the knee joints, in connective tissue, and in the medullary pyramids of the kidney. Treatment is directed toward lowering the concentration of serum uric acid and inhibiting its synthesis. *(Robbins et al, pp 1356–1361)*

516. The answer is D. A number of cell alterations can be produced or identified as a response to a variety of changes or stresses in the cell's environment. Hypertrophy refers to an increase in the size of cells—for example, myocardial fiber hypertrophy in response to increased demands in the setting of hypertension. Hyperplasia refers to an increase in the number of cells—for example, the increase in breast glandular epithelium in females at the time of puberty. Dysplasia refers to irregular, atypical proliferative changes of epithelial or mesenchymal cells in response to chronic inflammation or irritations—as is often seen, for example, in the uterine cervix. Atrophy is the loss of cell substance, producing a shrinkage in cell size—striated muscle response to disuse is an example. Metaplasia refers to the replacement of one type of adult cell, epithelial or mesenchymal, by another type of adult cell. The replacement of the normal type of adult ciliated columnar epithelium of the bronchial mucosa by the adult type of squamous epithelium in response to chronic irritation due to cigarette smoking is such an example. *(Robbins et al, pp 29–35)*

517. The answer is E. A wide variety of afflictions may be caused by vitamin deficiencies. Niacin deficiency, also known as pellagra, is associated with dermatitis, diarrhea, and dementia. Night blindness (nyctalopia), with or without keratomalacia, and papular dermatitis suggest vitamin A deficiency. Vitamin K deficiency may manifest itself as a bleeding diathesis due to the role of vitamin K in the formation of prothrombin and clotting factors VII, IX, and X. Scurvy, or vitamin C deficiency, results in the altered formation of connective tissues, such as collagen, osteoid, dentin, and intercellular cement substance. Vitamin B deficiency, or beriberi, occurs in three ways that generally overlap to some extent in any given patient. Neuromuscular signs and symptoms alone are known as "dry beriberi" but in association with edema are known as "wet beriberi." Heart failure, generally high-output failure, accounts for so-called cardiac beriberi. *(Robbins et al, pp 415–416)*

518. The answer is B. Adult polycystic disease of the kidneys is inherited by an autosomal dominant mechanism with almost complete penetrance. It is associated in a number of cases with polycystic change in the liver and to a lesser degree with polycystic change in the pancreas. Approximately 20 percent of patients with polycystic disease of the kidneys may have berry aneurysms in the circle of Willis, and sometimes it is rupture of these aneurysms that brings to attention the polycystic disease in general. There are some forms of childhood cystic disease of the kidneys that are autosomal recessive, but this is not true of adult polycystic disease. (Rubin and Farber, pp 838–842)

519. The answer is B. Vitamin C, ascorbic acid, is a water-soluble vitamin widely distributed in nature. Citrus fruits and fresh vegetables are particularly rich sources of the vitamin. Vitamin C plays a pivotal role in collagen synthesis through hydroxylation of proline and lysine residues. Hypovitaminosis C leads not only to a bleeding diathesis but also to poor wound healing, loose teeth, and in children, abnormalities of bone development. Subperiosteal hemorrhage and joint hemorrhage are particularly characteristic in scorbutic infants. Although bleeding is a significant component of hypovitaminosis C, the clotting factors themselves usually are normal in structure, function, and quantity. (Robbins et al, p 412)

520. The answer is C. Hepatocytes synthesize a diverse population of proteins, including albumin, blood clotting factors, and enzymes (lactate dehydrogenase, aminotransferases, glutamate dehydrogenase, ornithine carbamyl transferase, and isocitrate dehydrogenase). In chronic liver disease, albumin production is reduced, leading to a drop in serum albumin levels. Elevated albumin levels in chronic liver disease would be truly exceptional. Increased serum levels of hepatic enzymes (alanine aminotransferase, aspartate aminotransferase, and lactate dehydrogenase) are seen with chronic liver disorders as damaged or dying hepatocytes release these enzymes into the serum. Gamma globulin levels are increased in all chronic disease states, particularly in chronic liver diseases. (Kissane, pp 1096–1103)

521. The answer is C. In the photomicrograph, there is clearly a multinucleated giant cell surrounded by some monocytes and lymphocytes. This is the typical picture of a granulomatous form of inflammation without, in this illustration, any evidence of caseation. This is seen in such diseases as Crohn's disease, sarcoidosis, temporal arteritis, and some stages of tuberculosis. Ulcerative colitis is an inflammatory condition that may be acute or subacute and occurs predominantly in the colonic mucosa but does not extend into the submucosa and does not produce the granulomatous change seen in Crohn's disease or in the other granulomatous diseases mentioned. Tuberculosis is the only form of such granulomas that produces the breakdown characteristic of caseation, although this is not always seen, particularly in the early stages of the

disease. (Rubin and Farber, pp 692–700; Kissane, pp 44–46)

522. The answer is C. The constellation of dry eyes (keratoconjunctivitis sicca or xerophthalmia), dry mouth (xerostomia), and chronic arthritis constitutes the clinicopathologic entity known as Sjögren's syndrome. In the absence of arthritis, the symptoms are referred to as the sicca syndrome. Sjögren's syndrome primarily affects middle-aged women, either alone or in combination with other connective tissue disorders. About 50 percent of patients have rheumatoid arthritis. Large numbers of autoantibodies are seen in the serum of patients with Sjögren's syndrome. Symptoms are, in part, the result of the infiltration of salivary and lacrimal glands by lymphocytes, both B and T cell types. Over time, atrophy, fibrosis, hyalinization, and fatty change ensue. The lymphoid infiltrate may be heavy with the formation of lymphoid follicles with germinal centers and may mimic lymphoma. Of interest, however, is the finding that patients with Sjögren's syndrome show an increased tendency to develop lymphoma and so-called pseudolymphoma. Involvement of the respiratory tract, stomach, and kidneys (tubulointerstitial nephritis) also may occur. (Robbins et al, pp 189–190)

523. The answer is B. The human embryo is most susceptible to malformations caused by environmental factors during days 15 to 60 of gestation. This time period is referred to as the "organogenetic period." Although environmental factors acting during the first 2 weeks (days 1 to 15) after fertilization may interfere with implantation or the development of the early embryo, rarely do they produce congenital malformations. Instead, these very early disturbances usually result in death or abortion of the blastocyst or early embryo. Exposure to teratogenic agents during the described critical period (days 15 to 60) may lead to death or abortion of the same embryo but usually produces major malformation. (Robbins et al, pp 479–482)

524. The answer is B. All of the alternatives mentioned are forms of immune deficiency. DiGeorge's syndrome and thymic aplasia are associated with developmental abnormalities of the immune system. Hypocomplementemia and agammaglobulinemia may have many causes. However, AIDS has now been shown clearly to be caused by viruses of the HIV group, and antibodies to the viral antigens can be found in certain stages of the disease in a high proportion of infected patients. There are, however, times during the early phase of infection when some of the viral proteins may be present in the serum but there are no antibodies. This form of immune deficiency appears to be acquired, and the virus specifically attacks the target cell, the T lymphocyte. The resultant immune deficiency or derangement that occurs may mimic some of the other forms of immune deficiency mentioned but is characteristically different in the spectrum of the immune changes and the types of patients infected. The natural history of the disease is clearly different. *(Redfield and Burke, pp 90–98)*

525. The answer is A. DiGeorge's syndrome is a deficiency of T lymphocytes due to thymic hypoplasia. Developmental failure of the third and fourth pharyngeal pouches is responsible for total or partial thymic, parathyroid, thyroid, and ultimobranchial pouch abnormalities. These structural anomalies lead to the absence of the cell-mediated T lymphocyte immune response, tetany, and congenital heart and great vessel abnormalities. B lymphocyte and plasma cell populations tend to be normal, as do serum immunoglobulin levels. The syndrome appears to be the result of an intrauterine insult to the fetus sometime before the eighth week of gestation. The syndrome is not genetically determined. As the affected children grow older, T cell function improves so that by age 5 yr, many affected children fail to demonstrate a T cell deficit. Some patients have been treated successfully by transplantation of fetal thymic tissue. *(Robbins et al, pp 207,1250)*

526. The answer is E. Clinically detectable diverticulosis is seen in about 1 in 8 patients beyond 45 yr of age. In autopsy series, this incidence estimate appears to be higher. Diverticulosis occurs in the sigmoid colon in 99 percent of affected individuals. Other segments of the large bowel become involved by diverticulosis as follows: descending colon, 30 percent; transverse colon, 4 percent; entire colon, 16 percent. The sigmoid is the region of the colon exclusively involved in about 41 percent of cases. In underdeveloped and tropical countries and Japan, diverticulosis is rare, apparently partially because of the high-residue diets in these regions of the world. The most consistent abnormality seen in diverticulosis is an abnormality of the muscle wall, leading to herniation of the colonic mucosa and submucosa through the muscularis and eventually into the pericolic adipose tissue. Fecal material may become trapped in the diverticulum, leading to ulceration, inflammation, and rarely perforation. Cecal diverticula differ from those in the other segments of the colon in that they are generally solitary, are not necessarily associated with sigmoid involvement, and classically lack the muscle wall defect. Many reports, however, state that cecal diverticula also lack a muscle wall and thus resemble those seen elsewhere in the large bowel. *(Kissane, p 1057)*

527. The answer is B. The nephrotic syndrome is defined as a syndrome in which there are proteinuria, edema, and to a variable degree, hyper-

cholesterolemia. Whatever the cause, the common factor appears to be leakage of protein through the glomerular basement membranes, and the proteinuria is a characteristic finding. In interstitial nephritis, this is a chronic inflammatory change between the renal tubules, and only in a very late stage of disease does it alter glomerular function. There is no proteinuria. Unilateral hydronephrosis may cause complete disruption of the function of one kidney, but the other functions normally. In acute crescentic glomerulonephritis, which usually occurs after a streptococcal infection, there may be hematuria and a rise in blood pressure or even anuria, but proteinuria and edema, in the absence of these other findings so typical of the nephrotic syndrome, are not seen, particularly in the acute phase. Some forms of acute glomerulonephritis may progress to a chronic form that may have some elements of the nephrotic syndrome. Polycystic disease of the kidneys is associated with hypertension and some hematuria but not with the classic nephrotic syndrome. Membranous glomerulonephritis is the most typical form of glomerular disease associated with the nephrotic syndrome, particularly in adults, and can be recognized by both light microscopy and electron microscopy and immunofluorescence. *(Robbins et al, pp 1011–1021; Rubin and Farber, pp 845–847)*

528. The answer is B. All of the choices, except celiac sprue, usually occur as mass lesions in the duodenum. A mass lesion of the duodenum is a fairly common clinical problem. Ulcers, usually peptic in nature, are the most common cause. Benign tumors, such as ectopic pancreas, Brunner gland adenomas, adenomatous polyps, and lipomas, all occur in the duodenum as tumorous lesions. Malignant tumors of the duodenum are rare and would include adenocarcinomas, carcinoid tumors, and lymphomas. Celiac sprue is an immunologic disease characterized by marked loss of the villi. Females are more often afflicted than males. People with the disease usually have HLA-B8 or D/DR 3 or D/DR 7. Placing the patient on a gluten-free diet will alleviate acute symptoms. Long-term follow-up reveals that celiac sprue patients have an increased risk of developing bowel lymphomas or carcinomas. *(Robbins et al, pp 841–848)*

529. The answer is C. The pathognomonic lesion of gout is the tophus—a collection of crystalline or amorphous urates surrounded by an inflammatory response consisting of macrophages, lymphocytes, fibroblasts, and foreign body giant cells. In the photomicrograph that accompanies the question, the darker stellate deposits denote the center of the tophus. These urate deposits would appear golden brown, in contrast to the pink-staining tissue about them on the actual hematoxylin–eosin (H & E) glass slide. Gout is a systemic disorder of uric acid metabolism resulting in hyperuricemia. Urates precipitate out of the supersaturated blood and deposit in the joints and soft tissues. Rheumatoid arthritis, which includes ankylosing spondylitis, is characterized by a diffuse proliferative synovitis, suppurative arthritis by a prominent neutrophilic inflammation, and osteoarthritis by cartilaginous and subchondral bone changes. Additionally, the various types of arthritis are associated with different causes, symptoms, and extent and distribution of joint involvement. (Robbins et al, pp 1356–1361)

530. The answer is D. The photomicrograph shows a typical, chronic peptic ulcer with the loss of epithelial continuity, the ulcer bed with necrotic tissue, and fibrosis between the ulcer bed and the main muscle. These peptic ulcers are associated with increased acid and pepsin secretion, may well be complicated by hemorrhage, since the ulcer erodes major blood vessels in the submucosa and muscularis mucosa, and if the ulcer continues unabated, will perforate through into the peritoneal cavity. Although malignant change may occur at the edge of certain types of gastric peptic ulcers, the illustration shows the ulcer itself, and this is not a neoplastic process at this stage of the disease. Long-standing peptic ulcers that do not heal often produce such malignant transformations, which can be determined by biopsy. (Kissane, pp 40–41; Rubin and Farber, pp 648–655)

531. The answer is C. A choristoma is a collection of normal cells or tissues that occurs in an abnormal location. It usually consists of a mass of heterotopic tissue—for example, a focus of pancreatic tissue in the gastric wall or adrenal tissue in the lung. Occasionally, individual, normal-looking cells of one type are seen in an improper location. It is important to be aware of the existence of such tissues or cells so as not to confuse them with neoplasms or metastases. Only rarely do true neoplasms arise in such heterotopic rests. A hamartoma is a localized overgrowth of mature, normal cells or tissues in the appropriate organ (i.e., the organ that is normally composed of the given cell or tissue type). Adenomas and polyps are, for the most part, benign epithelial neoplasms. A chloroma is a mass of neoplastic myeloid cells most commonly seen in the bone in patients with myelogenous leukemia. (Robbins et al, pp 216,497)

532. The answer is E. The neuroblastoma, retinoblastoma, and medulloblastoma, as the suffix blastoma would imply, are primitive tumors ranging from and including the adrenal gland in origin, the retina, and the midline of the brain and characteristically are seen in early childhood. Astrocytomas may occur in all age groups, including childhood, whereas the meningioma is characteristically a neoplasm arising from the dura or its

invaginations and is typically seen in a much older population. (Kissane, pp 1915–1924)

533. The answer is A. Neuroblastoma is a common tumor of childhood, arising primarily in children younger than 5 yr of age and very rarely in adults. Tumors arising in patients younger than 1 yr old are often benign and regress spontaneously, whereas tumors discovered in older children may be highly malignant. These tumors are from neural crest derivatives and may arise in the adrenal medulla, near the retroperitoneum, in the posterior mediastinum, or along other derivatives of neural crest tissue, such as the sympathetic chains. Grossly, these tumors are large and bulky, and histologically, they are composed of small round cells, often in rosette patterns. Because of the neural crest origin of these tumors, they secrete catecholamines, principally norepinephrine. These secretory products cause the clinical symptoms of diarrhea and flushing. Neuroblastomas may grow rapidly and metastisize widely. (Robbins et al, pp. 498–500,1247–1248)

534. The answer is B. Benign tumors are designated by adding the suffix oma to their primary cell type. However, some malignant neoplasms have retained the oma suffix that was used in previous nomenclature schemes. Examples include hepatoma and melanoma, which are accepted names for hepatocellular carcinoma and melanocarcinoma, respectively. An adenoma is a benign epithelial neoplasm composed of glandular tissue. Cystadenomas form benign cystic masses, whereas papillomas form benign fingerlike projections. Sarcomas are malignant tumors arising from mesenchymal tissue Carcinomas are malignant neoplasms arising from epithelial cells—either endodermal, ectodermal, or mesodermal. A prefix such as adeno or squamous may further describe the microscopic growth patterns. Melanomas are malignant tumors derived from melanocytes. Leukemias are malignancies derived from hematopoietic cells, and lymphomas are malignant tumors with a lymphoid tissue origin. Teratomas are benign compound tumors derived from more than one germ layer, and teratocarcinoma is the malignant counterpart. (Robbins et al, pp 214–218)

535. The answer is B. The genotype (genetic makeup of an organism) is determined by the molecular structure of the DNA contained in its chromosomes. Pinocytosis refers to invaginations of the cell membrane useful in fluid movement. The lysosomal content, number of microvilli, and rate of metabolism of a cell are in part determined by the cell's genotype but do not themselves direct or define the genotype. Rather, they are outward expressions (phenotype) of the DNA structure. (Kissane, p 97)

536. **The answer is B.** Leukocytes are important in the first line of defense in acute inflammatory reactions. These WBCs normally are in the blood stream, with a small proportion marginating along the vessel walls. In response to inflammatory stimuli, they line up or marginate along the vessel wall, falling out of the normal flow. RBCs can also stagnate and sludge. These leukocytes become sticky and adhere to the endothelial cells. Normally the WBCs and endothelial cells repel each other, but by intrinsic changes, the WBCs adhere to the endothelial cells in the inflammatory response. Mechanisms for this cell stickiness include changes in the negative charges of the WBC surface coat, pseudopod formation, and the development of divalent cation bridges. The WBCs then emigrate from the blood vessels into the surrounding tissues. They use their pseudopods to crawl into the junctions between the endothelial cells and cause widening of the interendothelial junctions. They cross the basement membranes and escape into the perivascular tissue. This process is one of active mobility and requires considerable flexibility in the leukocytes. Unlike the changes that occur in vascular permeability, there is no contraction of endothelial cells to widen the gap between cells. Also, the emigration of leukocytes is so tight that there is no accompanying vascular leakage. Chemotaxis is the undirectional movement of WBCs toward the inflammatory stimulus. It is important in attracting leukocytes to the site of injury. The two main chemotactic factors for neutrophils are bacterial products (e.g., proteases) and complement factors. The complement compounds include C3, C5, and C$\overline{567}$, which can be generated both by immunologic reactions and by direct cleavages by bacterial and tissue enzymes. *(Robbins et al, pp 41–61)*

537. **The answer is C.** Although most bacteria invoke a polymorphonuclear leukocyte response and produce a characteristic form of inflammation, the organism causing typhoid fever produces a negative chemotaxis toward polymorphs. The cells of first response and those seen most characteristically in either the primary lesions in the Peyer's patches of the intestine or the regional lymph nodes are sheets of monocytes. Eosinophils tend to be attracted toward protozoal and fungal proteins and are not seen particularly in this type of infection. Multinucleated giant cells are characteristically seen in granulomatous disease, and typhoid fever is more in keeping with an acute bacterial infection. Plasma cells have an intermediate function and may be seen in small numbers. *(Kissane, pp 304–305)*

538. **The answer is C.** A fibrinous exudate is associated with many types of severe inflammation. The fluid that pours into the spaces has a large amount of plasma proteins, fibrinogen, and fibrin precipitates. The inflammatory responses are usually acute and severe, allowing these large protein molecules to escape. It accompanies rheumatic heart diseases, causing bread-and-butter pericarditis, and occurs in pneumococcal pneumonia. Histologically, fibrin strands and eosinophilic proteinaceous material are seen. These fibrinous exudates may stimulate fibroblastic and blood vessel proliferation, with organization of the proteinaceous precipitates and formation of fibrous connective tissue. The exudates also may resolve spontaneously. Serous exudates are fluids with a low protein concentration, arising from either the blood or the mesothelial cell secretions. They are seen early in acute inflammation or with mild injuries. Hemorrhagic exudates are a result of ruptured blood vessels. Suppurative exudates are seen in severe bacterial inflammation with massive neutrophil response and are characteristic of pus or abscess formation. *(Robbins et al, pp 41,277)*

539. **The answer is B.** Renal cell carcinoma is a characteristic tumor arising from renal parenchymal and probably renal tubular cells in adult life. In fact, the majority of cases occur after the age of 50, and it is seen more frequently in males. It invades the renal capsule and perinephric fat and has a marked propensity to invade the renal vein, with extension of the tumor into the vena cava. Although metastases may occur all over the body, bone and lung metastases are seen with a higher frequency. This tumor does not occur in infants or early childhood. The tumor that occurs in early infancy or childhood is the nephroblastoma, or Wilms' tumor, which is an embryonal malignant tumor of the kidney and distinctly different from renal cell carcinoma. *(Robbins et al, pp 1054–1057)*

540. **The answer is E.** About 1 in 11 women in the United States will have breast cancer in her lifetime. Many western nations (USA, Canada, Australia, western Europe, and New Zealand) have similar, high rates of carcinoma of the breast. Most Asian nations, including Japan, have a much lower incidence of mammary cancer. In one or two generations, Japanese women who emigrate to the United States develop the high rate of breast cancer of native-born American women. Factors other than geography that are associated with an increased rate of breast cancer include menarche at an early age, late age of menopause, a diet high in fat and calories, a family history of breast cancer, and atypical hyperplastic lesions of the breast. *(Kissane, pp 1554–1555)*

541. **The answer is D.** Hirschsprung's disease (idiopathic megacolon) usually appears soon after birth, with abdominal distention, failure to pass stool, and occasionally, acute intestinal obstruction. The pathogenesis involves abnormal functioning and coordination of the propulsive forces in the distal segment of the large bowel. This motility disorder occurs because of an absence of parasympathetic ganglion cells in the submucosal and myenteric plexus, the diagnostic histologic feature of Hirschsprung's disease. Hypertrophied, disorganized nonmyelinated nerve fibers are often identified in place of ganglion cells. The length of large bowel involved varies. Proximal to the involved segment, however, the colon may be dilated and hypertrophied. The mucosa often appears normal or inflamed. A full-thickness rectal biopsy is the standard procedure employed in diagnosis. Mucosal polyps are not associated with Hirschsprung's disease. (Robbins et al, pp 855–856)

542. **The answer is B.** Neonatal cholestasis in most cases results from bile duct obstruction, the most common cause (more than 90 percent of cases) of which is EBA. Clinically, EBA may mimic neonatal hepatitis, which is an abnormality of unknown cause and requires a diagnosis by exclusion. α_1-Antitrypsin deficiency, metabolic disorders, and infectious processes must be ruled out before a diagnosis of neonatal hepatitis can be made. Histologically, neonatal hepatitis and EBA may appear similar—in particular, both generally contain giant cells. EBA, however, usually can be identified by evidence of large biliary duct obstruction when examined microscopically. The cause of EBA is still undetermined. Originally, it was thought to represent a congenital anomaly. Some investigators consider it to be an acquired disorder secondary to neonatal hepatitis with cholangitis and sclerosis of large bile ducts, either in utero or in early neonatal life. Overall, few cases can be corrected with standard therapy. The natural history is progression to secondary biliary cirrhosis and death in early childhood. Liver transplantation is a viable alternative therapeutic approach in these patients. Neonatal cholestasis may also, but rarely be caused by intrahepatic biliary atresia, which is characterized by choledochal cysts and the absence of bile duct elements in the liver. Primary biliary cirrhosis is seen in middle-aged persons, typically females. The Budd-Chiari syndrome describes obstruction of the hepatic veins by a number of varied processes. (Kissane, pp 1162–1163)

543. **The answer is B.** Adult respiratory distress syndrome, or shock lung, is a disease characterized by diffuse alveolar wall damage. There is loss of surfactant, with subsequent atelectasis. Both endothelial and epithelial cells are damaged. Type I pneumonocytes are extremely vulnerable to injury and are lost early. Grossly, the lungs are filled with fluid and blood and are heavy, red, and meaty. There is congestion, exudation of pink proteinaceous fluid, and hyaline membrane formation along the alveolar walls. Repair and organization result in proliferation and hyperplasia of type II

pneumonocytes and fibroblast proliferation. The alveolar walls become thickened and fibrotic. This syndrome is described in multiple clinical settings, usually when hypotension, sepsis, and oxygen therapy are present. There is severe respiratory failure accompanied by hypoxia unresponsive to oxygen treatment. Physiologically, shock lung is thought to occur secondary to increased permeability of the alveolar capillary walls, with leakage of fluid and subsequent pulmonary edema and atelectasis. (Robbins et al, pp 714–717)

544. **The answer is B.** Red hepatization is the second stage in the course of bacterial lobar pneumonia. It is histologically described as filling and dilatation of the alveolar spaces with neutrophils, WBCs, fibrin strands, RBCs, and bacteria. There is preservation of the pulmonary architecture, but it is obscured by the massive cellular exudate. This stage of bacterial pneumonia is accompanied by a fibrinous pleuritis. It characteristically develops in untreated, debilitated patients and is caused by a strain of pneumococcus in 90 percent of all cases. (Robbins et al, pp 733–736)

545. **The answer is E.** Chronic granulomatous disease is most often X-linked and associated with a decreased ability of neutrophils and other phagocytic cells to kill ingested bacteria. As a result, by 2 yr of age, signs of chronic low-grade infections appear, such as lymphadenitis, splenomegaly, pneumonia and sinusitis. The NBT test shows a markedly decreased, not increased, chemical reduction and helps confirm the diagnosis, since lack of NBT reductive capacity correlates with poor bactericidal activity. (Kissane, p 157)

546. **The answer is B.** The effect of syphilis on the heart and great vessels is characteristically the result of an endarteritis obliterans of the vasa vasorum of the aortic arch, which produces ischemic change in the media resulting in stellate fibrous replacement of the elastic tissue. Similar changes may occur in the opening of the coronary arteries, giving rise to narrowing of the coronary ostia and possibly producing angina pectoris. The result of the fibrous replacement of the media results in saccular dilatation or aneurysm but does not produce a dissection, since the fibrous tissue makes the media even less likely to split apart. The characteristic appearance of dissection occurs when there is a breakdown of ground substance in the media, which is not a characteristic of syphilis. (Kissane, pp 707–711)

547. **The answer is B.** All connective tissue, valves, and muscle of the heart are affected to some degree in rheumatic carditis; hence the term "pancarditis." Certain areas are more selectively involved in a higher proportion of cases. In the early acute phase

of rheumatic carditis, the pericardium shows fibrinous pericarditis, and the valve rings, particularly the mitral valve, show thickening and swelling of the free margins, with small fibrinous vegetations on the free margins. The characteristic Aschoff nodules and fibrosis may occur throughout the other mentioned aspects of the heart, but the characteristic vegetation seen in the early phase of the disease is usually confined to the free margins of the mitral valve. It has been thought that, in some instances, if there are no further occurrences of rheumatic fever, these may even resolve. Often, however, with or without recurrence, these fine verrucous vegetations are converted into more dense fibrous tissue, leading to narrowing of the mitral valve. *(Robbins et al, pp 572–574)*

548. The answer is D. Edema is increased volume of extracellular extravascular fluid due to interference with the normal flow of fluids between blood, lymphatics, and tissue. The lymphatic circulation takes up a significant portion of fluid from the interstitial tissues, along with extravascular proteins, and returns it to the blood. If the lymphatic circulation is obstructed, the lymphatic drainage is interrupted. Affected areas have large accumulation of fluid and are edematous. The vascular system also aids in maintaining fluid volume. The endothelium is the lining of the vessels and serves as a semipermeable membrane for fluids and components, primarily by keeping proteins intraluminally. If the endothelium is damaged, there is increased permeability to proteins, reducing the intraluminal colloidal pressure and causing fluid leakage and edema. Capillary blood pressure (BP), or hydrostatic pressure, is the force in capillaries that drives fluids from the capillaries into the tissues. By increasing the hydrostatic pressure, fluids tend to be forced out of the capillaries into tissues, causing edema. Sodium and water also aid in maintaining fluid balance. Sodium retention causes water retention, leading to an expansion of the extracellular fluid volume both intravascularly and in the tissues with edema. Increased tissue colloid osmotic pressure can be an important factor in causing edema. The protein concentration of plasma also functions in the maintenance of fluid balance. The major protein involved is albumin. By decreasing the plasma protein concentrations, there is a decreased colloid osmotic pressure in the blood, so there is a decreased counterforce to the hydrostatic BP. Thus, there is increased fluid escaping from the capillaries and decreased resorption of fluid from tissues. Fluid tends to accumulate extravascularly, with generalized edema. *(Robbins et al, pp 85–88)*

549. The answer is B. Radiation energy is a well-documented carcinogen. The sources of the radiation include sunlight and occupational and therapeutic ex-

posure. Therapeutic radiation was previously used to treat many benign conditions as well as thyroid disease, and a 10- to 20-yr follow-up of patients who received this therapy shows an increased incidence of several types of cancer. People exposed to occupational irradiation also have a marked increase in carcinoma. Classic among these are employees who painted the faces of watches with radioactive paints and miners of radioactive ores. Survivors of atomic bombs show a markedly increased rate in the development of cancers and leukemias. The major biochemical theory of radiation-induced carcinogenesis is linked to damage of the cell's DNA. Radiation injures the DNA, inducing a mutation. The amount of cell damage is related to the dose, rate, quality, and length of total exposure to the radiation energy. Cells also have reparative capabilities for radiation damage, and they may repair or ignore the injured DNA. The exact mechanism of radiation-induced carcinogenesis is still unclear, but the existence of this phenomenon is well documented. *(Robbins et al, pp 241–243)*

550. The answer is E. High doses of radiation delivered in utero to the embryo during its susceptible period may be a potent teratogen. Recognized abnormalities associated with high-dose radiation include microcephaly, mental retardation, and skeletal malformation. It is also believed to cause genetic mutations in fetal germ cells. Diagnostic doses of radiation, although not conclusively responsible for malformations, must be cautioned against, since the developing CNS is particularly sensitive to radiation injury. Masculinization of the female fetus is generally associated with maternal use of androgenic agents (e.g., progestogens) during pregnancy, not with radiation. *(Kissane, pp 258–260)*

551. The answer is D. For any given area of skin, there is no significant difference in the number of melanocytes in blacks as compared with whites. Blacks do, however, have larger melanocytes that are reactive (as determined by dopa reactivity) and have more dendritic processes. In whites who are not exposed to UV light, melanocytic dopa activity is quite variable. After a single exposure to UV light, the melanocytes present demonstrate an increase in size and dopa activity. With repeated exposure to UV light, there is also an increase in the concentration of melanocytes. Studies of mice have shown sufficient mitotic activity in skin melanocytes repeatedly exposed to UV light to account for the increase in concentration. *(Lever and Schaumburg-Lever, p 16)*

552. The answer is A. Duchenne muscular dystrophy, also known as X-linked muscular dystrophy, is the most common of the muscular dystrophies. It usually occurs in early life, with symmetrical weakness and involvement of the pelvic girdle mus-

stasis. Hypercoagulable states include disseminated intravascular coagulation (DIC) and carcinomatosis. Treatment with warfarin, an anticoagulant, would inhibit clotting, making intravascular thrombogenesis unlikely. (*Robbins et al, pp 96–103*)

564. The answer is D. The Tzanck test is a cytologic smear obtained by scraping the base of an early, freshly opened skin vesicle. The scrapings are smeared onto a glass slide and stained by either the Wright or Giemsa method. This technique allows a rapid, although preliminary, diagnosis of a vesicular skin rash that appears to be of the herpesvirus group. Definitive diagnosis should still rely on culture or direct immunofluorescence (IF) of a lesion and skin biopsy. The Tzanck test is nonspecific within the group of skin lesions that are caused by herpesviruses. Varicella (chickenpox), herpes zoster, and herpes simplex skin lesions all demonstrate the same cytologic changes in the Tzanck smear. The smear is examined for the presence of multinucleated acantholytic balloon cells from the floor of the vesicle. It should be noted that the biopsy specimens of all skin lesions of the herpesviruses show the same histology and cannot be differentiated from one another by biopsy alone. The history, physical examination, and culture would all aid in subtyping a particular herpesvirus skin lesion. The Tzanck test is of no value in the diagnosis of the skin lesions listed as alternative choices in the question. (*Lever and Schaumburg-Lever, p 364*)

565–566. The answers are 565-B, 566-C. Light and electron microscopy (EM) and IF are complementary studies in the evaluation of renal biopsy specimens. The EM that accompanies the question demonstrates MGN. The changes to be noted include a thickened basement membrane (BM), subepithelial dense deposits (DD), and spike (SP) formation. The spike formation results from the remodeling of the basement membrane in response to the presence of the dense deposits. This remodeling may result in the eventual incorporation of the deposits into the substance of the basement membrane. The resultant projections of the basement membrane around the deposits give rise to the spiked appearance. Fusion of the epithelial foot processes is also noted. In general, all forms of glomerular disease listed in question 565, except AGN, may show fusion of the epithelial foot processes on EM. It is then necessary to evaluate the presence and distribution of electron-dense deposits to further classify the disease process. Of the entities listed in the question, MGN, MPGN, and AGN demonstrate dense deposits on EM. In MPGN, the deposits tend to be subendothelial in location. AGN renal biopsy specimens show subepithelial deposits described as "humps" but lack the fusion of the epithelial foot processes It should be noted that MGN is subclassified into

six stages depending on the extent of glomerular basement membrane reaction. In early (I) and late (VI) stages, the diagnosis may be difficult. MGN shows a male predominance of 2:1 or 3:1 and is most common between the ages of 50 and 70 yr. At the time of diagnosis, 70 to 80 percent of patients have nephrotic syndrome. MGN accounts for 20 to 30 percent of cases of nephrotic syndrome in the adult population and is usually idiopathic.

IF is evaluated on the basis of the pattern (diffuse, granular, or linear) and type (IgG, IgA, IgM, complement, and antiglomerular basement membrane) of staining, if any. Idiopathic MGN is the most common cause of MGN and is the most appropriate diagnosis for an MGN that demonstrates IgG and complement IF staining. MGN characteristically shows diffuse and granular IF for IgG along the capillary walls corresponding to the subepithelial deposits. Diabetic nephropathy may also demonstrate IgG on IF but usually in a diffuse, linear pattern without the accompanying dense deposits on EM. Goodpasture's syndrome typically shows linear IF staining but with antiglomerular basement membrane antibody, a specific IgG. IgA nephropathy is a focal glomerulonephritis with positive IF for IgA. AGN, despite its positive IF for IgG and complement, usually can be distinguished from MGN when the EM and clinical history are incorporated into the evaluation process. (*Kissane, pp 734–747*)

567. The answer is E. The most common pituitary neoplasm is the pituitary adenoma, which arises from the endocrine-producing cells of the anterior pituitary. These tumors occur in the area of the sella turcica. They are solid or cystic and characteristically are composed of sheets or papillary clusters of uniform, round, benign-appearing cells. Based on H & E staining, the tumors have been classified as chromophobes (no staining), acidophils, or basophils. By immunohistochemical staining, electron microscopy (EM), and biochemical studies, they can be classified according to the types of hormones they secrete. Each tumor usually is composed of one type of hormone-secreting cell. Seven percent of pituitary adenomas secrete ACTH and cause Cushing's syndrome. These tumors arise in the anterior lobe and are usually chromophobes. By immunohistochemical staining, these tumors have ACTH granules, as demonstrated in the photomicrograph that accompanies the question. EM shows large, dense, secretory granules and microfilaments in the cells. Other pituitary adenomas may secrete thyroid-stimulating hormone (TSH), prolactin, or growth hormone. Pituitary granulomas are rare diseases usually secondary to tuberculosis, sarcoidosis, or histiocytosis X. Parapituitary gliomas are parapituitary astrocytomas with no endocrine activity. Craniopharyngiomas are pediatric tumors of the suprasellar region, are derived from Rathke's pouch remnants, and have no endocrine activity. Adrenocortical carcinomas are primary tumors of the adrenal gland that may be functioning, secreting cortisol, and causing Cushing's syndrome. These tumors are very rare, and it is extremely unusual for them to metastasize to the pituitary. *(Kissane, pp 1385–1391)*

568. The answer is D. Auer rods are round, rod-shaped, or elongate cytoplasmic inclusions in the cytoplasm of immature, abnormal granulocytes or myeloblasts. They represent aberrant forms of the cytoplasmic azurophilic granules produced by abnormal cytoplasmic maturation in the leukemic blast cells. Although they may be seen in occasionally CML in blast crisis, they are most characteristic of AML. Erythroleukemia (DiGuglielmo's syndrome) is also considered one of the acute myeloid leukemias in the French-American-British classification (M-6) but is predominantly a disorder of erythroid precursors. At some stage of the disease, myeloid precursors may also be abnormal. In these instances, Auer rods may be seen when myeloblasts are present. ALL and CLL are leukemias of the lymphocyte cells and do not demonstrate Auer rod formation. *(Kissane, pp 1331–1332; Robbins et al, pp 674–685)*

569. The answer is E. T cell lymphocytes can be enumerated by their ability to form rosettes with sheep erythrocytes. They are the crucial element of cellular immunity. Mycosis fungoides is a T cell lymphoproliferative disorder with prominent skin lesions. Characteristic findings in the skin lesions include Pautrier's microabscesses and hyperchromic, atypical lymphocytes with marked convolutions called mycosis cells. Multiple myeloma and macroglobulinemia are lymphoproliferative disorders of B cells. AML and CML are neoplasms of nonlymphoid myeloid cells. *(Robbins et al, pp 158–159,1271–1272)*

570. The answer is D. CLL is common in the elderly population and uncommon in younger individuals. Affected patients may initially experience hepatosplenomegaly, lymphadenopathy, pancytopenia, malaise, and weight loss. Fever does not occur and is uncharacteristic of CLL unless there is a superimposed infectious process. About one fourth of patients are asymptomatic at the time of diagnosis, with the diagnosis having been made on the basis of an abnormal peripheral CBC. The diagnosis often can be made from the peripheral blood smear alone without the need for a bone marrow biopsy or aspirate. This tends to be true particularly when >15,000 mature lymphocytes are seen in the peripheral blood smear. The malignant lymphocytes are usually B cells that demonstrate small amounts of monoclonal surface immunoglobulin, usually IgM. Hypogammaglobulinemia affects at least 50 percent of patients and, in combination with neutropenia, may eventually render these patients susceptible to infection. Survival in CLL is long, with a median range of between 6 and 9 yr. Treatment is noncurative and is reserved for those patients who are symptomatic. Death is usually the result of infection, hemorrhage, or inanition. *(Robbins et al, pp 674–685; Kissane, pp 1336–1337)*

571. The answer is C. The anemias are classified morphologically on the basis of RBC appearance, mean corpuscular volume (MCV), and mean corpuscular hemoglobin concentration (MCHC). Classically, iron deficiency anemia is characterized by a hypochromic microcytic anemia with MCV <80 g/100 ml and MCHC <31 g/100 ml. Vitamin B_{12} and folic acid deficiencies both produce macrocytic (MCV >94 g/100 ml and MCH >31 g/100ml) megaloblastic anemia. Accelerated erythropoiesis also produces a macrocytic anemia, but of the non-megaloblastic type. Megaloblastic changes refer to abnormalities in the maturation of the cell, usually nuclear. Recent blood loss, when sufficient to produce anemia, is generally of the normochromic-normocytic (MCV 82 to 92 mg/100ml and MCHC >30 mg/100ml) type. *(Robbins et al, pp 422–423)*

572. The answer is D. LDH is the enzyme that catalyzes the conversion of pyruvate to lactate using nicotinamide adenine dinucleotide (NAD) as the cofactor. This enzyme is found in all tissues of the body and is a tetramer composed of two different peptic chains, identified as M and H. There are five different isoenzyme combinations of the M and H subunits. Various body tissues contain characteristic amounts of these isoenzymes, which can be separated and identified on the basis of different physical and chemical properties. Tissue damage and necrosis cause release of this intracellular enzyme into the circulating plasma. The amount and type of isoenzyme released reflect the organ or tissue injured. Normal circulating plasma contains primarily LDH_2, with small amounts of LDH_3, LDH_4, and LDH_5. The heart is primarily composed of LDH_1, the HHHH tetramer. With a myocardial infarct, there is a massive release of LDH_1, elevating its quantity in relation to LDH_2. An increase in total LDH with a relative increase in LDH_1 in relation to LDH_2 is consistent with a myocardial infarct—myocardial tissue injury. This pattern of elevated LDH_1 over LDH_2 is illustrated in the graph that accompanies the question. Liver and skeletal muscle are composed primarily of LDH_5, the MMMM tetramer, so their injury produces elevated serum LDH_5 levels. Pulmonary embolism is reflected in an increase in serum LDH_3 levels. Brain and cerebrospinal fluid contain relatively small amounts of LDH isoenzymes, so infection here is not correlated with increases in serum LDH levels. *(Tietz, pp 692–694)*

573–575.   The answers are 573-B, 574-A, 575-E. There are many compounds important chemically in mediating the acute inflammatory response. Histamine is an example of the vasoactive amines, which are principally important in the acute phase of increased vascular permeability. It causes vasodilatation and increased venular permeability. It is released from mast cells and platelets. The kinin system produces vasoactive peptides, of which bradykinin is the most potent. It causes vasodilatation, increased vascular permeability, smooth muscle contraction, and pain, but it is not chemotactic. It is derived from the clotting cascade from factor XII, the Hageman factor, through a kallikrein intermediate step. The complement system produces many compounds that help mediate the inflammatory response. These include C3 and C5a, which cause increased vascular permeability, and C5a and C$\overline{567}$, which are chemotactic factors. Prostaglandins are arachidonic acid derivatives that are important in the inflammatory response. Prostaglandin E potentiates the permeability effect of the other chemical mediators and is also important in the production of pain, fever, and vasodilatation. The neutrophils themselves also release into the media lysosomal enzymes that are important chemical mediators. These compounds are released during phagocytosis, reverse endocytosis, or with neutrophil death. They consist of neutral proteases, which degrade such extracellular material as collagen, fibrin, and cartilage, acid proteases, which digest proteins, and cationic proteins. *(Robbins et al, pp 52–58)*

576–578.   The answers are 576-A, 577-E, 578-B. Humans have 46 chromosomes. The normal male karyotype is 46,XY. The normal female karyotype is 46,XX. Klinefelter's syndrome is a cytogenetic disorder with an abnormal 47,XXY karyotype. Persons with Klinefelter's syndrome usually have testicular atrophy, azospermia, gynecomastia, mental retardation, female distribution of hair, and eunuchoid body habitus. Turner's syndrome, also called gonadal dysgenesis, is a cytogenetic disorder with an abnormal 45,XO karyotype. Turner's syndrome patients have primary amenorrhea, webbed necks, short stature, and infertility and are subject to increased risk of congenital cardiac abnormalities. Down's syndrome and Edwards' syndrome are cytogenetic disorders with trisomy of chromosomes 21 and 18, respectively. *(Robbins et al, pp 119–133)*

579–581.   The answers are 579-E, 580-B, 581-D. Tularemia, pertussis, and plague are examples of bacterial diseases. Tularemia is caused by *Francisella tularensis,* a small gram-negative pleomorphic coccobacilus. Affected animals and arthropods serve as the vectors, of which wild rabbits and squirrels are the most common in the USA. Pertussis is caused by *Bordetella pertussis,* a gram-negative coccobacillus, and is transmitted via airborne droplets to the respiratory tract. Plague is transmitted through a number of animal vectors, the major reservoir being squirrels. The causative agent is *Y. pestis,* an encapsulated, gram-negative, pleomorphic bacillus. Rocky Mountain spotted fever is among the rickettsial diseases, caused by obligate intracellular microorganisms smaller than bacteria and larger than viruses. The vector is an infected tick. Lymphogranuloma venereum is a disease attributed to *Chlamydia* microorganisms, specifically *C. trachomatis.* Chlamydiae are also obligate intracellular microorganisms intermediate between bacteria and viruses but are transmitted through sexual contact (a venereal disease). *(Robbins et al, pp 294–295,328–330)*

582–584.   The answers are 582-E, 583-D, 584-A. *Salmonella* species, *Shigella* species, and *V. cholerae* are all gram-negative rods that produce gastrointestinal disease. These organisms, however, may affect different sites and have various histologic manifestations. *Salmonella* species may produce typhoid fever, gastroenteritis, and septicemia. Typically, *Salmonella* species produce a marked reticuloendothelial hyperplasia in local, intestinal, and distant lymph nodes and in the spleen and liver. Erythrophagocytosis is highly suggestive of *Salmonella* infection, particularly of typhoid fever. *Salmonella* species may produce intestinal ulceration, generally in the small intestine. In contrast, *Shigella* species rarely produce bacteremia and elicit little, if any, reaction outside the intestinal tract. All *Shigella* species produce an endotoxin. Additionally, *Shigella dysenteriae* produces a potent exotoxin. The *Shigella* microorganisms tend to damage the colonic mucosa, producing mucosal ulcerations. Rarely, similar ulcerations may be seen in the ileum. *V. cholerae* produces both an endotoxin and an exotoxin. Voluminous amounts of watery diarrhea containing bits of mucus, ricewater stool, are the result of the effects of the exotoxin. The organism is essentially noninvasive, does not produce bacteremia, and therefore elicits few anatomic changes and no mucosal ulceration in the bowel mucosa. The intestinal biopsy specimen in such a case would reveal an intact mucosa and only mild, nonspecific submucosal inflammatory changes. *(Robbins et al, pp 318–323)*

585–587.   The answers are 585-C, 586-D, 587-B. Graves' disease and Hashimoto's disease are two diseases of the thyroid that have autoimmune causes. Both diseases are characteristically found in females, with Hashimoto's thyroiditis predominating in women older than 40 yr and Graves' disease occurring in young, emotional women. Hashimoto's thyroiditis is thought to be secondary to circulating antithyroglobulin antibody as well as other organ-specific antibodies. The clinical picture is one of atrophy and depletion of the thyroid gland, which is diffusely involved and shows significant infiltration by lymphoid tissue with germinal centers and small atrophic follicles. Degenerating follicles are classically composed of large pink cells, called Hürthle or Askanazy cells. Fibrosis of the thyroid also may be seen. Affected patients are either euthyroid or hypothyroid. Long-acting thyroid stimulator is an immunoglobulin that is found in most patients with Graves' disease. It acts as a thyroid stimulator, causing hyperthyroidism. The thyroid gland is vascularized and shows uniform follicular and epithelial hyperplasia. A lymphoid infiltrate may also be present in patients with Graves' disease. *(Kissane, pp 1401–1402,1405–1407; Robbins et al, pp 180,1206–1208,1210–1212)*

588–590.   The answers are 588-A, 589-B, 590-D. Cervical cancer is typically a disease of females between the ages of 40 and 50 yr, but an increasing frequency in young women has recently been noted. It is currently the sixth most frequent cause of death in women. It has an increased incidence in women who are prostitutes, are multiparous, have multiple sexual partners, began sexual relationships at an early age, and are of low socioeconomic status. Nuns and Jewish and Muslim women are seldom affected. Cervicitis and dysplastic changes in the cervical epithelium are findings related to the development of squamous cell carcinoma of the mucosal surface. Early detection of cervical cancer is possible by cytologic cancer screening (Pap smear), which has dramatically decreased morbidity and mortality. Carcinoma of the endometrium is a disease of older women and is associated with obesity, diabetes, hypertension, and infertility. Its incidence has been rising in the past 10 yr and now accounts for 10 percent of all cancers in women. Prolonged estrogenic stimulation and hyperplasias with atypia have been related to the later development of endometrial cancer. Histologically, endometrial cancer is an adenocarcinoma. Neither cervical cancer nor endometrial cancer has been associated with oral contraceptives or exposure to DES. *(Robbins et al, pp 1123–1128,1137–1139)*

591–592.   The answers are 591-C, 592-A. Hydatidiform mole and choriocarcinoma represent the benign and malignant forms, respectively, of the spectrum of disease known as gestational trophoblastic neoplasia. Common to both forms of the neoplastic process, which develops after pregnancy, is the proliferation of trophoblasts. In addition to trophoblastic elements, the hydatidiform mole contains edematous placental villi with decreased vasculature—the hydropic villi. Trophoblasts, in all forms of this disease entity, produce human chorionic gonadotropin (hCG), a hormone that can be readily assayed in the laboratory. hCG is, there-

fore, a valuable aid in the diagnosis of new cases and for the subsequent monitoring of patients after therapy for gestational trophoblastic neoplasia. *(Robbins et al, pp 1158–1162)*

593–595.   The answers are 593-A, 594-C, 595-C. Of all persons who suffer from congenital heart disease, 25 to 30 percent are afflicted with a ventricular septal defect, the most common form of these abnormalities. The defect in the ventricular septum is usually subaortic, secondary to incomplete closure of the membranous and muscular septum. It is accompanied by right ventricular hypertrophy, an enlarged pulmonary orifice, endocardial thickening of the right ventricle, left ventricular and atrial hypertrophy, and an enlarged mitral valve region. There is increased blood flow through the mitral, tricuspid, and pulmonary valve areas. These changes are all related to the left-to-right shunt of blood from the higher pressure of the left ventricle into the lower pressure of the right ventricle, with secondary increased blood flow to the pulmonary system and increased blood volume circulating through the left atrium and ventricle.

In the fetal heart, the ductus arteriosus (a derivative of the left sixth aortic arch) connects the pulmonary artery to the aorta, allowing oxygenated blood to bypass the lungs. In many cases, the duct may remain patent after birth, either as an isolated condition or accompanied by other congenital heart problems. A duct that is still patent after 3 mo of age is considered pathologic. Closure of the duct is thought to occur secondary to either muscle contractions of the wall, with narrowing and occlusion of the duct, or endothelial and fibroblastic proliferation from increased blood flow. The patent ductus arteriosus allows passage of blood from the aorta back into the pulmonary arteries and lungs, in a left-to-right shunt of blood. There is left atrial and ventricular hypertrophy secondary to increased blood flow and enlargement of the mitral and pulmonary valve regions. The pulmonary arteries and trunk are dilated and thickened due to the increased flow, and the endothelial surfaces may even show changes suggestive of atherosclerosis. The size and diameter of the patent ductus vary greatly. Females are affected considerably more often than are males.

Tetralogy of Fallot is the most common congenital heart disease associated with cyanosis and clubbing. This is a disease complex characterized by ventricular septal defect, overriding right-sided aorta, pulmonary stenosis, and right ventricular hypertrophy. There is a combination of obstruction to blood flow and shunting of blood. Affected persons may or may not be cyanotic, depending on the size of the defect and the amount of obstruction. The cyanotic form is accompanied by significant stenosis of the infundibulum (pulmonary valve region), with hypertrophy of the right atrium and right ventricle secondary to the obstruction to flow. Blood flow is decreased to the left atrium and ventricle, so they remain normal in size or even atrophic. With obstruction to blood flow from the right ventricle to the pulmonary artery, the blood is shunted through the ventricular septal defect into the left ventricle, with a right-to-left shunt. In the acyanotic form of tetralogy of Fallot, the ventricular septal defect is large, with less significant obstruction at the infundibulum. The ventricular septal defect favors a left-to-right shunt; the greater pressure of the left side causes blood flow into the right side. There is augmented blood flow and pressure on the right ventricle and atrium, accompanied by hypertrophic changes and increased pulmonary blood flow. The left side shows hypertrophic changes due to the greater blood volume through it. Enlarged mitral and aortic valve regions are characteristic. (Kissane, pp 663–683; Robbins et al, pp 585–592)

596–598.   The answers are 596-A, 597-C, 598-D. Both asbestos and beryllium are inorganic dusts found in the environment and may produce pulmonary disease. The pneumoconioses represent a spectrum of pulmonary disorders associated with some form of air pollution. Pulmonary fibrosis characterizes the collagenous pneumoconioses. In contrast, pulmonary fibrosis is less significant in the noncollagenous pneumoconioses except in the very severe forms of the disease. Both asbestos and beryllium produce a diffuse pattern of fibrosis and are examples of collagenous pneumoconioses. Although exposure to beryllium may produce an acute bronchopneumonia-like picture, more commonly there is a diffuse fibrosing pneumonitis due to chronic exposure to beryllium. Similarly, asbestosis demonstrates diffuse interstitial fibrosis containing asbestos or ferruginous bodies within lesions. Additionally, pleural fibrosis with plaque formation is a prominent feature. Asbestos exposure, in contrast to beryllium exposure, is associated with late-appearing carcinomas. Bronchogenic carcinoma and mesothelioma are the most common of these asbestosis-associated malignancies. Exposure to asbestos confers to an individual a twofold increased risk of tumors of the esophagus, stomach, and colon. It is suggested that asbestos exposure potentiates the carcinogenic effects of other hydrocarbons. However, the exact mechanism has not been determined. Exposure to asbestos is seen in persons involved with the mining and subsequent handling of asbestos and asbestos products. Beryllium exposure is associated with the space industry and the manufacture of fluorescent lights. Silica exposure, in contrast, produces nodular pulmonary fibrosis. Of note is the visualization of birefringent silica oxide particles within nodules that are examined under polarized light. This finding becomes significant in differentiating silicosis from other forms of nodular or granulomatous fibrosing pulmonary disease. (Robbins et al, pp 438–442)

599.   The answer is C (2,4). Goodpasture's syndrome is an autoimmune disease associated with renal failure and pulmonary hemorrhage. The renal lesions are characterized by damage to the glomerular basement membrane, resulting in glomerulonephritis. The pulmonary lesions show destruction and necrosis of the alveolar septa, with hemorrhage and hypertrophy of the alveolar lining cells. Immunofluorescence studies have categorized this disease as immunologically mediated by immunoglobulins directed against the glomerular basement membranes and pulmonary septal membranes, leading to the initial destruction. This is a disease of young people (20 to 40 yr of age), and there is a striking male predominance. (Robbins et al, pp 745–746,1010–1011)

600.   The answer is A (1,2,3). ARF is a systemic inflammatory disease caused by a hypersensitivity reaction to group A β-hemolytic streptococcus. It usually occurs after streptococcal pharyngitis. The most commonly affected individuals are children 5 to 15 yr of age, but the incidence and severity of ARF have been declining recently. The heart, joints, tendons, skin, respiratory system, and blood vessels are most often affected. ARF is not known to cause hepatitis. The classic pathologic findings in ARF are Aschoff bodies, which can be found in any involved site but are most common in the heart. They are regions of fibrinoid change surrounded by inflammatory cells, proteinaceous material, large mesenchymal cells called Anitschkow myocytes, and multinucleated giant cells. In the heart, ARF may involve the epicardium, myocardium, or endocardium. There is a fibrinous pericarditis, myocardial inflammation with Aschoff body formation, and a diffuse acute myocarditis and endocarditis. The endocardial reaction usually involves the valves, especially the mitral valve, causing vegetation formation on the leaflets. Healing of the valvular verrucae causes fibrosis and deformation of the valves, with formation of the characteristic fish-mouthed stenotic valves of rheumatic heart disease. Joint involvement by ARF is very common, causing synovial membrane thickening and ulceration with acute inflammation and Aschoff body formation. This disease is benign and transient. The skin lesions are either a rash (erythema multiforme) or subcutaneous nodules that contain Aschoff bodies. Blood vessels may show arteritis. The lungs and pleurae show changes of nonspecific acute pneumonitis and pleuritis. The most severe clinical problem with ARF is the development of carditis. Long-term follow-up is required of patients with carditis, since the healing of the endocardial lesions creates valvular deformation that can cause future cardiac problems. *(Robbins et al, pp 571–576)*

601. The answer is E (all). Concepts of the development of neoplasia describe first an initiation step that establishes an incipient neoplasia. This lesion has a variable neoplastic potential. Time and other stimuli combine to induce the development of various lesions. These lesions range from minor atypias and dysplasias to severe dysplasia, to CIS, to invasive carcinoma. CIS is a distinct entity that is described as severe dysplasia of an entire surface or mucosal lining without spread from its original location. The neoplastic cells are restrained by the basement membrane and do not invade the surrounding tissue. Invasive carcinoma involves very specific changes, not just a gradual progression over time and space. The life cycle of CIS may include regression and disappearance, persistence without any change, simple progression of the lesion without an increase in malignant potential, or invasion and progression. The last category includes changes to a more neoplastic tumor or to invasive carcinoma. *(Robbins et al, pp 1123–1128)*

602. The answer is A (1,2,3). Islet tumors of the pancreas are fairly rare and usually occurs in adults. The tumors may be single or multiple. Both hormonally functioning and nonfunctioning cases occur. Hormone products can include insulin (hypoglycemia), gastrin (gastrointestinal ulcers), glucagon (diabetes), somatostatin (diabetes, steatorrhea), and vasoactive intestinal peptide (watery diarrhea, hypokalemia). Symptoms of ectopic hormone production usually occur early in the course of the disease, not late. *(Robbins et al, pp 986–989)*

603. The answer is A (1,2,3). MEN IIa (Sipple syndrome) is a genetic disorder believed to be inherited in an autosomal dominant pattern with a high degree of penetrance. Expected findings include medullary carcinoma of the thyroid, pheochromocytoma, adrenocortical adenomas, or adrenocortical hyperplasia. Medulloblastoma is a brain tumor of childhood arising usually in the cerebellum and is not a feature of MEN IIa. *(Robbins et al, pp 988,1222–1223,1244–1247,1406–1407)*

604. The answer is B (1,3). Bacterial endocarditis is an infectious disease of the valvular tissues, creating vegetations on the valvular cusps or leaflets. The most commonly affected sites are the mitral and aortic valves, and the tricuspid and pulmonic valves are rarely affected. The two most common organisms responsible for bacterial endocarditis are *Streptococcus viridans* and *Staphylococcus aureus*. These vegetations are often large and friable and are composed of the organisms, necrotic debris, cellular material, and fibrin. They may erode into the underlying valve tissue or into the myocar-

dium, with abscess formation. The two major predisposing features are bacterial sepsis and underlying valvular heart disease. Damaged heart valves, either congenital in origin or a result of rheumatic heart disease, are at an increased risk for developing these thrombotic growths. These valvular vegetations are very friable and may break off and embolize to the systemic circulation, causing infarction and abscess formation. They also can cause myocardial degeneration with abscess formation from direct extension. With extensive disease, there is valvular destruction with incompetence, and congestive heart failure ensues. *(Kissane, pp 611–625)*

605. The answer is A (1,2,3). Disorders with autosomal dominant inheritance are characterized by the following: (1) diseased individuals have a diseased parent, (2) unaffected relatives do not transmit the disease, and (3) offspring of an affected person and a normal mate have a 50–50 chance of disease. Of the listed choices, achondroplasia, Huntington's chorea, and hereditary lymphedema have autosomal dominant inheritance. Achondroplasia, an abnormality of cartilage proliferation, is a form of dwarfism typified by a normal-sized head and body with short arms and legs. Huntington's chorea is a neurologic disorder with an age of onset at 20 to 50 yr, extrapyramidal or choreiform movements, and progressive dementia. Milroy's disease is present at birth and usually effects the lower extremities. Albinism is an autosomal recessive disorder characterized by an inability to synthesize melanin pigment. *(Robbins et al, pp 136–137,141,538,1321,1416)*

606. The answer is E (all). The organs most severely affected in patients with diabetes mellitus are usually the kidneys, with renal failure accounting for a large percentage of associated deaths. The glomeruli, tubules, blood vessels, or the pelves may be damaged. The glomeruli are most commonly affected, showing diffuse nodular and exudative lesions. The diffuse lesions affect 90 percent of all diabetic patients and show PAS-positive thickening of the basement membrane with proliferation of mesangial cells and eventual sclerosis. This is a nonspecific change. The nodular change known as Kimmelstiel-Wilson syndrome is diagnostic of diabetic glomerular disease and afflicts 15 to 30 percent of diabetic patients. This is a proliferative lesion, with the formation of ovoid laminar hyaline masses in the mesangial region of the glomeruli. The exudative lesions consist of fibrin capsular crescentic deposits between the endothelial cells and the basement membrane, or outside the basement membrane under the visceral epithelial cells. The vascular lesions consist of arteriolar and arterial sclerosis. Both acute and chronic pyelonephritis commonly afflict diabetic patients. Many diabetic persons suffer necrotizing papillitis and necrosis of the renal medulla. Glycogen and fatty material may accumulate in the tubular epithelial cells. (Robbins et al, pp 1022–1025)

607. The answer is E (all). AIDS is a disease of markedly impaired cellular immunity believed to be caused by the human immunodeficiency virus (HIV). Diseased individuals are susceptible to opportunistic infections by cytomegalovirus, Epstein-Barr virus, *Pneumocystis, Toxoplasma*, atypical mycobacteria, *Candida, Cryptococcus*, and *Aspergillus*. In addition, malignant lymphoma and Kaposi's sarcoma occur commonly. The infective viron is most easily contracted by parenteral avenues. Hence, intravenous drug users sharing needles and recipients of multiple blood transfusions are at risk. The virus is also capable of being transmitted to infants of known AIDS-positive mothers. The exact mode of venereal transfer in non-intravenous drug-using homosexual males with multiple partners and heterosexual partners is not entirely clear. (Robbins et al, pp 208–210)

608. The answer is B (1,3). Sarcoidosis is a multisystem granulomatous disease, the cause of which has yet to be defined. It demonstrates ethnic, regional, and age differences in its incidence, being 10 to 20 times more common in blacks than whites in the USA, 4 to 5 times more common in some northern Europeans (e.g., Scandinavians), and most common between the ages of 20 and 40 yr. Approximately 90 percent of cases are estimated to be asymptomatic or only mildly symptomatic, precluding a physician's visit. When symptoms prompt medical aid, they may mimic a variety of other diseases, including rheumatoid arthritis and Crohn's disease. Skin lesions, including erythema nodosum, may cause a patient to consult a dermatologist. Despite the presenting symptoms, most patients will have some degree of thoracic disease, which will be detected on x-ray in about 90 percent of cases. About 70 percent demonstrate bilateral hilar adenopathy (BHA), which is suggestive of, but not pathognomonic for, sarcoidosis. BHA may also occur in about 10 to 20 percent of lymphomas and less than 1 percent of pulmonary and metastatic malignancies. In sarcoidosis, approximately 80 percent of cases resolve spontaneously with or without therapy within 1 to 2 yr. Several factors generally are indicative of a favorable prognosis, including absence of x-ray evidence of thoracic disease. Corticosteroids, the therapeutic agents of choice, are generally used to treat symptomatic patients. (Robbins et al, pp 390–392)

609. The answer is C (2,4). Pernicious anemia is a form of megaloblastic anemia with defective absorption of vitamin B_{12} because of lack of intrinsic factor. Autoantibodies to gastric parietal cells, antibodies to intrinsic factor, or antibodies that block binding of vitamin B_{12} to intrinsic factor may all be present. The hematologic picture is macrocytic anemia, pancytopenia, and a bone marrow with megaloblastic maturation. The lack of vitamin B_{12} results in disordered DNA synthesis. The megaloblastic cells have immature nuclei with relatively normal cytoplasmic maturation. Treatment of pernicious anemia is achieved by parenteral vitamin B_{12} injections. (Robbins et al, pp 631–634)

610. The answer is A (1,2,3). *C. neoformans* is an encapsulated, yeastlike fungus that measures approximately 4 to 6 μm in diameter. It has a prominent polysaccharide capsule that characteristically stains with the mucicarmine stain and measures from 1 to 30 μm in diameter. Cryptococcal disease most often affects the CNS, producing meningitis or cystlike cavities full of organisms in the brain substance. Classically, in the brain, and to a lesser extent elsewhere, *Cryptococcus* elicits little if any inflammatory response and does not produce significant tissue damage or necrosis until the infection is severe. CNS disease is usually insidious, producing nonspecific symptoms during a period of weeks to months. Likewise, pulmonary infection may produce mild, vague symptoms. Skin lesions, usually painless, occur in about 10 percent of patients. In about 50 percent of patients with cryptococcosis, no obvious predisposing factors can be identified. However, there is an increased frequency of infection in some immunocompromised hosts, particularly those receiving corticosteroid therapy. Antibody to *Cryptococcus* is formed in response to infection but has no direct effect on the organisms. It exerts its influence in conjunction with the cell-mediated host response and is a useful serologic tool in the diagnosis of disease and the monitoring of therapy. (Robbins et al, pp 355–356)

611. The answer is B (1,3). The Stein-Leventhal syndrome is a disease of women primarily 20 to 40 yr of age who, after a normal menarche, develop progressive oligomenorrhea that leads to secondary amenorrhea. Bleeding or menorrhagia may precede the amenorrhea. Affected women are also sterile, secondary to anovulation, and they may be obese or hirsute. Breast development is usually normal but may be decreased. These patients have persistent anovulation, and examination may reveal enlarged ovaries with multiple cysts bilaterally. No consistent hormonal abnormalities have been found in these patients, but they do have normal follicle-stimulating hormone levels and normal estrogen secretion cycles. Recently, successful pregnancy and normal menstruation have occurred in some patients after bilateral wedge resections of the ovaries, but the exact mechanism is unknown. (Kissane, pp 1500–1502)

612. The answer is B (1,3). Hemolytic disease of newborn infants is an immunohematologic disease that is generally the result of a fetal–maternal incompatibility involving the Rh or ABO blood group system. In Rh incompatibility, the IgG class of antibodies crosses the placenta and gains access to the fetal RBCs, producing hemolysis. The symptoms in Rh incompatibility are more severe than in ABO incompatibility, may be life-threatening, and include anemia, congestive heart failure, hydrops, and death. Severe congenital deformities are not a feature of hemolytic disease of the newborn. In contrast, ABO incompatibility, although more common, tends to produce mild symptoms and is often asymptomatic. Rh incompatibility can now be prevented by the use of Rh hyperimmune globulin. *(Robbins et al, pp 486–490)*

613. The answer is E (all). Phagocytosis is the process of ingestion and digestion of foreign material by WBCs. The first step is cellular recognition of the foreign material. Normally, WBCs do not recognize all microorganisms and particles but only those that are coated with opsonins, which are serum immunologic products composed of IgG and C3. These serum components on foreign particles attach to specific receptors on the neutrophils, allowing for recognition. Next the foreign particle is engulfed by pseudopodia, with the formation of a cytoplasmic membrane around the material. This vacuole fuses with a lysosome, with release of the lysosomal granules. During degranulation, some of the hydrolytic enzymes and metabolites leak out into the external media. Within the phagolysosome, the foreign particles are killed and degraded by enzymatic action. There are oxygen-dependent and oxygen-independent mechanisms for digestion. The oxygen-dependent mechanisms involve the toxic compounds hydrogen peroxide with myeloperoxidase and superoxide radicals. The oxygen-independent mechanisms include the enzyme lysozyme, cationic proteins, and pH changes. All these degradation mechanisms are important, but it is still uncertain which are the crucial steps in killing bacteria. *(Robbins et al, pp 49–51)*

614. The answer is C (2,4). The striking histologic feature of the liver biopsy specimen shown in the question is that of multiple granulomas in the portal tracts. Granulomas are seen in 3 to 10 percent of liver biopsy specimens examined in general hospitals. The most common causes of granulomatous hepatitis are sarcoidosis, intrinsic liver disease (mainly primary biliary cirrhosis), and *Mycobaterium tuberculosis*. Additional causes include drug-induced lesions, neoplasms, and other infectious agents. The specimen shown was taken from a patient with sarcoidosis. Hepatoma and metastatic adenocarcinoma are both neoplasms but with very different histologies. Neither is characterized by a granulomatous process in the portal tracts in the liver. *(Kissane, pp 889–891)*

615. The answer is A (1,2,3). The major lesion of primary pulmonary tuberculosis is the Ghon complex, which is located classically in the lower part of the upper lobes or in the upper portion of the lower lobes of the lungs, subpleurally. Bilaterality is very rare in primary tuberculosis. This initial lesion is a well-defined, walled-off area of firmness in the lung, which on histologic examination shows granulomatous lesions. These granulomas have necrotic, cheesy, caseous centers and are composed of histiocytes, macrophages, and Langhans' multinucleated giant cells. With time, this initial lesion becomes fibrosed, but with lymphatic spread of the tubercle bacilli, the lymph nodes at the hilum of the lung are involved early. This combination of lobar and perihilar lymph node involvement by tuberculous granulomas is a Ghon complex. The lung is the first site of involvement, secondary to inhalation of minute particles of material containing the bacilli, which are inspired from the air and trapped in the respiratory mechanism. *(Robbins et al, pp 340–346,739–742)*

616. The answer is E (all). Amyloid is an abnormal protein compound produced by various types of cells. It is distributed throughout the body in a variety of pathologic states. Under the light microscope, amyloid is eosinophilic, amorphous, and hyaline appearing. With special stains, such as Congo red, it appears apple-green under polarized light. Amyloid is composed of nonbranching fibrils that are 7.5 to 10.0 nm in width and are arranged in bundles or in a meshwork. These fibrils are composed of amino acids, and the fibrils are arranged in antiparallel β-pleated sheets. Clinically, amyloidosis has been divided into primary and secondary forms (i.e., patients with and without an underlying chronic disease). Another categorization of amyloidosis is based on its two biochemical forms: AI, or amyloid B, is amyloid of immunologic origin; and AUO, or amyloid A, is amyloid of unknown origin. Amyloid B is systemic in origin and is found in patients with plasma cell abnormalities, such as multiple myeloma. In all these cases, the amyloid is thought to arise from plasma cells. Although in many cases no known plasma cell dycrasia is found, these forms are still designated AI. Amyloid A deposits also are systemic in their distribution, but the liver, spleen, kidneys, and adrenals are the most common sites. There is no hormology to immunoglobulins. Cases of secondary amyloid, or AUO, are found in patients with a wide spectrum of long-standing chronic infections, connective tissue diseases, and malignancies in which there is continuous, massive cell breakdown. Until the era of modern pharmacology, 50 percent of patients with tuberculosis had amyloidosis. Biochemically, amyloid A and B differ, but they do have some immunologic cross-reacting groups, indicating some similarities in origin. The exact pathology and cellular origin of amyloid are still unknown. *(Robbins et al, pp 195–205)*

617. The answer is B (1,3). A follicular adenoma is a common benign tumor of the thyroid. It is usually uninodular, well encapsulated, and composed of uniform, small, benign-appearing follicles that are dissimilar from the surrounding tissue. The nodule compresses the adjacent thyroid tissue, causing atrophy. These characteristics are in contrast to those seen in nodular hyperplasia, which is composed of multiple nodules that are only partly encapsulated and are similar histologically to the adjacent thyroid tissue. Adenomas may or may not be functional, with secretion of colloid. Malignant transformation of these tumors is very rare and is seen in fewer than 10 percent of all cases. *(Kissane, pp 1408–1410)*

618. The answer is C (2,4). With blood vessel injury, platelets are attracted to the newly exposed connective tissue and collagen and adhere at this site. This is called primary aggregation. These aggregated platelets form pseudopodia and have organelle redistributions. Granules that contain ADP, serotonin, histamine, and lysosomal enzymes are released into the circulation. ADP especially is a platelet-aggregating compound, and it initiates a secondary aggregation step in which more platelets are attracted to form the thrombus. Plasmin is a fibrinolytic enzyme that helps dissociate thrombi. Platelet aggregates in thrombi have no known relationship to megakaryocyte replication in the bone marrow. *(Robbins et al, pp 93–96)*

619. The answer is C (2,4). Granulation tissue is the specialized tissue of a healing wound or repaired inflammatory region. It first appears 24 hr after injury and is most pronounced after 3 to 5 days. Granulation tissue is pink and soft. Histologically, it is characterized by fibroblast proliferation and the formation of small young blood vessels. These blood vessels sprout, branch, and are composed of proliferating endothelial cells. These young vessels are dilated and leaky, with resultant edema of the granulation tissue. The fibroblasts may acquire characteristics of smooth muscle cells, accounting for the contractility of wounds. The end result of granulation tissue is a scar composed of dense inactive fibroblasts, collagen, extracellular matrix, and a few mature blood vessels. *(Robbins et al, pp 71–72)*

620. The answer is A (1,2,3). Chronic inflammation is a result of persistent inflammatory stimuli. The exact distinction between chronic and acute inflammation is unclear, but an inflammation that persists for weeks is described as chronic. Chronic inflammation may be caused by persistence of the irritant, repeated bouts of acute inflammation, or a smoldering mild inflammatory stimulus. Chronic inflammation is characterized by infiltration by mononuclear cells, such as histiocytes, lymphocytes, plasma cells, and macrophages, with proliferation of fibroblasts and small blood vessels with neovascularization. Macrophages, the classic cells of chronic inflammation, are derived from monocytes recruited from the blood and from local proliferation of macrophages. Macrophages also tend to stimulate fibroblastic and blood vessel proliferation. Abscess formation is characteristic of acute inflammation and does not accompany chronic inflammation. *(Robbins et al, pp 61–69)*

621. The answer is C (2,4). Carcinoma of the prostate is a common disease of elderly men, detected in more than 30 percent of all men. Many cases are occult or latent and are detected incidentally or not until autopsy. These tumors arise from the tubuloalveolar secretory ducts at the periphery of the prostate gland, usually in the posterior lobe. This peripheral origin contributes to their delay in diagnosis. Histologically, the tumors are usually adenocarcinomas, but rare cases arise from larger central ducts and may show squamous or transitional patterns. Many of these tumors are circumscribed, but they may spread into the adjacent gland and capsule or into lymphatics. The most common metastatic site is the vertebral skeleton. These tumors mimic normal glands, but their architectural pattern is diagnostic of cancer. They often show small, well-formed glands with little intervening stroma. Cytologically, they may or may not look malignant. Grossly, these tumors are rock-hard nodules. Carcinoma of the prostate may be treated with surgery if it is localized. Estrogen therapy and orchiectomy decrease androgen levels and may cause the tumor cells to regress. Chemotherapy and radiation treatment also have been attempted. *(Kissane, pp 824–829)*

622. The answer is B (1,3). Carbon monoxide binds almost irreversibly to hemoglobin to form carboxyhemoglobin. Carboxyhemoglobin cannot bind oxygen, and the lack of available oxygen-carrying capacity leads to systemic asphyxiation. The chemical properties of carboxyhemoglobin include a bright cherry-red color, which is imparted to the blood in cases of poisoning. Pneumonias and bacterial infections are not classic features of carbon monoxide poisonings. *(Robbins et al, p 450; Kissane, pp 214–216)*

623. The answer is C (2,4). Malignancy of the pleural cavity presents a common clinical problem of defining the exact cell type of the tumor. This must be known to determine the prognosis and before appropriate therapy can be initiated. The histology of certain malignant pleural tumors by routine hematoxylin and eosin stains is not always sufficient to identify the cell type of the tumor. Immunoperoxidase staining procedures can help to characterize antigens present on particular kinds of cells. The intermediate filament cytokeratin can be found in normal glandular and mesothelial epithelium. Its presence in this tumor would support the diagnosis of either metastatic adenocarcinoma (a glandular malignancy) or mesothelioma (a tumor of mesothelial cells). Leukocyte common antigen is a marker present on most white blood cells. Its absence in the tumor would make the diagnosis of lymphoma (a malignancy of white blood cell lymphocytes) highly unlikely. Similarly, the absence of S100, a marker of neurologic and melanocytic tissue, in the tumor would make the diagnosis of metastatic melanoma (a malignant tumor of melanocytes) highly unlikely. *(Robbins et al, pp 219–221)*

624. The answer is B (1,3). The carcinoid syndrome is related to the elaboration of secretory products from tumor cells that have metastasized to the liver. The primary lesion usually is a carcinoid tumor of the intestine or appendix. Common components of the syndrome include cramps, diarrhea, nausea, and vomiting, episodic flushing and cyanosis, cough, asthmatic wheezing, and dyspnea, and right-sided cardiac fibrosis involving valves and endocardium. Usually a massive tumor load is necessary in the liver to override the normal hepatic detoxifying deamination. Transitional cell carcinoma of the bladder and glioblastoma multiforme (a malignant brain tumor) are not features of the carcinoid syndrome. *(Robbins et al, pp 844–845)*

625. The answer is A (1,2,3). The biopsy specimen of the gastroesophageal junction shown in the question demonstrates the histologic changes characteristic of cytomegalovirus (CMV) infection. CMV is a member of the herpesvirus group and is responsible for a diverse spectrum of disease. Infection may be asymptomatic and subclinical or severe, with a variable morbidity and mortality. The latter characteristically occurs in neonates and in immunologically incompetent or debilitated adults. CMV is a member of the TORCH (Toxoplasmosis, Other, Rubella, CMV, Herpes) group of infectious agents, which may be responsible for severe congenital diseases. The mode of spread is diverse and includes intimate sexual contact, transmission in utero and during vaginal delivery, dissemination in respiratory droplets, blood transfusion, organ transplantation, and transmission through mother's milk. CMV, like other viral diseases, is resistant to antibiotic therapy. Histologically, the infected cells are markedly enlarged (epithelial and mesenchymal) with large, pleomorphic nuclei. Large intranuclear and smaller basophilic cytoplasmic inclusions are characteristic and represent the developing virions.

Focal necrosis is often identified. *(Robbins et al, pp 286–288)*

626. The answer is E (all). The immune system in the normal state reacts to substances that it recognizes as foreign to itself. Other determinants that influence a substance's antigenicity include all those listed in the question. Very small substances (e.g., amino acids) are nonimmunogenic. Substances with a molecular weight of <10,000 are poor antigens. The strongest immune response is seen against substances with a molecular weight of >100,000. Some small substances, known as haptens, become antigenic when coupled with large carrier molecules. Polypeptides consisting of a single amino acid sequence are poor immunogens, whereas those composed of several different amino acids are strong immunogens. Lipids, steroids, and nucleic acids are also poor immunogens. Some substances produce a strong antigenic response only when introduced to the host by a certain route in a certain dose range. The host's ability to react to various antigens has been shown to be genetically determined by immune response genes. *(Kissane, pp 449–459)*

627. The answer is E (all). Cystic fibrosis is a genetic disease with prominent pulmonary complications. Usually, the pulmonary complications are responsible for the early death of infants, children, and young adults who have the disease. Early pulmonary problems include bronchiectasis and repeated bacterial infections. Late lung disease is that of cor pulmonale. The exact genetic defect is obscure, but there are widespread abnormalities of exocrine gland secretion. *(Kissane, p 863)*

628. The answer is A (1,2,3). Vitamin A is a fat-soluble vitamin. Adequate dietary intake is necessary to maintain function and structure of certain epitheliums, particularly skin and retina. Deficiencies of vitamin A produce abnormalities of the skin (follicular hyperkeratosis) and eye (xerophthalmia, night blindness). Rickets is caused by a deficiency of vitamin D, not vitamin A. *(Kissane, p 500)*

629. The answer is C (2,4). Premature infants who are exposed to high concentrations of oxygen may develop retrolental fibroplasia or retinopathy of prematurity. The retinas of premature infants of 6 to 7 mo gestation are avascular around their periphery. On exposure to a high concentration of oxygen, the further development of the vessels that are already in the retina is inhibited because of their marked sensitivity to oxygen. This prevents the normal vascularization of the periphery of the retina. With prolonged oxygen exposure, retinal vessels may constrict and become obliterated. When oxygen exposure is eliminated, abnormal vascularization takes place. These abnormal, new vascular channels often enter the vitreous, bleed or ooze serum, and may eventually produce fibrosis, retinal detachment, or blindness. Retinal dysplasia is a congenital anomaly, and intraocular melanomas affect adults and are unrelated to oxygen exposure. (*Kissane, p 961*)

630. The answer is D (4). Exstrophy of the bladder describes a deformity of the anterior abdominal wall and bladder due to the failure of the mesoderm to migrate inferiorly over the anterior bladder wall. As a result, the abdominal and anterior bladder wall musculature does not develop, and there is abnormal formation of the symphysis pubis. The bladder, therefore, communicates with the external body surface through an abdominal wall defect or is left open. Exposure of the bladder mucosa renders it susceptible to infection, which may extend retrograde to other urinary structures. With time, the mucosa may become ulcerated and develop granulation tissue or undergo metaplasia into a stratified squamous epithelium. The risk of the development of carcinoma is increased in such bladders. Pyelonephritis and renal failure are the most common direct causes of death in affected individuals. However, since most cases can be treated successfully with corrective surgery, this deformity is not considered to be incompatible with life. (*Robbins et al, p 1067*)

631. The answer is E (all). Temporal arteritis, or giant cell arteritis, is a disease of elderly women that is characterized by an insidious onset of throbbing headaches and low-grade fever. Without treatment, the disease may progress to occlusion of the temporal artery, with obstruction of the ophthalmic artery and subsequent blindness. The disease usually involves the temporal artery or its tributaries, but rarely other systemic arteries may be involved. The cause is unknown. Progress of disease may be arrested by corticosteroid therapy. Diagnosis is based on a biopsy specimen, which shows a granulomatous reaction in the area of the internal membrane involving the entire arterial wall with proliferation of giant cells and histocytes. (*Kissane, pp 696–706*)

632. The answer is A (1,2,3). Wilson's disease, also called hepatolenticular degeneration, is an inherited autosomal recessive disorder of copper metabolism. Abnormal accumulation of copper within the liver, brain, and eye produces the most characteristic lesions. The liver lesions early in the disease have a hepatitic pattern. Later, cirrhosis occurs. The brain lesions include cavitation, atrophy, or brownish pigmentation of the lenticular nucleus and, rarely, the dentate nucleus. Kayser-Fleischer rings result from accumulation of brown copper granules in Descemet's membrane close to the limbus of the cornea. α_1-Antitrypsin levels are normal in Wilson's disease. (*Robbins et al, pp 932–933*)

633. The answer is A (1,2,3). Fluid homeostasis in the body can be thought of in terms of the Gibbs-Donnan equilibrium for fluids and components with a semipermeable membrane, the capillary endothelium. The fluid contains electrolytes and water, which are freely permeable, and proteins, which are not. Plasma has a higher concentration of proteins and ions than does the interstitial tissue. The osmotic pressure is dependent on the concentration of proteins. This pressure is much higher intravascularly than interstitially. This difference in colloid osmotic pressure tends to draw fluid into the vessels. The fluid or hydrostatic pressure is the force of the fluids themselves. In the capillaries, this force is great, tending to push the fluid out into the tissues, whereas in the tissues, this force is small. At the arterial end of capillaries, the hydrostatic pressure is less than the osmotic pressure, so fluid is reabsorbed intravascularly. Thus the presence of proteins, the colloid osmotic pressure, and the hydrostatic pressure of fluids interstitially and intravascularly determine fluid distribution. The fluid pressure intracellularly has no role in determining fluid homeostasis between plasma and tissue. (*Robbins et al, pp 85–88*)

634. The answer is A (1,2,3). Alzheimer's disease is a progressive chronic dementia that usually becomes clinically apparent between ages 50 and 65. Typically, the disease occurs with a loss of higher intellectual function, emotional lability, and episodic confusion. As the disease runs its 5- to 10-year course, a profound dementia develops. Death usually is caused by dehydration or pneumonia. Gross brains with Alzheimer's disease are moderately atrophied. The histologic findings include a constellation of senile plaques, granulovacuolar degeneration, neurofibrillary tangles, and Hirano bodies. Negri bodies are the hallmark of rabies, not Alzheimer's disease. (*Robbins et al, pp 1414–1416*)

635. The answer is E (all). Testicular tumors arise from both germ cell and sex cord–stromal elements. In large series of tumors, about 95 percent are of germ cell origin. Germ cell tumors occur in pure form (only one cell type) about 60 percent of the time and are divided histologically into seminoma, embryonal carcinoma, teratoma, and choriocarcinoma. Mixed tumors are composed of two or more of the pure forms. The sex cord–stromal tumors include Leydig tumors, Sertoli tumors, and various mixed and dedifferentiated forms. Other rare tumors of the testes include lymphoma and other sarcomas. (*Robbins et al, pp 1090–1097*)

BIBLIOGRAPHY

Kissane JM, ed. *Anderson's Pathology*. 8th ed. St. Louis: CV Mosby; 1985.

Lever W, Schaumburg-Lever G. *Histopathology of the Skin*. 6th ed. Philadelphia: JB Lippincott Co; 1983.

Man JM, Chin J, Piot P, Quinn T. AIDS—A special edition. *Sci. Am.* October 1988;82–89.

Redfield RR, Burke DS. AIDS—A special edition. *Sci. Am.* October 1988;90–98.

Robbins SL, Cotran RS, Kumar V. *Pathologic Basis of Disease*. 3rd ed. Philadelphia: WB Saunders Co; 1984.

Rubin E, Farber JL, eds. *Pathology*. Philadelphia: JB Lippincott Co; 1988.

Tietz NW, ed. *Textbook of Clinical Chemistry*. Philadelphia: WB Saunders Co; 1986.

Wirz D. Subarachnoid hemorrhage secondary to ruptured intracranial aneurysm. *Resident Staff Phys.* April 1983;85–95.

Subspecialty List: Pathology

Question Number and Subspecialty

509. Respiratory system
510. Cardiovascular system
511. Genetic syndromes and metabolic diseases
512. Inflammation
513. Circulatory disorders
514. Immunopathology
515. Genetic syndromes and metabolic diseases
516. Processes of neoplasia
517. Nongenetic syndromes
518. Kidney and urinary system
519. Hemostasis and coagulation
520. Alimentary system
521. Inflammation
522. Immunopathology
523. Abnormal growth and development
524. Immunology
525. Immunopathology
526. Alimentary system
527. Kidney and urinary system
528. Alimentary system
529. Cutaneous, osseus, and muscle systems
530. Alimentary system
531. Abnormal growth and development
532. Nervous system
533. Endocrine system
534. Processes of neoplasia
535. Miscellaneous
536. Inflammation
537. Inflammation
538. Inflammation
539. Processes of neoplasia
540. Processes of neoplasia
541. Alimentary system
542. Abnormal growth and development
543. Respiratory system
544. Respiratory system
545. Genetic syndromes and metabolic disorders
546. Circulatory system
547. Circulatory system
548. Circulatory system
549. Processes of neoplasia
550. Abnormal growth and development
551. Cell injury and response

552. Nervous system
553. Genital system
554. Genetic syndromes and metabolic diseases
555. Genital system
556. Genital system
557. Processes of infection
558. Immunopathology
559. Processes of neoplasia
560. Nongenetic syndromes
561. Inflammation
562. Healing and repair
563. Hemostasis and coagulation
564. Infectious diseases
565. Kidney and urinary system
566. Kidney and urinary system
567. Endocrine system
568. Blood and lymphatic system
569. Blood and lymphatic system
570. Blood and lymphatic system
571. Blood and lymphatic system
572. Miscellaneous
573. Inflammation
574. Inflammation
575. Inflammation
576. Genetic syndromes and metabolic disorders
577. Genetic syndromes and metabolic disorders
578. Genetic syndromes and metabolic disorders
579. Infectious diseases
580. Infectious diseases
581. Infectious diseases
582. Infectious diseases
583. Infectious diseases
584. Infectious diseases
585. Endocrine system
586. Endocrine system
587. Endocrine system
588. Genital system
589. Genital system
590. Genital system
591. Abnormal growth and development
592. Abnormal growth and development
593. Cardiovascular system
594. Cardiovascular system
595. Cardiovascular system
596. Nongenetic syndromes

597. Nongenetic syndromes
598. Nongenetic syndromes
599. Respiratory system
600. Cardiovascular system
601. Processes of neoplasia
602. Endocrine system
603. Endocrine system
604. Cardiovascular system
605. Genetic syndromes and metabolic disorders
606. Genetic syndromes and metabolic disorders
607. Immunopathology
608. Immunopathology
609. Blood and lymphatic system
610. Processes of infection
611. Genital system
612. Abnormal growth and development
     Blood and lymphatic system
613. Inflammation
614. Liver
615. Respiratory system

616. Genetic syndromes and metabolic diseases
617. Endocrine system
618. Circulatory system
619. Inflammation
620. Inflammation
621. Genital system
622. Miscellaneous
623. Miscellaneous
624. Nongenetic syndrome
625. Processes of infection
626. Immunopathology
627. Childhood diseases
628. Abnormal growth and development
629. Nongenetic syndromes
630. Abnormal growth and development
631. Cardiovascular system
632. Genetic syndromes and metabolic disorders
633. Circulatory system
634. Nervous system
635. Genital system

Pharmacology
Questions

DIRECTIONS (Questions 636 through 685): Each of the numbered items or incomplete statements in this section is followed by answers or by completions of the statement. Select the ONE lettered answer or completion that is BEST in each case.

636. A hypothetical drug, when given as a single-bolus dose of 1 g to a 70-kg (154-lb) patient, results in peak plasma level of 20 μg/ml. The apparent volume of distribution is

    (A) 0.05 L
    (B) 5.00 L
    (C) 14.20 L
    (D) 50.00 L
    (E) 500.00 L

637. A hypothetical drug follows first-order kinetics and has a half-life of 6 hr. A peak serum level obtained after a single IV dose of 100 mg is 8 μg/ml. After 12 hr, the serum level is expected to be

    (A) 6 μg/ml
    (B) 4 μg/ml
    (C) 2 μg/ml
    (D) 1 μg/ml
    (E) none of the above

638. Warfarin exerts its anticoagulant effect by

    (A) blocking calcium binding to clotting factors
    (B) forming a complex with clotting factors
    (C) breaking down thrombin
    (D) inhibiting the formation of active clotting factors
    (E) none of the above

639. All of the following sedatives have pharmacologically active metabolites EXCEPT

    (A) prazepam
    (B) chlordiazepoxide
    (C) diazepam
    (D) lorazepam
    (E) chlorazepate

640. All of the following are important side effects of glucocorticoids when used as anti-inflammatory agents EXCEPT

    (A) suppression of pituitary–adrenal function
    (B) masculinization of female patients
    (C) increased susceptibility to infections
    (D) osteoporosis
    (E) Cushing's habitus

641. Which of the following antineoplastic agents is associated with an increased incidence of severe pulmonary disease?

    (A) methotrexate
    (B) fluorouracil
    (C) bleomycin
    (D) vincristine
    (E) cisplatin

642. Which of the following laxatives is a bulk-forming agent?

    (A) docusate
    (B) cascara sagrada
    (C) magnesium citrate
    (D) psyllium hydrophilic mucilloid
    (E) bisacodyl

643. Use of magnesium-containing antacids is most likely to result in

    (A) constipation
    (B) diarrhea
    (C) nausea
    (D) headache
    (E) neurologic impairment

644. Potassium supplementation often is necessary for patients taking

(A) spironolactone
(B) triamterene
(C) furosemide
(D) amiloride
(E) captopril

645. Hormonal side effects of estrogen excess related to oral contraceptive use may include all of the following EXCEPT

(A) weight gain
(B) headaches
(C) amenorrhea
(D) edema
(E) breast tenderness

646. A patient experiencing an initial attack of acute gout is most likely to respond to treatment with

(A) indomethacin
(B) tolmetin
(C) phenylbutazone
(D) colchicine
(E) ibuprofen

647. Severe bone marrow suppression can result with the concurrent administration of 6-mercaptopurine and

(A) phenobarbital
(B) chloramphenicol
(C) allopurinol
(D) phenytoin
(E) metronidazole

648. Lidocaine

(A) is a short-acting local anesthetic because it is metabolized by pseudocholinesterases
(B) has direct vasoconstrictor activities
(C) is inappropriate for use as a topical anesthetic
(D) is a local anesthetic and thus is devoid of CNS effects
(E) appears to block nerve conduction by preventing the large transient increase in sodium permeability produced by depolarization

649. The ideal hypnotic should be absorbed rapidly so that its pharmacologic effect can occur, it should be eliminated rapidly, and it should not be biotransformed to long-acting metabolites to avoid

hangover effects. The hypnotic that most nearly achieves these criteria is

(A) triazolam
(B) temazepam
(C) flurazepam
(D) diazepam
(E) chlordiazepoxide

650. All of the following are fetal or neonatal side effects of β-sympathomimetic tocolytics EXCEPT

(A) tachycardia
(B) hyperglycemia
(C) ileus
(D) hypocalcemia
(E) hypotension

651. Cimetidine and ranitidine are pharmacologically classified as histamine receptor (H_2) antagonists. Which of the following disease entities is most likely to respond to the use of these agents?

(A) motion sickness
(B) seasonal rhinitis
(C) urticaria
(D) duodenal ulcer
(E) conjunctivitis

652. All of the following are factors that may increase the sensitivity of the myocardium to digoxin EXCEPT

(A) hypercalcemia
(B) hypoxia
(C) hypokalemia
(D) hyperthyroidism
(E) hypomagnesemia

653. Which of the following statements is correct regarding angiotensin-converting enzyme (ACE) inhibitors?

(A) chronic therapy with ACE inhibitors impairs hemodynamic response to exercise
(B) rebound hypertension after abrupt cessation of therapy is a frequent problem
(C) use of ACE inhibitors depresses renin activity
(D) therapy with ACE inhibitors appears useful in essential hypertension
(E) ACE inhibitors are of little value in therapy of congestive heart failure

654. All of the following drugs can decrease lower esophageal sphincter pressure EXCEPT

(A) dopamine
(B) morphine
(C) propranolol
(D) fentanyl
(E) theophylline

655. All of the following statements about rifampin are true EXCEPT

(A) it inhibits microbial RNA synthesis
(B) it is primarily excreted in the bile
(C) hepatotoxicity is a side effect
(D) it is used exclusively in the treatment of tuberculosis
(E) it reduces the effect of anticoagulants

656. Which of the following types of pulmonary dysfunction may follow heroin overdose?

(A) pulmonary fibrosis
(B) pulmonary edema
(C) bronchospasm
(D) pulmonary hypertension
(E) pneumonitis with eosinophilia

657. Which of the following statements regarding antidiuretic hormone (ADH) is correct?

(A) release of ADH is under the control of ADH-releasing factor, a hypothalamic hormone
(B) one of the main stimuli to ADH release is a decrease in plasma osmolality
(C) intranasal desmopressin (1-deamino-8-D-arginine vasopressin) is useful in treating diabetes insipidus
(D) ADH is one of at least 10 important hormones secreted by the anterior pituitary gland
(E) ADH can relax vascular smooth muscle

658. Of the following hypnotics, the safest is

(A) flurazepam
(B) chloral hydrate
(C) pentobarbital
(D) glutethimide
(E) paraldehyde

659. Since 1984, several new antiarrhythmic agents, including encainide, have become available for clinical use. Encainide is distinct from previous agents (procainamide or quinidine), since it is

(A) a member of the calcium channel blocker family

(B) useful in life-threatening sustained arrhythmia
(C) associated with prolonged repolarization (QT interval)
(D) capable of abolishing nonsustained ventricular arrhythmia with minimal cardiac toxicity [atrioventricular (AV) or sinoatrial (S-A) block]
(E) the only one available in a form for oral therapy

660. H_1 receptor antagonists are used to treat all of the following EXCEPT

(A) motion sickness
(B) allergic rhinitis
(C) sleep disorders
(D) bronchial asthma
(E) urticaria

661. All of the following are true about phenytoin EXCEPT that it

(A) is highly bound to plasma proteins
(B) is mainly excreted unchanged in the urine
(C) has dose-dependent elimination kinetics
(D) is effective in grand mal seizures
(E) induces the metabolism of certain drugs

662. Heparin anticoagulant therapy is associated with the following effects EXCEPT

(A) release of lipoprotein lipase
(B) breakdown of thrombin
(C) suppression of aldosterone secretion
(D) shortening of partial thromboplastin time (PTT)
(E) osteoporosis

663. Which of the following tricyclic antidepressants is most selective in blocking nerve reuptake of norepinephrine?

(A) doxepin
(B) desipramine
(C) amitriptyline
(D) imipramine
(E) nortriptyline

664. The onset and duration of sedative–hypnotic activity of the ultrashort-acting barbiturates may be influenced by all of the following EXCEPT

(A) serum elimination half-life
(B) lipid solubility
(C) cerebrovascular blood flow
(D) extent of tissue binding
(E) amount of body fat

DIRECTIONS (Questions 686 through 710): Each group of items in this section consists of lettered headings followed by a set of numbered words or phrases. For each numbered word or phrase, select the <u>ONE</u> lettered heading that is most closely associated with it. <u>Each lettered heading may be selected once, more than once, or not at all.</u>

Questions 686 through 689

For each laxative agent, select the group in which it is classified.

(A) bulk-forming
(B) lubricant
(C) stimulant
(D) stool softener
(E) osmotic

686. Psyllium

687. Bisacodyl

688. Docusate

689. Lactulose

Questions 690 through 692

(A) inhibits formation of the bacterial wall
(B) inhibits protein synthesis by binding to ribosomes
(C) causes misreading of mRNA at the ribosome
(D) inhibits nucleic acid synthesis
(E) prevents the incorporation of para-aminobenzoic acid (PABA) into folic acid

690. Rifampin

691. Tetracycline

692. Vancomycin

Questions 693 through 696

For each agent listed below, select the site or mechanism of action with which it is most closely associated.

(A) releases norepinephrine from storage sites
(B) direct α-adrenergic agonist
(C) blocks β-adrenergic receptors
(D) agonist of β-adrenergic receptors
(E) blocks α-adrenergic receptors

693. Isoproterenol

694. Propranolol

695. Amphetamine

696. Methoxamine

Questions 697 through 701

For each chemotherapeutic agent listed below, choose the unique side effect with which it is associated.

(A) neuropathies
(B) pulmonary fibrosis
(C) hemorrhagic cystitis
(D) congestive heart failure
(E) ototoxicity

697. Cyclophosphamide

698. Vincristine

699. Doxorubicin

700. Bleomycin

701. Cisplatin

Questions 702 through 704

For each agent listed below, select the physiologic response with which it is most closely associated after clinically relevant doses of the agent are administered.

(A) tachycardia
(B) cholinesterase inhibition
(C) decreased intraocular pressure
(D) muscle paralysis
(E) sedation

702. Pilocarpine

703. Atropine

704. Succinylcholine

Questions 705 through 710

For each antineoplastic agent listed below, select the pharmacologic class in which it belongs.

(A) plant alkaloid
(B) antimetabolite
(C) alkylating agent
(D) antibiotic
(E) antiestrogen

705. Vincristine

706. Methotrexate

707. 5-Fluorouracil

708. Cyclophosphamide

709. Bleomycin

710. Tamoxifen

DIRECTIONS (Questions 711 through 735): Each group of items in this section consists of lettered headings followed by a set of numbered words or phrases. For each numbered word or phrase, select
    A if the item is associated with (A) <u>only</u>,
    B if the item is associated with (B) <u>only</u>,
    C if the item is associated with <u>both</u> (A) <u>and</u> (B),
    D if the item is associated with <u>neither</u> (A) <u>nor</u> (B).

Questions 711 and 712
    (A) theophylline
    (B) isoproterenol
    (C) both
    (D) neither

711. Inhibits the enzyme that destroys cyclic AMP

712. Acts as a β-adrenergic receptor agonist

Questions 713 and 714
    (A) α-adrenergic receptors
    (B) β-adrenergic receptors
    (C) both
    (D) neither

713. Constriction of peripheral arterioles

714. Increased heart rate

Questions 715 and 716
    (A) diphenhydramine
    (B) cimetidine
    (C) both
    (D) neither

715. Inhibit gastric acid secretion

716. Useful in treatment of immediate hypersensitivity responses

Questions 717 through 721
    (A) cyclophosphamide
    (B) melphalan
    (C) both
    (D) neither

717. Must be activated by microsomal enzymes for its cytotoxic effect

718. Acts as an alkylating agent

719. Produces cystitis

720. S-phase specific

721. Produces alopecia

Questions 722 and 723
    (A) insulin
    (B) sulfonylureas
    (C) both
    (D) neither

722. Readily absorbed from the gastrointestinal tract

723. Useful in the treatment of diabetic ketoacidosis

Questions 724 through 727
    (A) nitroglycerin (glyceryl trinitrate)
    (B) nifedipine
    (C) both
    (D) neither

724. Relaxes vascular smooth muscle

725. In clinical doses, slows conduction through AV node

726. Associated with significant reflex tachycardia

727. Usually taken sublingually

Questions 728 through 731
    (A) aspirin (acetylsalicylic acid)
    (B) acetaminophen
    (C) both
    (D) neither

728. Analgesia

729. Antiplatelet effect

730. Antipyresis

731. Tinnitus

Questions 732 through 735
    (A) tetracycline
    (B) clindamycin
    (C) both
    (D) neither

732. Binds to the 50S ribosome of bacteria

733. May cause photosensitivity

		SUMMARY OF DIRECTIONS		
A	**B**	**C**	**D**	**E**
1, 2, 3 only	1, 3 only	2, 4 only	4 only	All are correct

760. According to the pH partition hypothesis, weak acids should be absorbed more rapidly from stomach (pH 3) than from the more alkaline intestine (pH 5 to 7). However, absorption of acids is always much faster from the intestine. Possible explanations for this discrepancy include

   (1) a considerably higher surface area in the small intestine than in the stomach
   (2) a high resistance epithelium in the intestine compared to the stomach
   (3) a much greater blood flow to intestines than to the stomach
   (4) avoidance of first-pass effects by the liver when drug is absorbed in the small intestine

761. Renal failure occurring during gentamicin therapy is characterized by

   (1) the inability to concentrate urine
   (2) the presence of protein and casts in the urine
   (3) rising trough concentrations of the drug
   (4) reversibility

762. Carbidopa is combined with levodopa in the treatment of Parkinson's disease because

   (1) lower doses of levodopa may be used
   (2) the peripheral side effects of levodopa are minimized
   (3) dosage titration is more rapid
   (4) levodopa is not effective alone

Answers and Explanations

636. **The answer is D.** In the example described in the question, the apparent volume of distribution is calculated as follows:

$$V_d = \frac{\text{total amount of drug in body}}{\text{concentration of drug in plasma}}$$

The total amount of drug in the body is the single-bolus dose of 1,000 mg and is calculated as follows:

$$V_d \neq \frac{1,000 \text{ mg}}{20 \text{ µg/ml}} = 50 \text{ L}$$

(Gilman et al, p 25)

637. **The answer is C.** The half-life for first-order kinetics is defined as the amount of time necessary for drug concentration to decrease by 50 percent. Six hours after a peak serum level of 8 µg/ml, the serum concentration of the drug described in the question should be 4 µg/ml. After 6 hr more (total of 12 hr), the serum level should be 2 µg/ml. *(Gilman et al, pp 25–28)*

638. **The answer is D.** Warfarin blocks the vitamin K-dependent step in the synthesis of clotting factors. Carboxylation of the molecule descarboxyprothrombin to form prothrombin requires the reduced form of vitamin K (KH_2), which, in the process, is converted to vitamin K epoxide (KO). KH_2 is regenerated by an epoxide reductase requiring NADH. It is this step that is blocked by warfarin. *(Gilman et al, p 1346)*

639. **The answer is D.** All benzodiazepines, with the exception of oxazepam and lorazepam, are converted via hepatic metabolic pathways. This usually occurs via *N*-alkylation or oxidation to metabolites that are pharmacologically active. This property may contribute to prolonged duration of action of the benzodiazepines. *(Gilman et al, pp 347–348)*

640. **The answer is B.** Glucocorticoids are valuable adjuvants in anti-inflammatory therapy and inhibit all phases of inflammation (vascular, cellular, and connective tissue repair). Usual therapy involves a synthetic derivative (e.g., prednisolone, triam-cinolone, desamethasone, betamethasone, beclomethasone) of the endogenous hormone, cortisol. Unfortunately, the biologic effects of glucocorticoids are myriad, and all effects aside from anti-inflammatory effects may become unwanted. Because of negative feedback from adrenal to pituitary gland, prolonged therapy with glucocorticoids can result in suppression of functions associated with this particular axis. Perhaps the most disasterous side effect is increased susceptibility to infection of all kinds secondary to effects of the drug on the immune system as well as inhibition of the inflammatory process. Decreased formation (decreased osteoblast activity) and increased resorption (secondary to elevated levels of parathyroid hormone due to decreased intestinal calcium absorption) of bone may lead to osteoporesis. Cushing's habitus, consisting of moonface, buffalo hump, enlargement of supraclavicular fat pads, central obesity, and other aspects of supraphysiologic affects of adrenal corticosteroids, also may occur. Masculinization of female patients is a common concern in androgen therapy. *(Gilman et al, pp 1478–1479)*

641. **The answer is C.** Ten to twenty percent of patients receiving bleomycin develop a pulmonary interstitial fibrosis that severely compromises gas exchange and reduces diffusing capacity. This condition is most prevalent in older patients or those receiving a total bleomycin dose above 400 units. *(Craig and Stitzel, p 816)*

642. **The answer is D.** Psyllium hydrophilic mucilloid, a bulk-forming laxative, exerts its therapeutic effect by increasing the mass and water content of stool and by speeding transit time in the colon. Bisacodyl and cascara sagrada are considered contact cathartics, which speed colonic transit time and alter water and electrolyte transport across the colonic mucosa. Magnesium citrate is a saline cathartic, which indirectly increases intestinal transit by its osmotic properties. Docusate, a stool-softening agent, is an anionic surfactant that presumably allows penetration of the fecal mass by water and fats. *(Gilman et al, pp 994–1003)*

643. The answer is B. The various magnesium salts act as saline cathartics and are sometimes used for this purpose. Hence, their use is commonly associated with the development of diarrhea. For this reason, various antacids contain an aluminum salt in addition to magnesium salts, which tends to counteract this effect. Neurologic sequelae develop when the small amount of absorbed magnesium cannot be excreted, as in moderate to severe renal insufficiency. *(Gilman et al, pp 994–1003)*

644. The answer is C. Spironolactone is a competitive antagonist of aldosterone and, therefore, may cause hyperkalemia if administered concomitantly with potassium supplements. Likewise, the potassium-sparing diuretics triamterene and amiloride cause potassium retention. Captopril inhibits production of angiotensin II and, therefore, inhibits aldosterone production. Furosemide promotes renal potassium excretion and often requires concomitant supplemental potassium administration. *(Gilman et al, pp 900–903)*

645. The answer is C. Oral contraceptive agents with a high estrogen content can produce adverse effects reflective of excess estrogen. These effects include weight gain, headache, edema, and breast tenderness. Amenorrhea is associated with estrogen deficiency. *(Katcher et al, pp 1251–1252)*

646. The answer is D. Colchicine is the drug of choice for an initial attack of acute gout because it provides symptomatic relief in more than 95 percent of cases. It also is a useful diagnostic tool because it is relatively specific for acute gout. The other choices listed in the question are nonsteroidal anti-inflammatory drugs that are used to treat acute gout if the side effects of colchicine are intolerable. *(Katcher et al, pp 1452–1455)*

647. The answer is C. Allopurinol often is used in conjunction with oncolytic therapy to reduce the elevated serum and urinary uric acid levels associated with the degradation of nucleoprotein. Allopurinol works by inhibiting xanthine oxidase. The antineoplastic agent 6-mercaptopurine can lead to excess accumulation of 6-mercaptopurine, resulting in severe bone marrow suppression. The remaining drugs listed in the question are all known to alter the hepatic mixed-function oxidase system, but they do not adversely interact with 6-mercaptopurine. *(Katcher et al, pp 945–946)*

648. The answer is E. Lidocaine is a potent local anesthetic that also is useful in treatment of ventricular dysrhythmia. In contrast to ester-type local anesthetics (procaine), lidocaine and other amides are metabolized slowly in the liver and have moderate to long durations of action. Unlike cocaine, which is a vasoconstrictor, lidocaine can cause vasodilatation that results in absorption of the drug away from its intended local site. Local administration can be achieved by injection or topical application. Inadvertent introduction of lidocaine in large doses intravenously may result in significant CNS effects. If administered properly, these concerns as well as cardiac effects are minimal. Although the mechanism of action is not completely understood, lidocaine appears to enter the nerve cell and attach to a receptor at a site within the sodium channel, leading to inhibition of sodium conductance after depolarization of the nerve. *(Covino)*

649. The answer is A. The benzodiazepine hypnotic triazolam most closely approximates the "ideal hypnotic" because of its rate of appearance in the blood after absorption, short elimination half-life, and lack of active metabolites. The other choices listed in the question are less than ideal. Temazepam has a slow onset, flurazepam has long-acting active metabolites, and diazepam and chlordiazepoxide have long half-lives and long-acting active metabolites. *(Craig and Stitzel, pp 500–501)*

650. The answer is B. β-Sympathomimetic agents, such as terbutaline and ritodrine, are used in the management of premature labor. Fetal and neonatal abnormalities secondary to these agents may include tachycardia, hypotension, hypocalcemia, and ileus. Hypoglycemia (not hyperglycemia) usually occurs because of increases in umbilical cord insulin caused by maternal hyperglycemia. *(Gilman et al, pp 942–943)*

651. The answer is D. Histamine receptor-blocking agents are classified as H_1 or H_2 blockers depending on what responses to histamine are prevented. H_2 receptors have been identified in numerous sites, including the stomach, uterus, ileum, and bronchial musculature. Gastric acid secretion involves activation of H_2 receptors, and disorders of acid secretion, such as duodenal ulcer, have responded to treatment with H_2 receptor antagonists. The remaining choices listed in the question do respond to conventional antihistamines (H_1-blocking drugs) but not to H_2 antagonists. *(Freston)*

652. The answer is D. Several factors are known to sensitize the myocardium to digoxin, predisposing patients to digoxin toxicity. These factors include hypercalcemia, hypokalemia, hypomagnesemia, and hypoxia. Hypothyroidism (not hyperthyroidism) also makes patients more sensitive to the effects of digoxin. *(Gilman et al, p 741)*

653. The answer is D. ACE inhibitors, such as captopril and enalapril, are effective agents in the treatment of systemic hypertension and congestive heart failure. Although initially perceived as being most useful for the therapy of renovascular disease and high renin hypertension, these drugs are now used routinely in many cases of essential hypertension. By inhibiting ACE, these drugs impair conversion of angiotensin I to angiotensin II while also prolonging the half-life of bradykinin, a vasodilator that normally is partially degraded by ACE. Accordingly, renin levels will rise as feedback inhibition via production of angiotensin II is removed. Unlike β-blockers, these drugs do not interfere with reflex sympathetic activity, and thus the response to exercise is unimpaired. Unlike centrally acting agents, such as clonidine, there is no indication of rebound hypertension. The drugs are being used more routinely as adjuvant therapy in congestive heart failure where a combination of decreased afterload and increased cardiac output is of great benefit to the patient. The mechanism underlying this effect is unclear. *(Lees)*

654. **The answer is C.** Certain drugs have been shown to decrease lower esophageal sphincter pressure and predispose patients to gastroesophageal reflux. These drugs include the anticholinergics, dopamine, isoproterenol, morphine, fentanyl, and theophylline. Propranolol has not been shown to decrease lower esophageal sphincter pressure. *(Craig and Stitzel, pp 165,371,598,602)*

655. **The answer is D.** Although rifampin is certainly a first-line drug in the treatment of tuberculosis, it is broadly antimicrobial and inhibits the growth of most gram-positive and gram-negative bacteria. More important, it is often part of the combined therapy used in the treatment of nontuberculous mycobacterial disease, where the causative organisms include *Mycobacterium leprae* or other species resistant to the other first-line antimycobacterial drugs, such as isoniazid. *(Gilman et al, p 1202)*

656. **The answer is B.** Heroin overdose often is associated with pulmonary edema and carries a mortality rate of about 10 percent. Treatment is primarily supportive, with respiratory and oxygen therapy. The other choices listed in the question represent other drug-induced pulmonary syndromes. *(Katcher et al, pp 373–377)*

657. **The answer is C.** ADH and oxytocin are the major peptide hormones secreted by the posterior pituitary gland. Osmoreceptors in the hypothalamus, close to nuclei that synthesize and secrete ADH, are stimulated by an increase in plasma osmolality. ADH binds to receptors in the basolateral membrane of cells of the distal tubule and collecting ducts of the nephron, increasing permeability to water and thus aiding in the formation of hypertonic urine. These ADH receptors are distinct from those found on vascular smooth muscle that result in ADH-induced vasoconstriction. ADH is rapidly metabolized by peptidases, and thus desmopressin is used as an intranasal spray for the treatment of diabetes insipidus. This derivative is less susceptible to peptidase digestion, and the intranasal route avoids some aspects of degradation within the gastrointestinal system. Other uses of vasopressin include treatment of esophageal varices, since the vasoconstrictor effects of ADH appear to be marked in splanchnic circulation. *(Rang and Dale, pp 366–369)*

658. **The answer is A.** Benzodiazepines (such as flurazepam) are considered the hypnotics of choice. In comparison with chloral hydrate, barbiturates (pentobarbital), and glutethimide, they have better therapeutic indices, less likelihood of interacting with other drugs, less abuse liability, and less effect on respiration. Paraldehyde usually is unacceptable because of its unpleasant taste and odor. Some persons may develop hypersensitivity to benzodiazepines or may be unable to tolerate the hypnotic effects. The relative costs of these various medications also may be a factor. The manufacture of glutethimide recently has been halted. *(Gilman et al, pp 357–367)*

659. **The answer is D.** Encainide is a structural analog of procainamide and is typical of the newly described class Ic antiarrhythmic drugs. Like quinidine or procainamide, it belongs to the family of drugs that block the fast inward sodium current in the heart. Unlike quinidine or procainamide, encainide does not alter the QT interval. Encainide is used for nonsustained arrythmia and is especially useful in conditions resistant to quinidine or procainamide, since encainide is without significant cardiac effects. Although some forms of life-threatening sustained arrhythmia may be treated with encainide, the drug has frequently been associated with exacerbation, rather than control, of these disorders. All three agents are available in oral form. Of note is that in many patients encainide is biotransformed to active metabolites under the control of a single hepatic cytochrome P_{450}. Encainide currently is under trial study to determine whether chronic antiarrhythmic treatment in postinfarction patients with arrhythmia reduces the risk of sudden death. *(Craig and Stitzel, pp 402–403)*

660. **The answer is D.** Although histamine release is likely to be a part of the pathophysiology of asthma, antihistamines are ineffective in treating the disease. Nevertheless, their ability to block histamine binding is used in treating a variety of hypersensitivity reactions, of which urticaria is one. H_1 antagonists have anticholinergic properties that make them useful secondary agents in treating motion sickness. Their sedative effect is used to treat sleep disorders. *(Craig and Stitzel, p 997)*

661. **The answer is B.** Phenytoin is effective therapy for most types of epileptic seizures except absence (petit mal) seizures. It is approximately 90 percent bound to plasma proteins. Phenytoin is eliminated mainly through metabolism that is saturable at attainable serum concentrations. The dose-dependent (nonlinear) elimination of phenytoin often presents a clinical problem, since small changes in dosage may result in large increases in serum concentration and toxicity. Dosage adjustment in an individual patient is best accomplished through careful monitoring of serum concentrations and close observation for early signs of toxicity that include nystagmus, vertigo, ataxia, and drowsiness. *(Craig and Stitzel, pp 560–561)*

662. **The answer is B.** Heparin inactivates thrombin; it does not cause its breakdown. Heparin achieves this effect in two ways: (1) by forming a complex with antithrombin III and the clotting factors, it promotes the action of antithrombin III in inhibiting the proteolytic conversion of prothrombin to thrombin, and (2) by directly and irreversibly inactivating thrombin. *(Gilman et al, p 1340)*

663. **The answer is B.** Tricyclic antidepressants block reuptake of aminergic neurotransmitters into the presynaptic neurons. The result is a net increase in the amount of neurotransmitter in the synaptic cleft. These agents are relatively selective for certain neurotransmitters. Desipramine is the most selective agent for blocking uptake of norepinephrine, and amitriptyline is the most selective agent for blocking reuptake of serotonin. Imipramine, nortriptyline, and doxepin are intermediate in their selectivity. *(Hollister, 1978)*

664. **The answer is A.** Barbiturates produce sedation through entry into the CNS. Ultrashort-acting agents are highly lipid soluble. The uptake of these agents by the CNS is rapid, with blood flow as the rate-limiting factor. The hypnotic activity of these agents is terminated by redistribution of drug from the CNS. Structural changes that affect various physiochemical properties of these agents influence the distribution of these agents into the CNS and, thus, their onset and duration of activity. Agents that are more lipid soluble (and are bound to tissues to a greater extent) have a rapid onset and short duration of action. Accumulation of these drugs in adipose tissue will affect the pharmacokinetics of these agents. Obese patients will require larger doses for sedative–hypnotic activity. Serum elimination half-life is not an important determinant of onset or duration of activity with ultrashort-acting agents. *(Gilman et al, p 356)*

665. **The answer is C.** Opiates act as agonists at specific receptor sites with the CNS and other tissues. Opiates influence many organ systems and may be responsible for undesirable effects as well as desirable effects, such as analgesia. Miosis is often a prominent effect of opiates. Effects on the gastrointestinal tract include nausea and emesis resulting from direct stimulation of the chemoreceptor trigger zone. Biliary spasm due to constriction of the Oddi's sphincter often results in elevation of serum amylase and lipase levels in patients receiving certain opiates. Increased muscle tone at the vesical sphincter of the bladder may make urination difficult and result in urinary retention. Opiates act to depress respiration by directly affecting brain stem respiratory centers, reducing the responsiveness to carbon dioxide content in blood. *(Levine)*

666. **The answer is D.** The metabolically active form of vitamin D (1,25-dihydroxycholecalciferol, or calcitriol) plays a major role in the control of calcium ion concentration in plasma. Calcitriol appears to enhance the intestinal absorption of calcium by stimulating formation of a calcium-binding protein that facilitates the absorption of calcium. Calcitriol also increases plasma calcium concentration through mobilization of calcium from bone. Parathyroid hormone appears to promote this action. Calcitriol's effect on the kidneys includes increased calcium and phosphate retention because of enhanced proximal tubular absorption. Negative feedback control of calcium homeostasis by calcitriol includes suppression of parathyroid hormone secretion and inhibition of renal activation of 25-hydroxycholecalciferol to calcitriol. Calcitriol has no effect on the formation or disposition of testosterone. *(DeLuca)*

667. **The answer is D.** Placental transport of maternal substances is established by the fifth gestational week. Passage of substances occurs by simple passive diffusion. Substances that are of low molecular weight, high lipid solubility, and un-ionized are able to cross the placenta more rapidly. Protein binding determines the amount of drug available for diffusion. Drugs that are highly protein bound exhibit low concentrations in fetal tissues. Maternal BP does not influence transplacental transport of drugs. *(Craig and Stitzel, pp 38–39)*

668. **The answer is A.** The un-ionized form of weak acids and bases undergoes passive reabsorption in the proximal and distal tubules. Because tubular cells are less permeable to the ionized form, reabsorption is pH dependent. When tubular urine is more acidic, weak bases are more ionized, passive reabsorption is reduced, and weak bases are excreted more rapidly. *(Craig and Stitzel, pp 23–24)*

669. **The answer is D.** Clonidine stimulates α-adrenergic receptors centrally, causing a decrease in sympathetic outflow and a resultant decrease in blood pressure. The major action of hydralazine is direct relaxation of resistance vessels, with a greater effect on the arterioles than on the veins. Prazosin is an α-adrenergic blocking agent that acts on vascular smooth muscle and produces both venodilatation and arterial dilatation. Nitroprusside has a direct effect on vascular smooth muscle and dilates both resistance and capacitance vessels. Minoxidil relaxes vascular smooth muscle and produces vasodilatation. *(Craig and Stitzel, pp 303–310)*

670. The answer is C. Spironolactone is a competitive antagonist of aldosterone. It binds to the receptor but evokes no response. Because aldosterone stimulates the reabsorption of Na+ in exchange for K+, the effect of the drug is to retain K+. It is often used in combined therapy with other diuretics likely to cause hypokalemia. Theophylline is the only one of the drugs listed that is not used primarily as a diuretic, although this is one of its actions. *(Gilman et al, p 900)*

671. The answer is E. High serum calcium concentrations may produce metastic calcifications, renal damage, electrophysiologic disturbances, and various other nonspecific symptoms. Calcium excretion may be enhanced through increased sodium excretion. This may be accomplished through administration of normal saline or diuretics that promote calcium as well as sodium excretion (e.g., furosemide). Corticosteroids, such as prednisone, may correct hypercalcemia through decreasing vitamin D–mediated calcium absorption from the gastrointestinal tract. Mithramycin, an antitumor agent, inhibits bone resorption as well as exerts an anti-vitamin D effect. Dihydrotachysterol is a synthetic form of vitamin D. This agent would increase serum calcium concentrations. *(Lindeman and Papper)*

672. The answer is D. Cocaine has two distinct pharmacologic actions. It is a potent local anesthetic as well as a CNS stimulant. Its local anesthetic activity makes this agent useful in surgical procedures involving the eyes and naso-oropharynx. Effects on the CNS progress from cortical excitement (resulting in euphoria, restlessness, and garrulousness) and respiratory stimulation with low doses to advanced stages of stimulation (e.g., tonic-clonic seizures) with high doses. Cardiovascular effects usually include a rise in blood pressure, particularly with higher doses. Mydriasis occurs presumably through potentiation of sympathetic stimulation. *(Gilman et al, p 309)*

673. The answer is C. The most common and distressing side effect of nonsteroidal anti-inflammatory agents is gastrointestinal complaints. Of those persons taking ibuprofen, 5 to 15 percent have symptoms referable to the digestive system. A similar incidence has been observed for naproxen. Toxic

amblyopia is an unusual complication of ibuprofen therapy. Edema formation and renal failure have uncommonly been associated with both drugs. Drowsiness is an extremely rare side effect. *(Craig and Stitzel, p 1030)*

674. The answer is C. In other respects, the action of levorphanol is similar to that of morphine. Thus, it depresses respiration, causes a histamine-mediated bronchoconstriction that makes it an inadvisable drug for asthmatics, produces a variety of allergic reactions, and like all opioid agonists, is blocked by naloxone. *(Gilman et al, p 491)*

675. The answer is A. Therapeutic plasma phenytoin levels range from 10 to 20 μg/ml. Above 20 μg/ml, dose-related cerebellar–vestibular effects occur. At concentrations of 20 μg/ml, nystagmus is initially observed. Ataxia is observed at levels of 30 μg/ml, and at 40 μg/ml, lethargy is noted. Increased frequency of seizures also has occured at very high plasma levels. *(Gilman et al, p 452)*

676. The answer is E. The use of cimetidine has been associated with a decrease in the hepatic metabolism of various drugs, including warfarin, diazepam, and theophylline. Cimetidine has been noted to cause gynecomastia, presumably by elevating prolactin levels. Suppressed spermatogenesis also has been observed. A broad range of CNS problems, including dizziness, confusion, lethargy, and coma, has been observed, particularly in patients with preexisting renal disease. Relapse of ulcer symptoms has prompted the use of low-dose maintenance cimetidine therapy in selected patients. *(Katcher et al, pp 411–412)*

677. The answer is E. Pharmacotherapy of the complex syndrome of bronchial asthma is aimed at reversing the bronchospasm, bronchial edema, and mucosal hypersecretion that are associated with the disease. Much of this pathophysiology is the result of altered autonomic control of the airways as well as contributions of chemical mediators from resident pulmonary and inflammatory cells. Airway smooth muscle appears to have a predominance of β2-receptors, and such agents as isoproterenol are useful in dilating constricted airways and relieving some of the symptoms. Propranolol, a nonselective β-antagonist, is contraindicated in asthma. Recently developed β-agonists with improved selectivity for β2-receptors include terbutaline and albuterol. Theophylline, or its more soluble derivative, aminophylline, also is useful in the treatment of asthma. Although xanthine derivatives are the drug of choice for many forms of asthma, their mechanisms remain obscure and probably involve (1) phosphodiesterase inhibition, (2) adenosine antagonism, (3) inhibition of other mediator release, and (4) increased sympathetic activity. Ipratropium bromide is a quaternary iso-propyl derivative of atropine, which when administered by inhalation, relaxes bronchial smooth muscle by virtue of its antimuscarinic effects. Cromolyn sodium (disodium cromoglycate) is not a bronchodilator but is effective in asthma by preventing the release of chemical mediators from various cell types, including the mast cell. Cromolyn is effective only when used prophylactically and thus is of no value for reversal of acute episodes of asthma. (Craig and Stitzel, pp 1014–1027)

678. The answer is A. In general, epinephrine decreases peripheral resistance because of the stimulation of β_2-receptors in skeletal muscle blood vessels, resulting in vasodilatation in these beds. Cardiac rate rises as a direct result of β_1 stimulation. Systolic blood pressure rises because of positive inotropic and chronotropic effects, as well as precapillary vasoconstriction. Myocardial stimulation increases oxygen consumption. Insulin secretion is inhibited as a result of β stimulation, and glucose levels rise. (Gilman et al, pp 151–156)

679. The answer is E. Since the depth of anesthesia varies directly with tension of the agent in the CNS and since, for most agents, tension in the brain is always approaching tension in the arterial blood, several kinetic factors will influence the uptake and distribution of inhalational anesthetics. The more soluble an anesthetic is in blood, the slower is the approach of blood tension to that of inhaled gases. Therefore, methoxyflurane levels will rise slower than enflurane levels. At equilibrium, the partial pressure of drug in the lung is near that in the brain, and conventional dosage comparisons are made using MAC (minimal concentration of anesthetic at 1 atm that produces immobility in 50 percent of patients). Accordingly, a lower MAC value is indicative of a more potent drug. As a sole agent, nitrous oxide is used to provide some degree of analgesia (e.g., in dental procedures). However, at concentrations that are not associated with intolerable levels of tissue hypoxia, nitrous oxide by itself is not an effective anesthetic. Halothane hepatitis is a highly unusual toxic effect of the drug, which appears to be greater during repeated administrations of halothane over a short period of time. The incidence is extraordinarily low and has not precluded the use of this standard halogenated hydrocarbon for anesthetic purposes. Indeed, there is little real choice among halothane, enflurane, isoflurane, and methoxyflurane. All are associated with significant dose-dependent decreases in systemic blood pressure. Enflurane was originally developed to avoid repeated administration of halothane and, for this and more subtle reasons, has become increasingly popular for anesthetic procedures. Isoflurane was introduced in 1981 and, aside from economic considerations, has become

popular in anesthetic procedures, since depth of anesthesia can be adjusted rapidly, cardiac output is well maintained, and arrhythmias are uncommon. (Gilman et al, pp 260–292)

680. The answer is B. Administration of glucocorticoids leads to an increase in the number of polymorphonuclear leukocytes in the blood, whereas the numbers of lymphocytes, eosinophils, monocytes, and basophils decreases. Neutrophilic leukocytosis is due to the release of mature neutrophils from the bone marrow. The lymphopenia associated with glucocorticoid use is due to a redistribution of the circulating lymphocytes to sites outside the intravascular compartment. Monocytopenia and eosinopenia are produced in the same fashion. (Craig and Stitzel, p 873)

681. The answer is C. The bioavailability of various oral ferrous salts is relatively similar, and the oral route is a reliable method of administration in most cases. Ferrous sulfate is less expensive than the other forms, however, and should be considered the treatment of choice. In those rare situations when the oral route cannot be used, parenteral iron dextran may be used. Its use is sometimes hampered by severe allergic and local reactions, precluding its routine use. (Gilman et al, pp 1315–1318)

682. The answer is E. The duration of action of various insulin preparations is related to the rate of absorption from the SC injection site. Binding with various proteins, such as protamine or globin, results in slower absorption of insulin. Preparations with large insulin crystals and high zinc content are also slowly absorbed. Ultralente insulin has a particularly long duration of action (approximately 36 hr) for the latter reasons. Regular insulin and semilente insulin are fast-acting insulins, with duration of action ranging from 6 to 14 hr. Intermediate-acting preparations with duration of action of approximately 24 hr include NPH insulin, lente insulin, and globin zinc insulin. (Gilman et al, p 1502)

683. The answer is C. Streptomycin is absorbed poorly by the gut mucosa and is usually administered by IV or IM injection. In the treatment of existing tuberculosis, a combination of drugs is used to offer continued protection should mycobacterial strains develop that are resistant to one drug. Although streptomycin has bacteriostatic, possibly even bactericidal, effects on the tubercle bacillus, its mode of administration is a negative feature and, in long-term therapy, can lead to poor patient compliance. (Gilman et al, p 1160)

684. The answer is C. Lovastatin (Mevinolin) is a recently approved drug that is a fungal inhibitor of cholesterol biosynthesis. It is a competitive, reversible, highly specific antagonist of HMG-CoA reductase, and in patients with heterozygous familial hypercholesterolemia, lovastatin lowers plasma low-density lipoprotein (LDL) by enhancing receptor-mediated degradation of lipoprotein. Nicotinic acid decreases the production of very low-density lipoprotein (VLDL), which in turn reduces production of its daughter particle, LDL. The mechanism by which this occurs is unclear and may be related to inhibition of lipolysis in adipose tissue, decreased esterification of triglycerides in the liver, and increased activity of lipoprotein lipase. Regardless, nicotinic acid does not affect synthesis of cholesterol or alter excretion of bile acids. Clofibrate reduces plasma triglyceride levels by lowering levels of VLDL. Although sites of action of clofibrate are only partially established, its primary effect is to increase the activity of lipoprotein lipase. Gemfibrozil is a congener of clofibrate that lowers VLDL in an undetermined manner but perhaps by hastening its secretion, since gemfibrozil does not affect lipoprotein lipase activity. Regardless of this lack of information, the net effect of gemfibrozil is to raise, not lower, HDL concentrations. Cholestyramine is a bile acid-binding resin that reduces the concentration of cholesterol in plasma by lowering the level of LDL. These resins are limited to an intestinal disposition where they hasten the excretion of neutral sterols as well as bile acids. Loss of these two substances results in compensatory changes in hepatic metabolism, including increase in number of cell-surface LDL receptors. This compensatory increase accounts for reduction in circulating concentrations of LDL. *(Gilman et al, pp 834–842)*

685.   The answer is D. The calcium in calcium disodium edetate is readily displaced by heavy metals, such as lead, forming stable complexes (chelates), which are excreted in the urine. Calcium disodium EDTA will bind in vivo any available divalent or trivalent metal that has a greater affinity for EDTA than has calcium. Mobilization and excretion of lead indicate that the metal is accessible to EDTA. Mercury poisoning does not respond to EDTA in vivo. *(Gilman et al, pp 1620–1621)*

686–689.   The answers are 686-A, 687-C, 688-D, 689-E. Proprietary laxatives are traditionally classified into bulk laxatives, lubricants, stimulants, stool softeners, and osmotic laxatives. Bulk-forming preparations, which expand and soften the stool via their ability to retain water, include such preparations as bran and psyllium. Lubricants, such as mineral oil, have no pharmacologic effect on the gut and simply lubricate the passage of stool. Bisacodyl is a stimulant-type laxative. Its effect was believed to be due to the initiation of peristalsis in the colon but may be more closely related to the intraluminal accumulation of water. Additional stimulant-type laxatives include phe-

nolphthalein, senna, cascara, danthron, and castor oil. Docusate is an anionic detergent that softens the stool by net water accumulation in the intestine. Osmotic laxatives are believed to hold water in the lumen by an osmotic action. Lactulose is a disaccharide compound that is broken down by colonic bacteria to form osmotically active molecules. Magnesium salts (magnesium sulfate and magnesium citrate) also act as osmotic laxatives. *(Thompson)*

690–692.   The answers are 690-D, 691-B, 692-A. Rifampin inhibits DNA-dependent RNA polymerase and thus blocks RNA synthesis. The mechanism is only effective in prokaryotes, since nuclear RNA polymerase from eukaryotic cells does not bind rifampin. The tetracyclines bind to the 30S subunit of the ribosome and prevent access of tRNA to the mRNA–ribosome complex. Vancomycin inhibits formation of the bacterial cell wall by binding to the terminal carboxyl group on the D-alanyl-D-alanine terminus of the N-acetylglucosamine N-acetylmuramic acid peptide and prevents polymerization of the peptidoglycan. *(Gilman et al, pp 1170, 1202; Craig and Stitzel, p 704)*

693–696.   The answers are 693-D. 694-C, 695-A, 696-B. Effector cells that are stimulated by the sympathetic nervous system contain α and β receptors. Agonists that affect these receptors themselves are termed direct agonists. Methoxamine is a direct agonist of α-adrenergic receptors. Isoproterenol is a direct β agonist. Some sympathomimetic agents act indirectly by displacing norepinephrine onto adrenergic receptors from storage sites in adrenergic nerve endings. Amphetamine acts in this way. α-Adrenergic and β-adrenergic blocking agents bind to adrenergic receptors and, therefore, interfere with the effects of sympathomimetic agents. Propranolol is the prototype β blocker, and phenoxybenzamine is an α blocker. *(Gilman et al, pp 145–174)*

697–701.   The answers are 697-C, 698-A, 699-D, 700-B, 701-E. Cyclophosphamide causes hemorrhagic cystitis in 5 to 10 percent of users. This is probably caused by chemical irritation, and it is recommended that persons who take this drug have ample fluid intake and void frequently. The toxicity associated with vincristine characteristically involves neuropathies, including paresthesias, neuritic pain, loss of deep tendon reflexes, muscle weakness that may cause footdrop and inability to walk, headache, and double vision. Doxorubicin causes either acute or chronic cardiomyopathy. The acute form is characterized by abnormal ECG changes, including ST-T–wave alterations and arrhythmias. The chronic toxicity is a cumulative, dose-related toxicity manifested by congestive heart failure that is unresponsive to digitalis. The unique toxicity associated with bleomycin is pulmonary fibrosis, the incidence of which increases with doses larger than 400 units and in patients older than 70 yr who suffer underlying pulmonary disease. Cisplatin may cause unilateral or bilateral hearing loss or tinnitus. (Gilman et al, pp 1247–1291)

702–704.   The answers are 702-C, 703-A, 704-D. The agents listed affect cholinergic transmission in different manners, and their clinical use is in large part a manifestation of their cholinergic effect. Pilocarpine is a naturally occurring alkaloid that is cholinomimetic in effect and acts predominantly at muscarinic sites. In mimicking the effect of acetylcholine, it will cause pupillary constriction, spasm of accommodation, and a transient rise in intraocular pressure that is followed by a prolonged and greater decrease in intraocular pressure. Small doses of pilocarpine are associated with bradycardia and arousal. Atropine is the prototypic antimuscarinic agent, and by competitively blocking the effect of acetylcholine at muscarinic receptors, atropine usually is associated with tachycardia. Central effects of low doses of atropine usually include excitation. Atropine causes mydriasis and cycloplegia but does little to intraocular pressure, with the exception of increasing it in patients with narrow-angle glaucoma. Succinylcholine is the typical depolarizing neuromuscular blocker that produces fasciculation of muscle followed by total paralysis. Succinylcholine may raise intraocular pressure by contracting extraocular muscles and may cause bradycardia because of stimulation of vagal ganglion. Although tachycardia is possible (via stimulation of sympathetic ganglion) after succinylcholine, it is unlikely. None of the drugs listed have appreciable effects on the activity of acetylcholinesterase, the enzyme responsible for hydrolysis of acetycholine as well as pilocarpine and succinylcholine. Typical inhibitors of cholinesterase are physostigmine, neostigmine, edrophonium, and diisopropyl fluorophosphate. (Gilman et al, pp 105–107, 130–137, 222–235)

705–710.   The answers are 705-A, 706-B, 707-B, 708-C, 709-D, 710-E. Antineoplastic agents are divided into several pharmacologic classes. The plant alkaloids are derived from the periwinkle plant, and they impair the synthesis of cellular microtubules. Vincristine and vinblastine are two clinically useful plant alkaloids. Antimetabolites interfere with the synthesis of new nucleic acids in actively dividing cells. Methotrexate, 5-fluorouracil, and 6-mercaptopurine are examples of antimetabolites. Alkylating agents form covalent bonds with nucleic acids, thus interfering with their action. Mechlorethamine, cyclophosphamide, chlorambucil, melphalan, and dacarbazine are examples of alkylating agents. Antibiotics, such as doxorubicin,

mithramycin, and bleomycin, are useful anticancer agents because they can inhibit DNA and RNA synthesis. Tamoxifen is an antiestrogen used in treating breast cancer. (Gilman et al, pp 1247–1291)

711–712.   The answers are 711-A, 712-B. Bronchodilator drugs are the mainstay of therapy for patients with bronchial asthma. Bronchodilators exert their antibronchoconstrictor effect via differing mechanisms. A definite relationship between the increase in cyclic AMP and the degree of bronchial smooth muscle relaxation has been demonstrated. The formation of cyclic AMP is mediated by adenylcyclase, an enzyme whose activity can be increased by β-adrenergic receptor stimulants, such as isoproterenol. In contrast, theophylline is a methylxanthine derivative that inhibits the enzyme (phosphodiesterase) that destroys cyclic AMP. Both theophylline and isoproterenol are useful bronchodilators for the treatment of asthma and chronic obstructive pulmonary disease. (Craig and Stitzel, pp 1015–1019)

713–714.   The answers are 713-A, 714-B. Postsynaptic adrenergic receptors of the autonomic nervous system may be classified as two types—α_1 and β receptors. Agents that stimulate peripheral α_1 receptors located in the peripheral arterioles provoke vasoconstriction. β receptors located on the postsynaptic membrane may be described as β_1 or β_2 receptor types. Stimulation of β_1 receptors in the heart results in a positive chronotropic (increased heart rate) and inotropic (increase in myocardial contractility) response. Isoproterenol stimulates both β_1 and β_2 receptors. Epinephrine stimulates both α and β receptors. (Gilman et al, pp 72–73)

715–716.   The answers are 715-B, 716-A. The agents listed are important examples of antihistamines. Cimetidine was the first H_2 receptor antagonist clinically available and gained widespread use in the treatment of duodenal ulcers and other gastric hypersecretory conditions. Although H_2 receptors exist in many biologic locations in most species, stimulation of gastric acid secretion by histamine is the most important H_2 receptor-mediated process, and accordingly, cimetidine (and other drugs, such as ranitidine) is relatively specific in producing a reduction in volume of gastric juice produced as well as its pH. This process is unaffected by H_1 receptor-mediated effects. Diphenhydramine is the prototype of this latter group of antagonists. Among its prominent roles is the ability to reduce edema formation and itch as well as minimize hypotension that may occur in humans during anaphylactoid and allergenic responses. Diphenhydramine is unable to antagonize endogenous (or exogenous) histamine's effect on gastric acid secretion. (Gilman et al, pp 618–627)

717–721.   The answers are 717-A, 718-C, 719-A, 720-D, 721-C. Cyclophosphamide must be activated by the P450 mixed function oxidase system in the liver to form 4-hydroxycyclophosphamide, which is in a steady state, and the acyclic tautomer, aldophosphamide. In cells, the latter is thought to convert to phosphoamide mustard and acrolein. Melphalan does not require activation. Both cyclophosphamide and melphalan are alkylating agents of the nitrogen mustard subgroup. They form an electrophilic ethylenimonium ion that can react with a nucleophilic site, such as the N7 position of guanine. The resulting alkylation of guanine disrupts the nucleic acid molecule. Cystitis is a side effect unique to cyclophosphamide. It is thought that the injury to the bladder mucosa is caused by acrolein, one of the metabolites of cyclophosphamide. Like all alkylating agents, cyclophosphamide and melphalan are not cell cycle specific. As is typical for the nitrogen mustards, administration of both cyclophosphamide and melphalan often results in alopecia, loss of scalp hair. The effect is somewhat greater with cyclophosphamide. *(Gilman et al, pp 1252,1254, 1256,1257)*

722–723.   The answers are 722-B, 723-A. The sulfonylureas are hypoglycemic agents that must be administered orally, whereas insulin is degraded by proteolytic enzymes when administered orally and must be given by either SC, IM, or IV injection. Diabetic ketoacidosis is a condition that is characterized by glycosuria, hypovolemia, ketonuria, ketonemia, metabolic acidosis, and often coma. This constitutes a life-threatening situation, and successful treatment requires the use of effective doses of insulin and appropriate fluid therapy. Sulfonylureas would not be indicated in this situation, since they are not useful in patients with insulin-dependent diabetes. *(Gilman et al, pp 1490–1512)*

724–727.   The answers are 724-C, 725-D, 726-C, 727-A. Nitroglycerin (actually a misnomer for glyceryl trinitrate) and nifedipine (calcium channel blocker) are used extensively, alone and in combination, in the pharmacotherapy of angina. Both agents are potent relaxers of vascular (and other) smooth muscle. Nitroglycerin relaxes smooth muscle by being metabolized to nitric oxide, with subsequent activation of intracellular guanylate cyclase. Nifedipine and other calcium channel blockers relax vascular smooth muscle by blocking the movement of extracellular calcium through voltage-dependent calcium channels, thereby interfering with electromechanical coupling of smooth muscle. Although nifedipine can reduce the slow inward current of calcium in the AV node, it does not prolong conduction time or the refractory period in clinical doses. Nitroglycerin is without significant direct inotropic effects on the heart. Accordingly, neither agent would be predicted to slow conduction through the AV node. This is in contrast to other antiangina agents, such as the calcium channel blocker verapamil or β blockers. Since both agents are capable of relaxing systemic arterioles and reducing systemic blood pressure (afterload), potential exists for reflex tachycardia. Reflex tachycardia (and increased contractility) may exacerbate symptoms of angina and should be avoided. This may be accomplished by careful titration of either agent or by using propranolol in concurrent therapy. Both nitroglycerin and nifedipine are highly lipid-soluble compounds that are well absorbed from most sites of administration and are both extensively degraded by the liver. Although nitroglycerin may be given orally, IV, by ointment, or transdermally, the usual route is sublingual to avoid first-pass effects and to ensure convenient rapid onset of action. In contrast, large doses of nifedipine usually are given orally in spite of first-pass effects. *(Craig and Stitzel, pp 360–367, 373–380)*

728–731.   The answers are 728-C, 729-A, 730-C, 731-A. Aspirin and acetaminophen have similar analgesic effects when administered in equivalent doses. With salicylates, this effect appears to be mediated through both a CNS and a peripheral effect. Antipyresis also is produced by both aspirin and acetaminophen. A potent anti-inflammatory effect is associated with aspirin only. This appears to result from the ability to block endogenous prostaglandin synthesis. Tinnitus (ringing in the ears) is a toxic side effect of high concentrations of salicylates. *(Hollister, 1981)*

732–735.   The answers are 732-B, 733-A, 734-A, 735-C. Clindamycin, like erythromycin and chloramphenicol, bonds to the 50S subunit of bacterial ribosomes. In contrast, tetracycline binds to the 30S ribosome subunit. Both agents are regarded as bacteriostatic (i.e., they only inhibit bacterial growth) at concentrations acceptable for humans. Plasmid-mediated resistance by reduction of permeability through bacterial cell membranes is responsible for the decline of susceptibility of many bacteria to the tetracyclines. Some patients taking certain types of tetracyclines may experience photosensitivity and may become more susceptible to sunburn. *(Jawetz et al, pp 117–144)*

736.   The answer is C (2,4). PSVT can result from reentry within the atrioventricular node. Pharmacologic treatment of PSVT is accomplished by increasing refractoriness in the antegrade slow pathway. Agents, such as edrophonium, phenylephrine, metaraminol, digoxin, propranolol, and verapamil, can be effective in terminating PSVT. Antiarrhythmic drugs, such as procainamide and quinidine, increase refractoriness in the retrograde fast pathway. (Craig and Stitzel, pp 381–413)

737. **The answer is C (2,4).** Thiabendazole has a high degree of activity against a wide variety of nematodes, including those of the genera *Ascaris, Enterobius, Strongyloides,* and *Trichuris.* Although thiabendazole is useful in treating patients with multiple infections, it would not be the agent of choice in treating single infections with either *Ascaris* or *E. vermicularis* because of its potential for adverse reactions. Pyrantel pamoate is also a broad-spectrum anthelmintic that is effective against these nematodes. Side effects, which occur only occasionally, include gastrointestinal upset, headache, or dizziness. Tetrachloroethylene is useful in the treatment of hookworm but is seldom used, since more effective and less toxic agents are available. Mebendazole is a highly effective agent against these nematodes and others. Systemic toxicity from mebendazole is rare, probably because of its limited absorption. (Gilman et al, pp 1009–1026)

738. **The answer is A (1,2,3).** Both vestibular and auditory toxicity have been reported as side effects of the administration of aminoglycosides. The toxicity is thought to be the result of sensory cell destruction. Although early toxicity may be reversible, once sensory cells are lost, regeneration does not occur. High concentrations of aminoglycosides accumulate in the renal cortex. Prolonged therapy with excessively high trough concentrations correlates with the development of both ototoxicity and nephrotoxicity. Nephrotoxicity usually is expressed as acute tubular necrosis, which first becomes detectable after 5 to 7 days of administration. Nephrotoxicity, unlike ototoxicity, is usually reversible. Neuromuscular blockade has been reported following intrapleural and intraperitoneal instillation as well as IV, IM, and oral administration. It is most common in association with anesthesia or other neuromuscular blocking agents. Calcium appears to overcome the effect of aminoglycosides at the neuromuscular junction. Although transient elevations in transaminases and bilirubin associated with aminoglycosides have been reported, hepatic failure has not. (Gilman et al, pp 1157–1160)

739. **The answer is B (1,3).** Propranolol blocks both β_1- and β_2-adrenergic receptors competitively. Orally administered propranolol undergoes an extensive first-pass effect, so that only about one third of an oral dose reaches the systemic circulation. Therefore, much lower doses are needed when propranolol is administered IV. Adrenergic bronchodilation is mediated by β_2 receptors, which may be blocked by propranolol, leading to increased airway resistance and perhaps precipitating an asthma attack. (Gilman et al, pp 194–199)

740. **The answer is A (1,2,3).** Pharmacologic relief of angina is directed at improving the imbalance between the oxygen supply and the oxygen used by the myocardium. This can be accomplished by increasing the supply of oxygen to ischemic myocardium by direct, selective dilatation of coronary vasculature or by decreasing the oxygen demand by reducing cardiac work. Nitrates appear to cause selective dilatation of large epicardial vessels, resulting in a redistribution of coronary blood flow to ischemic subendocardium. This redistribution is not characteristic of all vasodilators. Dipyridamole dilates resistance vessels in a nonselective manner and is not of benefit in patients with angina. (Gilman et al, pp 806–822)

741. **The answer is B (1,3).** Propranolol is a nonselective competitive β-adrenergic receptor blocker useful in the treatment of hypertension, cardiac arrhythmias, hyperthyroidism, and angina pectoris. Included among the mechanisms proposed to explain its antihypertensive action are blockade of cardiac β receptors, with a resultant reduction in cardiac output, decreased sympathetic outflow from the CNS, and blockade of renin release from the juxtaglomerular apparatus of the kidney. Although propranolol blocks the stimulus for release of norepinephrine from adrenergic nerve terminals, it does not deplete the nerve of its supply of amines. (Gilman et al, p 794)

742. **The answer is C (2,4).** Barbiturates and rifampin have similar effects in inducing P450 microsomal enzymes of the liver and, thereby, increasing the clearance of anticoagulants. Aspirin and phenylbutazone, in contrast, both increase the response even to the extent of risking severe hemorrhage. (Craig and Stitzel, p 425)

743. **The answer is A (1,2,3).** The six major manifestations of plumbism (chronic lead poisoning) are gastrointestinal, neuromuscular, CNS, hematologic, renal, and miscellaneous symptoms. Intestinal symptoms consist of anorexia and constipation. Lead palsy, as the neuromuscular syndrome is sometimes called, is progressive, initially resulting in muscle weakness and fatigue and eventually producing paralysis. Encephalopathic symptoms, more common in children, include loss of motor skills, vertigo, ataxia, insomnia, restlessness, and, progressively, seizures. Punctate basophilic stippling is the hematologic hallmark of chronic lead ingestion. Progressive and irreversible renal insufficiency may result as well. Miscellaneous symptoms, such as pallor, gingival lead line, and emaciation, have been observed. Skin rashes are not noted. (Craig and Stitzel, p 121)

744. **The answer is E (all).** Although the mathematical relationship predicting the concentration of drug X during multiple dosing therapy may be complex, it is important to bear in mind all of the above correct statements in predicting the direction of change of drug. Specifically the rate at which a new plateau is reached is independent of dose administered and solely a function of the half-life of the drug. The actual plateau concentration depends only on clearance and the dosage administered per dosing interval and is independent of the half-life of the drug. Fluctuations in concentration during given intervals are proportional to the ratio of dosage interval to half-time; halving both the dose and dosage interval will produce a smoother rise to plateau concentration with blunted fluctuations but the actual plateau concentration will be unchanged. Many situations exist in which the clinician is interested in reaching a predicted therapeutic level but cannot wait a requisite interval to achieve a new steady-state. In these conditions, a loading dose is used followed by a new regimen of multiple dosage. *(Gilman et al, p 29)*

745. **The answer is E (all).** The major advantage of combining a decarboxylase inhibitor (carbidopa) with levodopa is that the total daily dosage of levodopa is available for CNS penetration. In addition, far fewer gastrointestinal effects are observed, and interference by pyridoxine is avoided. The time required for dosage titration is reduced, since the limiting gastrointestinal side effects are diminished. Adverse cardiovascular effects of levodopa (arrhythmias) also are decreased. *(Gilman et al, p 481)*

746. **The answer is A (1,2,3).** Prostacyclin is a short-lived product of arachidonic acid metabolism. Most clinical and experimental measurements of prostacyclin are indirect in that the stable metabolite, 6-keto-PGF$_1$-α, usually is measured. Prostacyclin is a very potent vasodilator in most systemic vascular beds as well as an inhibitor of platelet aggregation. Since vascular endothelium is capable of synthesizing PGI$_2$, it has been suggested that it plays a critical role in maintaining vascular patency via these two mechanisms. In addition, PGI$_2$ is cytoprotective and is capable of inhibiting gastric ulceration by inhibiting volume of secretion, acidity, and pepsin content. This effect is useful in counteracting the gastrointestinal ulcerative effects of nonsteroidal anti-inflammatory drugs. *(Gilman et al, pp 666–671)*

747. **The answer is B (1,3).** ECG effects of digitalis glycosides include prolongation of the PR interval, T wave inversion, ST segment depression, and shortening of the QT interval. The QRS complex duration does not increase, even during toxicity. If this should occur, other causes, such as conduction defects, should be sought. *(Gilman et al, p 739)*

748. **The answer is B (1,3).** Peptidoleukotrienes are thiolether-linked lipoxygenase metabolites of arachidonic acid. Although their chemical identity has been realized only in the last few years, they appear to play a critical role in the bronchospasm, edema, and mucous hypersecretion common to many forms of asthma. Among their profound cardiovascular effects are their ability to constrict coronary arteries, supporting a potential role for leukotrienes in shock and myocardial ischemia. Most commonly used nonsteroidal anti-inflammatory drugs, such as aspirin, do not affect lipoxygenase activity, and there are suggestions that by inhibiting cyclooxygenase activity, aspirin's net effect is to direct arachidonic acid through lipoxygenase pathway. Platelets do not contain 5'-lipoxygenase (although they do contain 12'-lipoxygenase), and leukotrienes are not stored in platelet granules. The cyclooxygenase product of arachidonic acid, TXA$_2$, is critical in platelet physiology, and acetylation of this enzyme by aspirin accounts for the effect of this drug in inhibiting platelet function. *(Gilman et al, pp 660–673)*

749. **The answer is D (4).** Agents used in the treatment of gout may be classified by their ability to decrease the production of uric acid or increase its excretion. Allopurinol and its metabolite oxypurinol inhibit the enzyme xanthine oxidase. This enzyme is responsible for the conversion of hypoxanthine and xanthine to uric acid. Probenecid and sulfinpyrazone are uricosuric agents that promote renal excretion of uric acid. Colchicine inhibits the migration of granulocytes into acutely inflamed gouty tissue. *(Craig and Stitzel, pp 1007–1013)*

750. **The answer is D (4).** α-Adrenergic blocking effects frequently are observed after therapy with the phenothiazines or the butyrophenone antipsychotic agents. Chlorpromazine may cause orthostatic hypotension or reflex tachycardia because of the combination of α-adrenergic blockade and central actions of the drug. Meprobamate and the benzodiazepines have little or no α-adrenergic blocking activity. *(Gilman et al, pp 349, 365, 402)*

751. **The answer is A (1,2,3).** Methotrexate competitively inhibits the binding of folic acid to the enzyme dihydrofolate reductase. Cellular resistance to the drug can occur by amplifying the gene for the enzyme, thus increasing the number of enzyme molecules within the cell, by development of mutant forms of the enzyme that exhibit reduced affinity for the drug or by a reduction in the carrier-mediated uptake of the drug. Enhanced efflux is the mechanism underlying pleiotropic or multidrug resistance common to the anthracyclines, vinca alkaloids, dactinomycin, and podophyllotoxins but not methatrexate. *(Craig and Stitzel, pp 807–809)*

752. **The answer is D (4).** Streptokinase forms a complex with plasminogen, activating the protease to form plasmin. Thus, it does not itself bring about this conversion. Free plasmin degrades other molecules, in particular fibrin, but it can also cause the depletion of α_2-antiplasmin. *(Gilman et al, p 1354)*

753. **The answer is A (1,2,3).** GABA is the major inhibitory molecule in the CNS. Diazepam enhances the action of GABA in a number of ways. It increases the binding of GABA to its receptor. This receptor and the binding site of diazepam are both associated with the GABA-gated chloride channel and modulate it, causing an influx of chloride ions that results in a hyperpolarization of the cell. By these mechanisms and possibly by others, diazepam reduces repetitive neuronal firing. It has no action on serotonin binding. *(Swinyard et al)*

754. **The answer is E (all).** Oral anticoagulants interfere with hepatic synthesis of the vitamin K-dependent clotting factors. These factors (II, VII, IX, and X) appear in the form of their biologically inactive precursors after the administration of oral anticoagulants. In this precursor form, they are unable to bind to calcium or phospholipid, which is the usual site of activation. *(Gilman et al, p 1345)*

755. **The answer is D (4).** Most bacterial resistance to aminoglycosides occurs by enzymatic inactivation by multiple enzymes located in the bacterial membrane. These enzymes inactivate aminoglycosides by phosphorylation, acetylation, or adenylylation. Amikacin, however, is resistant to inactivation, with acetylation being the only mechanism of bacterial enzymatic resistance. *(Gilman et al, pp 1153, 1164)*

756. **The answer is B (1,3).** The duration of action of a local anesthetic is proportional to its contact time with nerves. Therefore, if the drug can be localized at the nerve, the period of analgesia should be prolonged. Using a vasoconstrictor, such as epinephrine, decreases the systemic absorption of the local anesthetic. Once the absorption of a local anesthetic is decreased, the anesthetic remains longer at the desired site and is systemically absorbed at a slower rate, which allows destruction by enzymes and less systemic toxicity. *(Gilman et al, p 306)*

757. **The answer is D (4).** In an individual severely poisoned by antihistamines, the central effects, both the depressant and stimulant actions, cause the greatest danger. There is no specific therapy for poisoning, and treatment is usually supportive. In a child, the dominant effect is excitation, and hallucinations, ataxia, incoordination, athetosis, and convulsions may occur. Symptoms such as fixed and dilated pupils, a flushed face, and fever are common and markedly resemble those of atropine poi-

soning. Deepening coma and cardiorespiratory collapse characterize terminal poisoning. Fever and flushing generally are not manifestations of antihistamine poisoning in adults. *(Gilman et al, p 626)*

758. **The answer is A (1,2,3).** The course of acute acetaminophen overdose follows a fairly consistent pattern. During the initial 24 hr, nausea, vomiting, anorexia, and abdominal pain occur. Indications of hepatic damage become evident biochemically within 2 to 6 days of ingestion of toxic doses. Prominent increases in the transaminase enzymes and lesser increases in alkaline phosphatase are common. The hepatotoxicity may precipitate jaundice and coagulation disorders and progress to encephalopathy, coma, and death. Tinnitus, or ringing in the ears, is a feature of chronic salicylate intoxication and is not encountered in acetaminophen overdose. *(Gilman et al, pp 694–695)*

759. **The answer is A (1,2,3).** Chronic abuse of sedative–hypnotics (e.g., barbiturates) results in drug tolerance to other agents within this class by (1) enhanced metabolism of similar agents and (2) cross-pharmacodynamic tolerance. Cross-tolerance by a pharmacodynamic mechanism has implications in the clinical management of withdrawal symptoms or detoxification. Patients who chronically abuse short-acting barbiturates, benzodiazepines (e.g., secobarbital, diazepam), or alcohol may undergo detoxification using a longer-acting agent, such as phenobarbital. Cross-tolerance does not extend to opiates. Sedative–hypnotics may be useful in symptomatic management of symptoms associated with withdrawal from opiates. *(Khantzian and McKenna)*

760. **The answer is B (1,3).** The movement of drug from one compartment (gastrointestinal tract) to another (blood) depends on several factors. Since most drug absorption from the gastrointestinal tract is via passive processes, the pH partition concept (as outlined in the question) predicts that a weak acid will exist in its nonionized form in the acidic environment of the stomach to a greater extent than in the more alkaline intestine and thus one would predict that absorption should be faster from the stomach. However, other important factors need to be considered, and since both surface area (200 vs 1 m²) and blood flow (1.0 L/min vs. 0.15 L/min) to exchanging sites are at least an order of magnitude greater in the intestine than in the stomach, the rate of absorption of drug from the intestine (even when the drug is ionized) will always be greater than from the stomach. The epithelium of the intestine has a low electrical resistance compared to that of the stomach, and this tends to offset the experimental and clinical observation noted in the question. Furthermore, a considerable portion of intestinal drainage enters the portal circulation, where first-pass liver effects may occur. *(Rowland and Tozier, p 22)*

761. **The answer is E (all).** Nephrotoxicity associated with gentamicin therapy resembles acute tubular necrosis. Manifestations include the inability to concentrate urine, proteinuria, and casts in the urine. Rising trough concentrations appear to be an early indicator of renal damage. If gentamicin is discontinued, damage is reversible. *(Gilman et al, p 1162)*

762. **The answer is A (1,2,3).** Parkinson's disease appears to be caused by a relative deficiency of dopamine in the basal ganglia of the brain. Levodopa, a precursor of dopamine, is transported into the CNS, where it is decarboxylated to form dopamine. Peripheral decarboxylation wastes a significant amount of absorbed levodopa and also causes peripheral side effects (e.g., cardiac arrhythmias, nausea, vomiting). Although levodopa is effective when used alone, peripheral conversion to dopamine may be inhibited by administration of carbidopa, a dopa-decarboxylase inhibitor. Carbidopa does not cross the blood–brain barrier and thus has no effect on conversion of levodopa to dopamine. Inhibition of peripheral destruction of levodopa allows a larger and more predictable proportion to enter the brain. *(Boshes)*

BIBLIOGRAPHY

Boshes BB. Sinemet and the treatment of Parkinson's. *Ann Intern Med.* March 1981; 364–370.

Covino BJ. Pharmacology of local anesthetics. *Rational Drug Ther.* 1987; 21:1–8.

Craig CR, Stitzel RE, eds. *Modern Pharmacology.* 2nd ed. Boston: Little, Brown and Co; 1986.

DeLuca HF. Vitamin D metabolism and function. *Arch Intern Med.* 1978; 138:836.

Freston JW. Cimetidine. I. Developments, pharmacology, and efficacy. *Ann Intern Med.* October 1982; 573–580.

Gilman AG, Goodman LS, Rall TW, Murad F, eds. *The Pharmacological Basis of Therapeutics.* 7th ed. New York: Macmillan; 1985.

Hollister LE. Treatment of depression with drugs. *Ann Intern Med.* July 1978; 78–84.

Hollister LE. Perspectives and summary of aspirin/acetaminophen symposium. *Arch Intern Med.* February 23, 1981; 404–406.

Jawetz EJ, Melnick L, Adelberg EA. *Review of Medical Microbiology.* 14th ed. Los Altos, Calif: Lange Medical Publications, 1980.

Katcher BS, Young LY, Koda-Kimble MA. *Applied Therapeutics: The Clinical Use of Drugs.* 3rd ed. San Francisco: Applied Therapeutics, Inc, 1983.

Khantzian EJ, McKenna GJ. Acute toxic and withdrawal reactions associated with drug use and abuse. *Ann Intern Med.* 1979; 90:361.

Lees KR. Angiotensin-converting enzyme inhibitors. *Rational Drug Ther.* 1988; 22:1–6.

Levine J. Pain and analgesia: The outlook for more rational treatment. *Ann Intern Med.* February 1984; 269–276.

Lindeman RD, Papper S. Therapy of fluid and electrolyte disorders. *Ann Intern Med.* January 1975; 64–70.

Rang HP, Dale MM, eds. *Pharmacology.* Edinburgh: Churchill Livingstone; 1987.

Rowland M, Tozier TN. *Clinical Pharmacokinetics: Concepts and Applications.* Philadelphia: Lea & Febiger; 1980.

Swinyard EA, White HS, Wolf HH. Mechanisms of anticonvulsant drugs. *ISI Atlas Sci Pharmacol.* 1988; 2:95–98.

Thompson WG. Laxatives: Clinical pharmacology and rational use. *Drugs.* January 1980; 49–58.

Subspecialty List: Pharmacology

704. Autonomic nervous system
705. Chemotherapeutic agents (topical and systemic)
Antineoplastic and immunosuppressive drugs
706. Chemotherapeutic agents (topical and systemic)
Antineoplastic and immunosuppressive drugs
707. Chemotherapeutic agents (topical and systemic)
Antineoplastic and immunosuppressive drugs
708. Chemotherapeutic agents (topical and systemic)
Antineoplastic and immunosuppressive drugs
709. Chemotherapeutic agents (topical and systemic)
Antineoplastic and immunosuppressive drugs
710. Chemotherapeutic agents (topical and systemic)
Antineoplastic and immunosuppressive drugs
711. Respiratory system
712. Respiratory system
713. Autonomic nervous system
714. Autonomic nervous system
715. Autacoids, histamine, and antagonists
716. Autacoids, histamine, and antagonists
717. Chemotherapeutic agents
Antineoplastic drugs
718. Chemotherapeutic agents
Antineoplastic drugs
719. Chemotherapeutic agents
Antineoplastic drugs
720. Chemotherapeutic agents
Antineoplastic drugs
721. Chemotherapeutic agents
Antineoplastic drugs
722. Endocrine system
723. Endocrine system
724. Cardiovascular and respiratory systems
725. Cardiovascular and respiratory systems
726. Cardiovascular and respiratory systems
727. Cardiovascular and respiratory systems
728. Nonnarcotic analgesia
729. Nonnarcotic analgesia
730. Nonnarcotic analgesia
731. Nonnarcotic analgesia
732. Antibiotics
733. Antibiotics
734. Antibiotics
735. Antibiotics
736. Cardiovascular and respiratory systems
Antiarrhythmic agents
737. Chemotherapeutic agents
738. Chemotherapeutic agents
739. Cardiovascular and respiratory systems
740. Cardiovascular and respiratory systems
741. Cardiovascular system
742. Blood and blood-forming organs
743. Poisoning and therapy of intoxication
744. General principles
745. Central and peripheral nervous systems
746. Autacoids and prostaglandins
747. Cardiovascular and respiratory systems
748. Autacoids and prostaglandins
749. Kidneys, bladder, fluids, and electrolytes
Uricosurics
750. Central and peripheral nervous systems
751. Chemotherapeutic agents
752. Blood and blood-forming organs
753. CNS agents
754. Blood and blood-forming organs
755. Chemotherapeutic agents
756. Central and peripheral nervous systems
757. Poisoning and therapy of intoxication
758. Poisoning
759. CNS agents
760. General principles
761. Chemotherapeutic agents
Antibacterial drugs
762. CNS agents

CHAPTER 7

Behavioral Sciences
Questions

DIRECTIONS (Questions 763 through 792): Each of the numbered items or incomplete statements in this section is followed by answers or by completions of the statement. Select the ONE lettered answer or completion that is BEST in each case.

763. A patient who is afraid of insects is first shown a picture of a butterfly. Next session, he is put in the same room as a bottle containing ants. This procedure may be an example of

    (A) biofeedback
    (B) shaping
    (C) desensitization
    (D) operant conditioning
    (E) stimulus generalization

764. The functions of the ego include all of the following EXCEPT

    (A) psychologic defense mechanisms
    (B) reality testing
    (C) thinking
    (D) perception
    (E) instinctual drives

765. In a prospective randomized study comparing drug A to placebo, by the luck of the draw, 80 of the 120 patients assigned to placebo were young and had relatively minor disease severity, whereas 80 of the 120 patients in the group assigned to drug A were older and more severely diseased. The authors report that 95 placebo-treated patients and 98 patients treated with drug A are alive at the end of 5 yr. They calculate chi-square and report that drug A is no better than placebo. Which of the following statements is true?

    (A) drug A is no more effective than placebo
    (B) matched pair analysis might demonstrate that drug A is better than placebo
    (C) since the patients were assigned by random allocation, it is not possible that the two groups would vary so much in baseline characteristics

    (D) stratified analysis of the data might demonstrate that drug A is more effective than placebo
    (E) this is an example of β error

766. In general, medical students experience all of the following EXCEPT

    (A) increasing identification with the medical profession
    (B) exposure to students from diverse backgrounds
    (C) increasing idealism throughout medical school
    (D) anxiety concerning evaluations and examinations
    (E) tendency for specialization

767. Which of the following statements concerning psychotherapy is correct?

    (A) psychotherapy can be performed only by professionals with special training in an accredited psychoanalytic institute
    (B) reliving childhood experience is the fundamental objective of psychotherapy
    (C) physical examination may be psychotherapeutic
    (D) giving advice is countertherapeutic
    (E) insight is always the goal in psychotherapy

768. A delusion may be distinguished from a hallucination on the basis of

    (A) consensual validation
    (B) perceptual experience
    (C) grandiosity
    (D) laboratory tests
    (E) intelligence tests

769. All of the following statements concerning the drug treatment of elderly patients is true EXCEPT

 (A) drug clearance may be delayed because of increased fat/muscle ratio
 (B) there may be increased toxicity due to decreased plasma albumin levels
 (C) excretion half-life of drugs may be increased because of decreased liver function
 (D) there may be decreased extrapyramidal side effects with neuroleptics because of decreased nigrostriatal dopamine
 (E) there may be increased sensitivity to anticholinergic drugs due to decreased CNS cholinergic functioning

770. Goslings that are exposed to humans early in life may follow them as if humans were their mothers. This conduct is an example of

 (A) instrumental conditioning
 (B) imprinting
 (C) cognitive map
 (D) instinctual behavior
 (E) counterphobic behavior

771. The double line of authority in the hospital is most likely to cause a conflict between professional and administrative roles for

 (A) physicians
 (B) hospital administrators
 (C) nurses
 (D) patients
 (E) hospital security officers

772. Assuming that 98 percent of all people with a particular illness, such as depression, will have positive results on a hypothetical new screening test and that 90 percent of all people without the illness will have a negative result, which of the following statements will be true when the test is used to screen a general population?

 (A) someone having a positive result has a 98 percent chance of having the illness
 (B) someone having a negative result has a 2 percent chance of having the illness
 (C) someone having a positive result has a 90 percent chance of having the illness
 (D) ten percent of the people with negative results will have the illness
 (E) none of the above

773. During human development, the capacity to discriminate between different sounds can first be demonstrated

 (A) in the newborn
 (B) at 3 mo
 (C) at 6 mo
 (D) at 9 mo
 (E) at 12 mo

774. Approximately what percentage of deaths among persons between 15 and 24 yr of age is attributable to accidents, murder, and suicide?

 (A) 10
 (B) 20
 (C) 40
 (D) 60
 (E) 75

775. The suicide rate is highest among

 (A) boys between the ages of 11 and 14 yr
 (B) girls between the ages of 15 and 19 yr
 (C) boys between the ages of 15 and 19 yr
 (D) girls between the ages of 11 and 14 yr
 (E) women between the ages of 20 and 25 yr

776. Thirty seventh-grade students who scored in the lowest tenth percentile of their class on a reading examination are assigned to a special education class in reading for a year. At the end of the year, the reading scores of these students are significantly improved in comparison with the rest of the class. Which of the following threats to internal validity is most likely to account for the improvement?

 (A) history
 (B) testing
 (C) statistical regression
 (D) instrumentation
 (E) maturation

777. Among children who are severely retarded, the percentage that shows some type of psychiatric disorder is

 (A) 10
 (B) 20
 (C) 30
 (D) 50
 (E) 75

778. In a case-control study of the relationship between exposure to a suspected toxic substance and the development of a rare type of cancer, 16 of 20 cases were exposed to the substance, whereas only 20 of 80 controls were exposed. The relative risk of developing the cancer among exposed subjects is best estimated to be

(A) 0.32
(B) 3.20
(C) 12.00
(D) 12.80
(E) none of the above

779. The most effective antidepressant therapy is

(A) tricyclic antidepressants
(B) monoamine oxidase inhibitors
(C) lithium carbonate
(D) psychotherapy
(E) electroconvulsive therapy (ECT)

780. All of the following are examples of biofeedback EXCEPT

(A) electric shock given to a person when antisocial behavior is manifested
(B) electronic display of skin temperature
(C) a physician's telling a patient that, as a result of a diet, the patient's blood pressure (BP) is reduced
(D) electroconvulsive therapy (ECT) given to a depressed patient
(E) tension headache treated with electromyogram

781. Tardive dyskinesia may be caused by all of the following EXCEPT

(A) perphenazine
(B) amoxapine
(C) trifluoperazine
(D) clorazepate
(E) haloperidol

782. A 38-year-old woman tells her physician that for several months she has been experiencing palpitations, shortness of breath, and a feeling of impending doom. She also has episodes of dizziness and a feeling that she is going to drop dead. The physician's first course of action should be to

(A) provide psychotherapy
(B) treat the patient with benzodiazepines
(C) perform a physical examination
(D) refer the patient to a psychiatrist
(E) teach the patient self-hypnosis

783. A patient is convinced that an IV injection he received has made him immortal. This is an example of

(A) illusion
(B) delusion
(C) hallucination
(D) delirium
(E) euphoria

784. Drugs used in the treatment of schizophrenia have in common their ability to

(A) block α-adrenergic receptors in the locus ceruleus
(B) block dopamine receptors in the brain
(C) sensitize the dopamine receptors in the locus ceruleus
(D) increase functional levels of norepinephrine in the synapses
(E) increase serotonin synthesis in the CNS

785. All of the following have been implicated as possible neurotransmitters EXCEPT

(A) norepinephrine
(B) endorphins
(C) γ-aminobutyric acid (GABA)
(D) serum pepsinogen
(E) glycine

Questions 786 through 789

A 35-year-old man is admitted to the hospital for an elective operation. After a week's stay in the hospital, during which various examinations are performed, he receives general anesthesia for an abdominal operation. Two days after the operation, he becomes agitated, visibly tremulous, and seems to be hallucinating. He also accuses the nurses of being unsympathetic and uncaring, just like his own mother.

786. In relation to this patient's agitation and hallucination, a history of which of the following would have most immediate relevance in management plans?

(A) schizophrenic family members
(B) alcoholism
(C) LSD use
(D) depression
(E) traumatic early childhood

787. This patient's accusatory behavior toward the nurses may be attributed to all of the following EXCEPT

    (A) transference
    (B) displacement
    (C) sublimation
    (D) regression
    (E) organic brain syndrome

788. If this patient's hallucinations are predominantly visual, the likelihood of which of the following diagnoses is increased?

    (A) organic brain syndrome
    (B) schizophrenia
    (C) depressive syndrome
    (D) anxiety neurosis
    (E) transference neurosis

789. Which of the following is LEAST likely to be essential in formulating effective management plans for this patient?

    (A) laboratory studies, e.g., electrolytes, blood urea nitrogen (BUN)
    (B) chart review to determine intraoperative complications
    (C) interview with the patient's mother to determine the quality of interaction in childhood
    (D) interview with the patient to get a good description of the hallucinations
    (E) interview with the patient's girl friend to determine drug and alcohol history

790. In the Isle of Wight study, the percentage of children who scored more than 2 standard deviations below the norm on the Wechsler Intelligence Scale for Children (WISC) was

    (A) 1.25
    (B) 2.51
    (C) 5.12
    (D) 8.40
    (E) 12.05

791. An example of rapid-eye-movement (REM) sleep disorder may be

    (A) narcolepsy
    (B) epilepsy
    (C) catalepsy
    (D) polydipsia
    (E) cachexia

792. All of the following are examples of biologic rhythms EXCEPT

    (A) rapid-eye-movement (REM) sleep
    (B) menstrual cycle
    (C) vernal equinox
    (D) basic rest–activity cycle
    (E) depressive mood swings

DIRECTIONS (Questions 793 through 837): Each group of items in this section consists of lettered headings followed by a set of numbered words or phrases. For each numbered word or phrase, select the ONE lettered heading that is most closely associated with it. Each lettered heading may be selected once, more than once, or not at all.

Questions 793 through 801

For each item listed below, choose the brain wave or phenomenon with which it is usually associated.

    (A) α wave
    (B) β wave
    (C) Δ wave
    (D) rapid-eye-movement (REM) sleep
    (E) cataplexy

793. Concentrating on mental arithmetic

794. Sudden loss of muscle tone

795. Non-REM (NREM) sleep

796. Sleepwalking

797. Irregular pulse rate and respiration

798. Visual dreams

799. Narcolepsy

800. Comatose state

801. Relaxed, awake state

Questions 802 through 804

For each study design described below, choose the major flaw or bias in its construction.

  (A) selection bias or confounding
  (B) Berkson's bias
  (C) overmatching
  (D) recall bias
  (E) no bias, no flaws

802. In a case-control study of toxic shock syndrome (TSS) demonstrating that Brand X tampons were a cause of TSS, controls were age-, race-, and gender-matched community controls (neighbors).

803. In a case-control study of the relationship between diethylstilbestrol (DES) use during pregnancy and the subsequent development of vaginal cancer in the offspring, controls were chosen from the birth records (controls were the next recorded female birth from the same hospital at which the patient was born). Use of DES during pregnancy was ascertained by inspection of the medical records of prenatal and obstetric care. During the period under study, DES was used for high-risk pregnancies or threatened abortions.

804. In a case-control study investigating the reputed importance of exposure to benzene as a cause of leukemia, controls were chosen from the workmates of cases.

Questions 805 through 808

For each experiment or research design described below, select the statistical test that would be most appropriate for the analysis of the data.

  (A) correlation coefficient
  (B) chi-square
  (C) Student's t-test
  (D) paired Student's t-test
  (E) Wilcoxon matched-pairs signed rank test

805. Sixty patients with a certain disease are randomly assigned to receive treatment A or placebo. Condition after 1 yr for each patient is rated as improved, no change, or deteriorated.

806. Two surgically similar wounds were inflicted on each of 10 rats. One wound was sutured; the other was taped. At the end of 10 days, tensile strength was measured using a spring scale that was judged to be accurate to about 10 lb/in².

807. To determine whether there is any relationship between blood pressure (BP) and serum cholesterol levels, BP and serum cholesterol levels are mea-

sured in a cross-sectional study of hypertensive patients.

808. Forty patients with hypertension are treated with active drug for 1 mo and placebo for 1 mo using a sophisticated cross-over design and washout period (to mitigate against the effects of secular trend or drug carryover). Blood pressure (BP) for each patient is determined during treatment with active drug and placebo according to a prearranged plan.

Questions 809 through 815

For each description below, choose the defense mechanism with which it is most closely associated.

  (A) repression
  (B) projection
  (C) isolation
  (D) regression
  (E) identification

809. A patient described, without showing any emotion, the details of an automobile accident in which his closest friend died.

810. A 6-yr-old child was brought to the doctor for bed-wetting. He had been successfully toilet trained previously. The mother is expecting a baby soon.

811. Free association may be effective against this.

812. Paranoid patients often manifest this.

813. Persons who had been abused as children often become child abusers.

814. May explain why so many people think the old days were so good.

815. A psychotic patient is found in bed in the fetal position.

Questions 816 through 823

For each description below, choose the neurotransmitter with which it is usually associated.

  (A) serotonin
  (B) norepinephrine
  (C) dopamine
  (D) acetylcholine
  (E) γ-aminobutyric acid (GABA)

816. Much of this substance in the brain is produced by the locus ceruleus

817. This substance opens the chloride channel

818. Blockers of this substance are effective in schizophrenia

819. An indoleamine

820. Decreased in Alzheimer's disease

821. Ingestion of L-tryptophan increases the levels of this substance in the brain

822. Dryness of mouth, constipation, and blurred vision are side effects of many antidepressants caused by the blocking of the effects of this substance

823. A depletion of this substance in the brain often results in muscular rigidity and tremors

Questions 824 through 827

For each developmental phase described below, select the age at which it is most likely to occur.

(A) 0 to 2 mo
(B) 2 to 8 mo
(C) 9 to 10 mo
(D) 10 to 17 mo
(E) 18 to 36 mo

824. Normal autistic phase

825. Separation-individuation phase

826. Normal symbiotic phase

827. Object constancy

Questions 828 through 831

For each of the following studies or problems, choose the most appropriate multivariable method of analysis.

(A) discriminant function analysis
(B) log linear modeling
(C) factor analysis
(D) analysis of variance
(E) analysis of covariance

828. One hundred mildly to severely hypertensive patients are randomly assigned to one of two treatment regimens. Blood pressure (BP) is determined for each patient before treatment and after 1 mo of treatment. Treatments are to be compared.

829. It is necessary to determine two indices, one measuring demoralization and the other measuring somatization, based on the information obtained from four separate questionnaires that were administered to 200 people and that initially were de-

signed to assess depression, anxiety, anger, and psychophysiologic symptoms.

830. It is to be determined which items measured on a 21-item life stress checklist predict the onset of illness during the 6 mo following health screening.

831. It is necessary to evaluate the effects of gender, socioeconomic status, and marital status on a happiness scale.

Questions 832 through 835

For an investigation of each situation described below, choose the study design that is most appropriate.

(A) retrospective case control
(B) randomized controlled clinical trial
(C) observational cohort
(D) cross-sectional survey
(E) prospective single-case study

832. The causes of or risk factors for a rare disease

833. An association between two diseases

834. The efficacy of a new intervention

835. The hazards of occupational or environmental exposure

Questions 836 and 837

For each of the following hypothetical situations, choose the most appropriate control population.

(A) community control
(B) hospital control
(C) matched control
(D) historical control
(E) no control necessary

836. A new case-control study designed to rebut criticisms that a previous study was flawed by Berkson's bias.

837. Investigation of a new treatment for a uniformly fatal disease.

DIRECTIONS (Questions 838 through 854): Each group of items in this section consists of lettered headings followed by a set of numbered words or phrases. For each numbered word or phrase, select

A if the item is associated with (A) only,
B if the item is associated with (B) only,
C if the item is associated with both (A) and (B),
D if the item is associated with neither (A) nor (B).

Questions 838 through 845

(A) oral stage
(B) anal stage
(C) both
(D) neither

838. Pregenital

839. Sucking

840. Parsimony

841. Sadism

842. Dependency

843. Fixation

844. Freudian developmental scheme

845. Penis envy

Questions 846 through 854

(A) endorphins (enkephalins)
(B) morphine
(C) both
(D) neither

846. Action blocked by naloxone

847. Synthesized endogenously

848. Tolerance develops

849. Analgesic effect

850. Behavioral change

851. Peptide

852. Effect on respiration

853. Neurotransmitter/neuromodulator

854. Catecholamine

DIRECTIONS (Questions 855 through 889): For each of the items in this section, ONE or MORE of the numbered options is correct. Choose the answer

A if only 1, 2, and 3 are correct,
B if only 1 and 3 are correct,
C if only 2 and 4 are correct,
D if only 4 is correct,
E if all are correct.

855. Depressive symptoms often are associated with

(1) hypothyroidism
(2) propranolol
(3) cancer of pancreas
(4) levodopa

856. A 30-yr-old woman complains of episodic faintness, tingling sensation in her hands, shortness of breath, and severe anxiety. Thorough medical workup reveals no pathologic condition. During an episode of these symptoms, chemical analysis of the serum will probably reveal

(1) decreased chloride
(2) increased blood urea nitrogen (BUN)
(3) decreased protein
(4) increased pH

857. Most children with emotional disorders are thought to

(1) grow up to become normal adults who do not have a neurosis
(2) develop neuroses or depressive states if their emotional disorder persists into adulthood
(3) have an ominous prognosis if they show antisocial behavior between 6 and 11 yr of age
(4) develop a psychosis if their emotional disorder persists into adulthood

Questions 858 through 862

A 42-yr-old widow complains of persistent burning pain in her right forearm. The patient has a history of recurrent depression. Her husband died of a myocardial infarction within the past year.

858. Possible diagnoses include

(1) causalgia
(2) depressive equivalent
(3) psychogenic pain
(4) myocardial infarction

859. If the patient described has difficulty falling asleep and frequently awakens from sleep because of the pain, which of the following may be true?

    (1) depression is possible

    (2) causalgia is possible

    (3) the symptoms are indicative of anxiety

    (4) the pain is likely to be organic

860. The nerve fibers conducting this patient's pain are likely to be

    (1) large myelinated fibers

    (2) those that carry vibration sense

    (3) sensory efferent fibers

    (4) C fibers

861. If the patient described is an exacting, orderly kind of person, which of the following approaches may be helpful?

    (1) give general reassurance to the patient

    (2) refrain from prescribing tranquilizers

    (3) give explanations that are nonspecific and general

    (4) administer pain medication on a "reverse prn" schedule

862. If this patient had her right arm amputated 6 mo previously, which of the following statements could be true?

    (1) the patient is obviously malingering

    (2) depression may be related to the pain

    (3) the symptoms are indicative of severe psychopathology

    (4) the gate-control theory may be relevant

863. According to a study by J. E. O'Malley and colleagues, children who have survived for more than 60 mo with cancer

    (1) frequently used denial as a coping mechanism

    (2) in most instances felt they had the right to know the diagnosis

    (3) would have liked to have had some form of psychosocial intervention during their illness

    (4) tend to have psychologic difficulties

864. Children's imaginary companions may serve as

    (1) an auxiliary conscience for the child's use

    (2) a scapegoat when the child commits some forbidden act

    (3) a vicarious means of gratifying some impulse

    (4) an adaptive mechanism to help master anxiety

865. Which of the following statements may be true concerning the development of seizures in children who are diagnosed as having autism?

    (1) about one fifth will develop seizures either in childhood or adolescence

    (2) the risk of developing seizures varies as age increases

    (3) the highest risk occurs between the ages of 11 and 14 yr

    (4) the rate for developing seizures is higher than for children in the general population

866. An attention deficit disorder may be present if a child shows

    (1) excessive activity, restlessness, fidgetiness, or an inability to sit still

    (2) difficulty in sustaining attention, disorganization, apparent forgetfulness, or poor independent performance

    (3) impulsive behavior, sloppy work, speaking out of turn, difficulty in waiting, or a low frustration tolerance

    (4) a preference for homosexual choices in peer relationships, excessive masturbation, and gender identity problems

867. According to a study by L. H. Robins, serious antisocial behavior in children between the ages of 6 and 11 yr is often

    (1) a predictor of violence in adolescence

    (2) the result of febrile seizures during infancy

    (3) later associated with a high risk of schizophrenia

    (4) the cause of parental divorce

868. According to a study by Dorothy Lewis and colleagues, when very violent incarcerated delinquent adolescents are compared with their less violent counterparts, they are more likely to

    (1) have been severely abused and to have witnessed violence at home

    (2) be paranoid and have loose, illogical thought processes

    (3) have major neurologic impairment

    (4) have soft neurologic signs and severe learning disabilities

869. According to Winnicott, the transitional object may

(1) represent the breast
(2) represent feces
(3) eventually develop into a fetish object
(4) be used again at a later age when deprivation threatens

870. According to Thomas et al, temperament in children includes such descriptive categories as

(1) activity level
(2) rhythmicity of biologic functions
(3) approach or withdrawal responses
(4) adaptability to change

871. Attachment behavior in infancy includes

(1) crying
(2) smiling
(3) vocalizing
(4) clinging

872. Infants at 1 wk of age appear to be visually attracted to

(1) moving objects
(2) distinctive patterns
(3) facelike mosaics
(4) the human breast

873. Alzheimer's disease

(1) is the most common dementing disease of the elderly
(2) is caused by aluminum deficiency
(3) is associated with Down's syndrome (trisomy 21)
(4) has physostigmine as the treatment of choice

874. True statements concerning information that is required for evaluating a patient include

(1) the patient's current state helps determine the immediate needs
(2) the patient's personality helps determine how the physician should approach the patient
(3) recent changes in the patient's environment may disclose contributing factors to illness
(4) psychologic defense mechanisms should be treated immediately

875. Placebo is characterized by its

(1) lack of observable effects
(2) ability to release endorphins
(3) usefulness in diagnosing psychogenic pain
(4) ability to produce side effects

876. The cognitive functions include

(1) memory
(2) orientation
(3) abstraction
(4) affect

877. Which of the following statements may describe the physician–patient relationship?

(1) it is an example of a contractual relationship
(2) placebo effects may occur
(3) it involves "unconscious" psychotherapy
(4) problems therein may lead to a tort

878. Methods used in treating premature ejaculation include

(1) stop–start
(2) free association
(3) squeeze technique
(4) sensate focusing

879. Which of the following factors may increase morbidity and mortality from physical illness?

(1) depression
(2) psychiatric impairment
(3) bereavement
(4) heredity

880. The fight–flight reaction described by Walter Cannon is characterized by

(1) sympathetic arousal
(2) activation of hypothalamus
(3) pituitary–adrenocortical activation
(4) conservation–withdrawal reaction

881. Concerning cocaine

(1) speedball contains cocaine
(2) symptoms of cocaine abuse include depression and anhedonia
(3) crack or freebase is the alkaloid form of cocaine
(4) symptoms of cocaine withdrawal include depression and fatigue

882. In the USA, opiate addiction is more common among

(1) lower socioeconomic groups than higher socioeconomic groups
(2) racial minorities than racial majorities
(3) psychiatrically disturbed persons than normal persons
(4) physicians than the laity

SUMMARY OF DIRECTIONS				
A	**B**	**C**	**D**	**E**
1, 2, 3 only	1, 3 only	2, 4 only	4 only	All are correct

883. Signs and symptoms of opiate intoxication include

(1) decreased respiratory rate and depth

(2) miosis

(3) scratching

(4) increased blood pressure (BP) and pulse

884. Signs and symptoms of phencyclidine (PCP) overdose include

(1) nystagmus

(2) hypertension

(3) sweating

(4) fever

885. Treatment for PCP-induced psychosis includes

(1) talking down

(2) benzodiazepines

(3) phenothiazines

(4) ammonium chloride

886. The *Diagnostic and Statistical Manual of Mental Disorders*, 3rd ed. rev. (*DSM-III-R*) diagnostic criteria for schizophrenia include the following characteristic psychotic symptoms in the active phase

(1) delusions

(2) hallucinations

(3) catatonic behavior

(4) flat or grossly inappropriate affect

887. Physicians, as compared with the general population, have a higher prevalence of

(1) drug addiction

(2) suicide

(3) alcoholism

(4) troubled marriage

888. *DSM-III-R* uses a multiaxial diagnostic scheme. Which of the following are correct?

(1) clinical syndromes are recorded in axis I

(2) developmental disorders are recorded in axis II

(3) physical diseases are recorded in axis III

(4) axis I may include conditions that are not attributable to a mental disorder

889. According to *DSM-III-R*, somatoform disorders include

(1) conversion disorder

(2) body dysmorphic disorder

(3) hypochondriasis

(4) malingering

Answers and Explanations

763. The answer is C. Desensitization is a procedure in which a phobic object (insect, in this case) is presented to the patient repeatedly in a nonthreatening way in gradual increments so that extinction to the conditioned response (fear) might occur. *(Leigh and Reiser, pp 41–76; Kaplan and Sadock, pp 184–198, 903–904)*

764. The answer is E. The ego functions include emotions, defense mechanisms, cognitive and perceptual functions, movement, and so forth. The ego is the agent of the personality system that mediates between the demands of the id, which is the reservoir of instinctual drives, and the demands of the superego, which represents parental and societal values. The ego also mediates between the personality system and external reality. *(Kaplan and Sadock, pp 386–391)*

765. The answer is D. Despite randomization, the two groups described in the question differed in baseline susceptibility, and drug A may be more effective than placebo. Matching must be performed before randomization and is probably logistically impossible. Stratified analysis would allow comparison of groups stratified according to equivalent baseline susceptibility—outcome for young and relatively healthy patients in one group would be compared with outcome for young and relatively healthy patients in the other group. Similarly, outcome for older and more severely diseased patients would be compared for each treatment. β Error (or type II error), which refers to the failure to reject the null hypothesis when the experimental hypothesis is true, results from not having a large enough sample size to demonstrate a particular level or magnitude of difference. *(MacMahon and Pugh, pp 278–281)*

766. The answer is C. Medical students experience an increasing identification with the medical profession. The student is exposed to persons from different backgrounds. There is generally much anxiety concerning evaluations and examinations. Unfortunately, the idealism that students originally brought into the medical school seems to fade. There is also a tendency for medical students to decide on specialization, although they may originally have intended to remain in general practice. *(Simons, pp 423–440)*

767. The answer is C. Physical examination is a potent psychotherapeutic tool in that it can reduce the patient's anxiety and provide effective reassurance. Psychotherapy may be performed by any clinician, knowingly or not. Whereas insight is the goal of depth psychotherapy, increase in coping ability is often the goal in supportive and other types of psychotherapy. *(Leigh and Reiser, pp 385–399)*

768. The answer is B. Both hallucination and delusion lack consensual validation. Delusion is a fixed idea or belief that is not based on reality. Hallucinations are perceptual experiences that are not based on stimulus from reality and that cannot be substantiated by normal observers. *(Leigh and Reiser, pp 143–175)*

769. The answer is D. With increasing age, there is decreased nigrostriatal dopamine, resulting in an increase rather than decrease in extrapyramidal side effects with neuroleptics. Other age-related changes include delayed absorption because of the antacids, milk of magnesia, or anticholinergic drugs that many elderly patients take, decreased first-pass effect with age and congestive heart failure, decreased hepatic function in general, decrease in renal function causing decreased lithium clearance and delay in reaching steady-state of lithium, and increased CNS sensitivity to benzodiazepines. *(Leigh and Reiser, pp 194–195)*

770. The answer is B. Imprinting refers to early learning that occurs during a critical period. It is characterized by rapidity and specificity. Instinctual behavior refers to preprogrammed, unlearned behavior. *(Kaplan and Saddock, pp 424–443)*

771. The answer is C. The nurses in a hospital are directly responsible to the hospital administration and also to the physicians concerning clinical matters. The physicians are responsible only to other physicians in a hierarchy usually apart from the administrative hierarchy of the hospital. Other staff personnel, including clerks and security guards, are responsible only to the hospital administration. *(Leigh and Reiser, pp 365–383)*

772. The answer is E. The percentage of people having positive (or negative) test results who have (or do not have) an illness (e.g., depression) will depend on the prevalence of that illness in the population studied. For example, if the prevalence of depression is 1 in 10,000 and 1,000,000 people are studied, 100 people will have the illness, 10 percent of the 999,900 people without it will have positive results (99,990 false positives), and 98 percent of the 100 people affected will have positive results (98 true positives). In this situation, only 98 of 100,088 people with positive results will have depression (less than 1 percent). Alternatively, if the population consisted only of people with the illness, 100 percent of the people with positive results would have depression. *(Feinstein, pp 215–226)*

773. The answer is A. Infants appear to be programmed to move in rhythm to the human voice. Observations have shown that they will orient with eyes, head, and body to animated sound stimuli. Within a few weeks after birth, infants are able to differentiate between sounds and make more appropriate responses. Obviously, this ability increases with maturity during the first year. *(Friedlander)*

774. The answer is E. Deaths due to violent causes are more common in the age group between 15 and 24 yr than among younger persons. Accidents and homicides constitute the major portion of these deaths, followed by suicides. Children younger than 12 yr rarely commit suicide, but thereafter the incidence increases through age 24 yr. *(Department of Health and Human Services)*

775. The answer is C. The ratio of attempted suicide increases by a factor of 10 between the ages of 15 and 19 yr, compared with the rate between the ages of 10 and 14 yr. At the same time, the ratio of boys to girls who commit suicide is 3 : 1. In 1979, suicide was the fourth cause of death among adolescents and rose to the second cause of death in 1982, surpassed only by accidents. *(Committee on Adolescence, American Academy of Pediatrics)*

776. The answer is C. A variety of random factors, including measurement error, transient illness, or random sloppiness, might account for low reading scores of many of the students assigned to a special education class. Since these random factors might account for the low scores, on retesting 1 yr later,

the group would be expected to regress toward the mean score, even in the absence of any intervention. Although historical factors, changes in the test (instrumentation), testing (learning from the test), and maturation might all affect performance on the second test, these factors would be likely to affect both the students who received special education and those who did not. *(Campbell and Stanley)*

777. The answer is D. The rate of psychiatric disorders among mentally retarded children is 50 percent. The rate found among the general population is 37 percent. There is nothing particularly characteristic about the kind of psychiatric disorder found among retarded children. *(Rutter et al)*

778. The answer is C. In a case-control study, the odds ratio serves as a good estimate of the relative risk. The odds ratio is defined as the ratio of cases to controls in the exposed group divided by the ratio of cases to controls in the unexposed group (in this example, $[16/20]/[4/60] = 12$). Since incidence rates of the disease for the exposed and nonexposed population are not calculated, the true relative risk can only be estimated. *(MacMahon and Pugh, pp 269–273)*

779. The answer is E. Although antidepressant drugs usually are used before ECT is considered, ECT remains the most effective (meaning that the response rate to ECT is higher than to other modalities) treatment for depression. ECT is indicated for patients who fail to respond to drug treatment. *(Leigh, p 134)*

780. The answer is D. Although biofeedback usually involves modern electronic instrumentation, the essence of the technique is the feedback of biologic information. ECT does involve the use of an electrical instrument, but there is no feedback element in this treatment. Although no sophisticated instrumentation is involved, a physician's telling the patient that the BP has been reduced entails all aspects of biofeedback, including a reward for desirable behavior (diet). *(Kaplan and Sadock, pp 1467–1473)*

781. The answer is D. Tardive dyskinesia is caused by neuroleptics that are dopamine receptor blockers (phenothiazines and butyrophenones). Amoxapine is an antidepressant that has dopamine-blocking function and has similar side effects as neuroleptics. Clorazepate is a benzodiazepine and is a muscle relaxant antianxiety agent. *(Leigh and Reiser, pp 401–418; Kaplan and Sadock, pp 1537–1553,1151–1152)*

782. The answer is C. The symptoms of the patient described in the question may result from anxiety alone, but a number of other causes must be ruled out first. These include hyperthyroidism, drug-induced states, and CNS-depressant withdrawal states. Physical examination and routine laboratory tests must be performed on all patients with anxiety symptoms before a specific course of treatment can be considered. *(Leigh and Reiser, pp 39–69)*

783. The answer is B. Delusion is a fixed idea or belief that does not correspond to reality. Hallucination is perception without stimulus. Illusion is distorted perception in the presence of stimulus. Delirium involves an alteration of the sensorium, with confusion and disorientation. Euphoria refers to expansive, exalted mood. *(Leigh and Reiser, p 145)*

784. The answer is B. All antipsychotic agents except rauwolfia alkaloids block dopamine receptors in the brain. Locus ceruleus is the site of most noradrenergic neurons in the brain. The dopaminergic neurons in the brain are primarily found in three areas—the basal ganglia (nigrostriatal tract), the midbrain (mesolimbic tract), and the hypothalamus. *(Leigh and Reiser, pp 412–414)*

785. The answer is D. Putative neurotransmitters include biogenic amines, such as norepinephrine, dopamine, and serotonin. Peptides such as endorphins are also neurotransmitters. GABA is a general inhibitory neurotransmitter. Glycine and substance P are also neurotransmitters. Serum pepsinogen is an enzyme. *(Leigh and Reiser, pp 58–60)*

786. The answer is B. The tremor and hallucinations experienced by the patient described in the question indicate the presence of delirium tremens. Physicians should be aware that alcoholic patients often do drink in the hospital. Following an operation, however, the patient is often allowed nothing by mouth, which may precipitate an alcoholic withdrawal state. *(Leigh and Reiser, pp 375–381)*

787. The answer is C. Transference may play a role in accusatory behavior, especially since the patient described in the question accused the nurses of being like his own mother. Regression results in the patient's feeling and thinking as though he were a child, which may in turn contribute to impulsiveness and increased transference feelings. His feelings concerning the nurses may be displacements from his mother. Organic brain syndrome, through reduction of higher cortical inhibitory functions, may increase distortion and impulsive behavior. Sublimation is the channeling of unacceptable impulses into acceptable and creative channels. *(Leigh and Reiser, pp. 77–98)*

788. The answer is A. Visual hallucinations are more common in patients with organic brain syndrome as opposed to schizophrenia. Visual hallucinations are particularly common in delirium tremens. Schizo-

phrenia usually is characterized by auditory hallucinations. *(Leigh and Reiser, p 165)*

789. The answer is C. Intraoperative factors may be important in causing postoperative organic brain syndrome. Laboratory tests may document a metabolic derangement that may account for the organic brain syndrome. Drug and alcohol history are important in considering withdrawal states. The patient's own description of the hallucinations is important in determining the possible cause of the syndrome; patient interview also is important to document the mental status. Early developmental history is of secondary importance in the management of acute organic brain syndrome. *(Leigh and Reiser, pp 177–207, 293–331)*

790. The answer is B. In the Isle of Wight study, 2.51 percent of children aged 9, 10 and 11 yr were found to be intellectually retarded. Among these children, 30 to 100 percent also were found to be behaviorally disturbed. This rate of disturbance is three to four times greater than the rate found in a control group. *(Rutter et al)*

791. The answer is A. Narcolepsy may be an REM sleep disorder. Hypnagogic hallucinations and cataplexy (sudden loss of muscle tone), often seen in patients with narcolepsy, may be caused by the dissociation of REM phenomena from sleep. Catalepsy refers to the waxy flexibility seen in patients with catatonic syndrome. *(Leigh and Reiser, pp 241–269)*

792. The answer is C. Biologic rhythms include ultradian, diurnal, and circadian rhythms. REM–nonREM (NREM) cycles, hormonal cycles (e.g., cortisol), and even pathologic cycles such as manic-depressive cycles are examples of biologic rhythms. Biologic rhythms are a subset of periodic phenomena, such as the vernal equinox, which is related to the earth's rotation around the sun. *(Leigh and Reiser, pp 241–269)*

793–801. The answers are 793-B, 794-E, 795-C, 796-C, 797-D, 798-D, 799-E, 800-C, 801-A. α waves are associated with a relaxed, awake state in which the subject's eyes are closed. Concentration, as during mental arithmetic, is associated with faster, β waves. Δ Waves (3 or less cycles per sec) are associated with NREM sleep (stages 3 and 4). Sleepwalking and night terrors occur during Δ wave sleep. Δ Waves are also prominent in comatose patients (the EEG tracing may be flat in very deeply comatose patients). REM sleep is characterized by visual dreams, relaxation of skeletal muscles, irregular respiration and pulse, and physiologic arousal, such as erection. Cataplexy is the sudden loss of muscle tone that occurs in narcolepsy. *(Leigh and Reiser, pp 241–269)*

802–804.   The answers are 802-D, 803-A, 804-C. The major flaw in the study design of question 802 is the possibility that women with TSS will be more likely to remember using a particular brand of tampon (especially one that the news media have already implicated) than will women who did not have TSS. Reports about the brand of tampon used need to be validated, although this may be quite difficult to accomplish. Berkson's bias, which refers to the differential rate of detection of disease in patients with and without the reputed risk factor, and confounding would not be problematic in this study.

In the study design of question 803, recall bias was avoided by the use of hospital records. The major flaw is the possibility that high-risk pregnancy or threatened abortion may be the cause or marker for the subsequent development of vaginal cancer as well as the cause of DES use. Rather than overmatched, the controls were undermatched, since they were less likely to have been high-risk pregnancies or threatened abortions.

In an attempt to avoid selection bias or possible confounding, the investigators in question 804 have ensured that the controls will have the same occupational exposure as the cases. Because both groups were exposed to benzene, benzene exposure could not be demonstrated as a risk factor for the occurrence of leukemia in this design, even if it were a significant risk factor (which it is). Controls should have an equivalent susceptibility to the development of the disease as the cases and an equivalent susceptibility to exposure as the cases, but they should not be overmatched to ensure that they have the same exposure history. *(MacMahon and Pugh, pp 207–282)*

805–808.   The answers are 805-B, 806-E, 807-A, 808-D. Chi-square is a nonparametric statistic that is particularly useful for analysis of categorical data (data measured nominally). In the situation described in question 805, outcome was measured in one of three categories. Chi-square is calculated by determining the difference between the observed frequency for each category (e.g., placebo-improved) and the expected frequency under the assumption that the treatment does not affect outcome.

Since the scale described in question 806 is not a true interval scale but is an ordinal scale and since we do not know anything about the underlying distribution of scores on the test, a nonparametric test should be used to analyze the data. The Wilcoxon matched-pairs signed rank test can be used on matched pairs in which measurements are made on an ordinal scale. The test is based on a ranking of the difference between scores obtained for each matched pair.

The correlation coefficient is particularly useful to describe the degree of association between two mutually dependent variables, as in question 807. The correlation coefficient (the product moment correlation or Pearson's coefficient of correlation) is unitless and varies between -1 and $+1$. A perfect correlation ($+1$ or -1) implies that the two variables are completely interdependent, whereas a zero correlation indicates that none of the variance of one variable can be explained by the other variable.

As described in question 808, each patient serves as his or her own control so that a paired Student's t-test is appropriate and has the greatest statistical power to demonstrate an association. Both the paired Student's t-test and the Student's t-test for independent samples compare the mean scores of the two groups and determine the probability of obtaining as large a difference (or larger) between the means if the two groups actually come from the same population. The probability will depend on the magnitude of the difference and the variance of the scores. *(Colton, pp 101–230)*

809–815.   The answers are 809-C, 810-D, 811-A, 812-B, 813-E, 814-A, 815-D. Isolation is the process by which painful emotions are selectively detached from factual memory, which may allow for factual report of a very traumatic event, such as an accident, without an emotional outburst. Regression is a pervasive change in personality to assume the attributes of an earlier age and, in severe form, is characteristic of severely ill schizophrenic patients. In less severe form, a child may unconsciously use this mechanism for increased attention. Repression relegates memories of conflictual or painful experiences into the unconscious, thus making the past appear to be better than it was. Free association may reveal the unconscious material by decreasing the alertness of the critical or sensoring function (superego) of the mind. Projection is a distortion of perception in which a characteristic of the self is attributed to someone else. Exaggerated projection leads to feelings of persecution (projected hostility) and paranoid symptoms. Identification is a process by which a person becomes like the person who is either admired or hated ("identification with the aggressor" as in case of a child abuser.) *(Leigh and Reiser, pp 77–98)*

816–823.   The answers are 816-B, 817-E, 818-C, 819-A, 820-D, 821-A, 822-D, 823-C. The amino acid L-tryptophan is the precursor for serotonin, which is a neurotransmitter needed for non-rapid-eye-movement (NREM) sleep as well as for mood and pain modulation. Up to 70 to 90 percent of brain norepinephrine is produced in the pontine nucleus, locus ceruleus. Dopamine is implicated in schizophrenia and also is an important neurotransmitter for the extrapyramidal system. Depletion of this substance, as in parkinsonism, causes muscular rigidity and tremors. Acetylcholine is the neurotransmitter associated with higher cortical functioning and is depleted in Alzheimer's disease. Acetylcholine also is an important neurotransmitter for the autonomic nervous system (parasympathetic system and the sympathetic nerves to the sweat glands). Many antidepressants have an anticholinergic action, thus dryness of mouth, constipation, and blurred vision. GABA is an important inhibitory transmitter that opens the chloride channels directly associated with the GABA receptors, hyperpolarizing the cell. *(Simons, pp 555–564; Leigh and Reiser, 58–62, 112–118, 154–160)*

824–827. The answers are 824-A, 825-C, 826-B, 827-E. The stages listed in the question form part of the developmental line that psychoanalytic theorists describe as occurring from dependency to adult object relationships. This sequence leads from the newborn's dependence on maternal care to the adult's emotional and material independence and self-reliance. The following eight steps, or stages, are described: period of biologic unity, part-object stage, stage of object constancy, preoedipal ambivalent stage, object-centered phallic-oedipal stage, latency period, preadolescent period, and adolescent stage. *(Freud)*

828–831. The answers are 828-E, 829-C, 830-A, 831-D. Analysis of covariance is used to describe the relationship between a dependent variable and one or more nominal independent variables, controlling for other continuous variables. Analysis of covariance might be used to demonstrate that post-treatment BP, when adjusted for pretreatment BP, is significantly less for one treatment than for another.

Factor analysis is a multivariable method that is used to reduce or explain the relationships among many intercorrelated variables to a few meaningful and relatively independent factors. In the example, four separate scales were reputed to measure four separate factors, but when the scales were administered to the same 200 individuals, they were found to be highly intercorrelated. By the use of factor analysis, two relatively independent factors could be identified that summarized the four original scales.

Discriminant analysis is used to determine how one or several independent variables can differentiate (or distinguish) among the different categories of a dependent variable. Discriminant analysis will provide a "discriminant function" that allows the prediction of illness onset based on knowledge of the values of the independent variables.

In question 831, analysis of variance is used to assess how several nominal independent variables (gender, socioeconomic status, marital status) affect a continuous dependent variable. In effect, analysis of variance compares the mean value of

the dependent variable (happiness) for each of the cross-classified independent variables (i.e., compares the mean happiness for single males of one socioeconomic status to the mean happiness for married males of the same socioeconomic status, and so forth). *(Kleinbaum and Kupper)*

832–835. The answers are 832-A, 833-D, 834-B, 835-C. Retrospective case-control studies are particularly well suited for the investigation of the causes of rare diseases. If a disease is sufficiently rare, the odds ratio determined from a retrospective case-control study provides a good approximation of the relative risk. Prospective studies would require extremely large initial populations in order to ensure an adequate number of cases, especially if the disease occurs rarely. Cross-sectional surveys will not provide information regarding causes, since associations are measured only at one point in time. Under certain circumstances, observational cohorts could be used to investigate the significance of a risk factor for the subsequent development of a disease, but the initial cohort would have to be very large, and the logistics of the investigation would be difficult.

Cross-sectional surveys measure two or more variables at a single moment in time. The strength of association between two variables can be determined, but temporality of the relationship (does the occurrence of variable 1 precede the occurrence of variable 2) cannot be determined from a cross-sectional survey. Relative risk may be determined on the basis of a cross-sectional survey, but causality cannot be inferred.

Randomized controlled clinical trials are state of the art for demonstrating the efficacy of a new intervention. Randomization helps ensure that the groups are equivalent, so that outcome is less likely to be biased by initial susceptibility. Randomized controlled trials may be costly and time-consuming and are not always feasible to use.

Observational cohorts, studied either retrospectively or prospectively, allow an estimation of the incidence or rate of occurrence of a specified outcome in a group with special exposure. Although retrospective case-control studies can be used also to investigate the relationship between prior exposure and disease onset, case-control studies start by identifying cases of specific disease (rather than exposed persons) and are less useful than observational cohorts for determining the effects of a given exposure. Classic examples of observational cohort studies are the numerous studies of occupational exposures (e.g., bladder cancer in workers exposed to dyes or scrotal cancer in chimney sweeps). *(MacMahon and Pugh, pp 207–300)*

836–837. The answers are 836-A, 837-D. Berkson's bias, a form of selection bias, may result when the exposure factor or other characteristic of interest differentially affects the probability of admission to a hospital for those persons with the disease and those without the disease. Berkson's bias occurs when cases are hospitalized patients with the disease of interest and controls are hospitalized patients with another illness (with a different rate of admission than that for the disease of interest) and when the exposure factor affects these rates of admission. In order to avoid Berkson's bias, controls could be drawn from the community.

The situation described in question 837 is one in which the use of historical controls may provide compelling evidence for the efficacy of a new treatment. Usually, historical controls are considered inadequate to demonstrate efficacy, since numerous factors (including the severity of the illness in the patients studied or other changes that have occurred over time in the management or treatment of patients) are not adequately controlled. If a disease has been fatal in nearly 100 percent of all previous cases, successful treatment of a small series of patients with the disease is extremely unlikely unless the new treatment is efficacious. The value of insulin in treating diabetic coma was demonstrated in comparison with historical controls. *(Lilienfeld and Lilienfeld, pp 199–202, 260–268)*

838–845. The answers are 838-C, 839-A, 840-B, 841-B, 842-A, 843-C, 844-C, 845-D. The oral stage of development, during the first year of life, is characterized by gratification related to the activities of the mouth. Sucking and biting are important activities associated with pleasure during this stage. A fixation in this stage results in dependent character traits. The anal stage of development occurs during the second year of life, with toilet training. Issues concerning autonomy and control are important. A fixation in this stage results in parsimony, rigidity, sadistic tendencies, and obsessive-compulsiveness. Both oral and anal stages are pregenital stages of development, as opposed to the phallic phase that appears between the ages of 3 and 6 yr and is characterized by penis envy, according to the freudian scheme of psychosexual development. *(Leigh and Reiser, pp 323–329)*

846–854. The answers are 846-C, 847-A, 848-C, 849-C, 850-C, 851-A, 852-C, 853-A, 854-D. Endorphins and enkephalins are endogenous substances that have opiate-like activities. Enkephalins are pentapeptides, and endorphins are larger peptides whose structures contain enkaphalins. Both opiates and endorphins are blocked by naloxone. All of these substances have similar effects on behavior and physiologic activities, including respiration. Both opiates and endorphins have analgesic effect, and addiction and tolerance develop with prolonged administration. *(Leigh and Reiser, pp 209–240)*

855. The answer is A (1,2,3). Endocrinopathies such as hypothyroidism, β blockers such as propranolol, and neoplasms, especially cancer of the tail of pancreas and other visceral tumors, are frequent medical reasons for depression. Levodopa, used in the treatment of parkinsonism, often is associated with manic symptoms and psychosis but not with depression. *(Leigh and Reiser, pp 99–141)*

856. The answer is D (4). Faintness, tingling of the hands, shortness of breath, and severe anxiety are indicative of the hyperventilation syndrome, which causes respiratory alkalosis due to the loss of carbon dioxide. This in turn causes vasoconstriction that may cause dizziness and decreased ionization of calcium, which may produce paresthesia and, in some cases, tetany. *(Leigh and Reiser, pp 63–64)*

857. The answer is A (1,2,3). Although some emotional disorders of childhood are precursors of adult neuroses, others often appear to be different types of conditions that usually carry a very good prognosis. In those persons whose emotional disorders persist into adulthood, the most common disorders are neuroses or depressive disorders rather than psychoses. Antisocial personality disorder is predated by antisocial behavior from a very young age, usually between the ages of 6 and 11 yr. *(Rutter and Hersov, p 449)*

858. The answer is A (1,2,3). The patient described in the question may be experiencing either organic or psychogenic pain. In view of her history of depression, depression occurring with pain cannot be ruled out. Pain associated with myocardial infarction usually is experienced as chest pain that radiates to the unlar surface of the left arm. Causalgia is a burning pain in the arm; its cause is unknown. *(Leigh and Reiser, pp 209–240)*

859. The answer is E (all). Difficulty falling asleep may be caused by anxiety and pain. Pain that awakens patients from sleep is more likely to be organic in origin. Depression may contribute to the pain and vice versa. *(Leigh and Reiser, pp 259–260)*

860. The answer is D (4). The fibers that transmit burning pain sensation are small, unmyelinated C fibers. The large myelinated fibers carry tactile and vibration sense. Pricking pain is transmitted by small myelinated fibers. *(Leigh and Reiser, pp 213–223)*

861. The answer is C (2,4). The exacting, orderly kind of patient has a need for autonomy that must be respected. Blanket and general reassurances are likely to be viewed with suspicion by these patients. Such patients appreciate specific and detailed explanations of diagnoses and procedures. A schedule in which pain medications are offered to the patient but may be refused if not needed facilitates the patient's sense of autonomy. *(Leigh and Reiser, pp 347–383)*

862. The answer is C (2,4). Phantom pain may be explained by the gate-control theory of pain, in which pain perception depends on a balance of stimuli that include pain and other sensations such as position and vibration. Phantom pain is not indicative of severe psychopathology. Depression may increase the perception of any pain, including phantom pain. *(Leigh and Reiser, pp 209–240)*

863. The answer is E (all). Increasingly, children with such conditions as neuroblastoma, Wilms' tumor, bone tumors, miscellaneous sarcomas, Hodgkin's disease, non-Hodgkin's lymphomas, and acute lymphocytic leukemias are surviving more than 5 yr past the initial diagnosis in a disease-free state and without treatment. Most of these children learned of the diagnosis from a parent and experienced shock or relief. Others felt angry or sad. More than half the children in this study of 115 patients had at least some mild psychiatric symptoms, and 12 percent seemed to be severely impaired. Psychosocial intervention would probably have been helpful to them. *(O'Malley et al)*

864. The answer is E (all). Imaginary companions are under conscious control of the child and are usually benign (ego-syntonic). They are often evoked at times of loneliness or stress. The child can easily differentiate fantasy from reality. The imaginary companion may persist throughout latency. *(Nagera)*

865. The answer is E (all). In normal children, there is no evidence to suggest that puberty is a high-risk period for developing seizures. Yet there is an increase in the incidence of seizures at puberty among children who are autistic. This difference suggests a unique cause of seizures in childhood autism. The added risk may be because of progressive brain pathology or the stress of maturational factors at adolescence. *(Deykin and MacMahon)*

866. The answer is A (1,2,3). In order to diagnose an attention deficit disorder, multiple symptoms, such as those listed in the question, must have been present for at least a year. Other disorders that may have concomitant hyperactivity and must be ruled out include cerebral palsy, childhood autism, psychosis, and mental retardation. Few individual children have every feature of the disorder. Learning difficulties and behavior problems also may be associated with an attention deficit disorder. *(Weiss and Hechtman)*

867. The answer is B (1,3). Robins compared 52 children seen in a child guidance clinic with 100 matched normal controls and followed up on them 30 yr later. Children referred for antisocial behavior differed from the control group, and the more severe the early antisocial behavior during childhood, the more disturbed was the later adjustment. *(Robins)*

868. The answer is E (all). A study of 97 incarcerated serious juvenile offenders between 11 and 17 yr of age with an average age of 15 yr found that when the cohort was divided into two groups, one more violent and the other less violent, 78.6 percent of the more violent group had witnessed extreme violence compared with 20 percent of the less violent group ($p<0.001$). They had similarly suffered more abuse, 75.4 percent compared with 33.3 percent ($p<0.003$). Similar differences were found in the other categories listed in the question. *(Lewis et al.)*

869. The answer is E (all). Transitional phenomena may appear any time between 4 and 12 mo of age. Out of these phenomena emerges some soft object, such as the corner of a blanket, to serve as the transitional object, which becomes an important item for the infant. The use of transitional objects may persist into childhood, particularly at bedtime or when the child is lonely or depressed. *(Winnicott, pp 229–242)*

870. The answer is E (all). Thomas et al identified the nine following categories constituting the temperament of the child: (1) activity level, (2) rhythmicity of such functions as hunger, elimination, and the sleep–wake cycle, (3) approach or withdrawal responses (e.g., to a person), (4) adaptability to an altered environment, (5) intensity of any given reaction, (6) threshold of responsiveness, (7) quality and quantity of moods, (8) degree of distractibility, and (9) persistence in the face of obstacles. This temperament, although in part genetically determined, shows much plasticity during the course of development. *(Thomas et al.)*

871. The answer is E (all). Attachment behavior in infancy facilitates proximity to the person to whom the child is attached. In general, attachment behaviors include signals (crying, smiling, vocalizing), locomotions (looking, following, approaching), and contacts (clambering up, embracing, clinging). Ainsworth herself described at least 15 kinds of such behaviors. *(Caldwell and Ricciuti, pp 1–94)*

872. The answer is A (1,2,3). Infants appear to respond most strongly to visual stimuli that include horizontal stripes, concentric circles, and facelike mosaics. Pattern is often preferred over color or brightness or size. The human face not only responds to the infant's own behavior but also comprises those characteristics most attractive to infants and to which they respond with interest and visual fixation. *(Bornstein and Kessen, pp 83–114)*

873. **The answer is B (1,3).** Alzheimer's disease is the most common dementing disease in the elderly, with a prevalence rate of approximately 6 percent. An increase in the brain aluminum levels has been reported in some Alzheimer's cases. Down's syndrome (trisomy 21) patients who survive to adulthood eventually develop Alzheimer's disease. Physostigmine, a cholinesterase inhibitor, may cause transient improvement in memory but is not effective on a long-term basis. *(Leigh and Reiser, pp 182–185)*

874. **The answer is A (1,2,3).** Information concerning the patient's current state determines the immediate needs and constraints for patient care. Information about recent changes provides clues to factors possibly contributing to illness, such as stress and life changes. Background information concerning the patient's personality and defense mechanisms helps the physician determine how best to approach the patient. Defense mechanisms, even if they are pathologic, cannot be treated immediately. Many defense mechanisms are adaptive. *(Leigh and Reiser, pp 273–291)*

875. **The answer is C (2,4).** Placebo is by no means inert—and it may have side effects. Since placebo analgesia is reversed by naloxone, the analgesic effect of placebo probably occurs through the release of endorphins. Placebos should never be used as a differential diagnostic tool, since severe pain due to organic causes may respond dramatically to placebo. *(Leigh and Reiser, pp 226–230)*

876. **The answer is A (1,2,3).** Cognitive functions have to do with thinking processes. Memory, orientation, abstraction, judgment, concentration, comprehension, perception, and logical thinking are aspects of cognitive function. Affect refers to the feelings evoked by a stimulus or the emotions associated with a mental state. *(Leigh and Reiser, pp 295–304)*

877. **The answer is E (all).** The physician–patient relationship is a contractual one, whether or not there is a written contract. There are placebo effects in the relationship as well as psychotherapeutic ones. The psychotherapeutic aspects are often "unconscious"—that is, not stated—and often occur without the awareness of either the physician or the patient. Tort is a legal term for a wrong for which damages may be awarded. *(Holder, pp 1–42)*

878. **The answer is B (1,3).** The stop–start and squeeze techniques are specific treatment methods for treating premature ejaculation. Free association is a psychoanalytic tool and is nonspecific. Sensate focusing is a standard routine exercise used by

Masters and Johnson to treat all types of sexual dysfunctions. *(Simons, pp 364–375)*

879. **The answer is E (all).** Psychiatric impairment judged on the basis of interview alone was a significant predictor of mortality following illness, according to the Midtown Manhattan study, discussed by Simons. According to Leigh and Reiser, depression is a significant factor in mortality and morbidity following medical diseases and procedures. Bereavement also increases mortality. Genetic factors, such as hyperlipidemia, are also important in predicting vulnerability to disease and mortality. *(Simons, pp 35–36; Leigh and Reiser, pp 106–110)*

880. **The answer is A (1,2,3).** The fight–flight reaction involves activation of the ergotropic areas of the hypothalamus, resulting in sympathetic arousal and activation of the pituitary–adrenocortical axis with an increase in the corticosteroid secretion. Conservation–withdrawal was postulated as an opposite reaction to fight–flight, with activation of the parasympathetic system. *(Simons, pp 92–99; Leigh and Reiser, pp 41–73)*

881. **The answer is E (all).** Speedball is a mixture of heroin and cocaine. When cocaine alkaloid is extracted from the hydrochloride form, it is called freebase or crack or rock and may be smoked. Symptoms of cocaine abuse, as well as withdrawal, include depression, anhedonia, fatigue, irritability, and paranoia. *(American Psychiatric Association, pp 142–143, 177–179)*

882. **The answer is E (all).** Opiate addiction is more common among persons in lower socioeconomic classes than higher socioeconomic classes and among the minority populations (who often tend to belong to low socioeconomic classes). Psychiatric disturbances, such as emotional instability, depression, and personality disorders (e.g., antisocial personality), commonly are observed in addicted individuals. Health care personnel, including physicians, also have a high incidence of opiate addiction. *(Leigh, pp 265–294)*

883. **The answer is A (1,2,3).** Opiate intoxication is characterized by miosis, decreased respiratory rate and depth, and decreased BP and pulse. Scratching, usually a slow and sensuous act, is also common. Euphoria and drowsiness also are present. *(Leigh, pp 265–294)*

884. **The answer is E (all).** Phencyclidine (PCP, angel dust, peace pill) intoxication is characterized by horizontal and vertical nystagmus, analgesia, tachycardia, increased deep tendon reflexes, muscle rigidity, ataxia, flushed skin, sweating, blank stare, apathy or excitement, body image distortion, floating feeling, hostility and possible violence, and fever. In overdose, additional symptoms include

coma and delirium, miotic but reactive pupils, hypertension, convulsions, decreased or absent reflexes, hypersalivation, inability to speak, labile affect, hallucinations, amnesia, and fever. *(Leigh, pp 265–294)*

885. **The answer is C (2,4).** Talking down is helpful in treating bad trips caused by LSD and other hallucinogens but is more likely to increase the agitation and violence in patients with PCP psychosis. Benzodiazepines are useful to treat PCP psychosis, whereas phenothiazines are not. Ammonium chloride or ascorbic acid can be useful in acidifying the urine, increasing excretion of PCP in the urine. *(Leigh, pp 265–294)*

886. **The answer is E (all).** The *DSM-III-R* diagnostic criteria for schizophrenia include at least two of (1) delusions, (2) prominent hallucinations, (3) incoherence or marked loosening of association, (4) catatonic behavior, or (5) flat or grossly inappropriate affect, or bizarre delusions, or prominent auditory hallucinations that are not affect-congruent for at least 1 wk. In addition, there are other criteria, including duration (continuous symptoms for 6 months), decline of function, and others. *(American Psychiatric Association, pp 194–195)*

887. **The answer is E (all).** More than 4,000 physicians (1.5 percent) in the USA are known drug addicts (30 to 100 times the rate in general population). About 2.3 to 3.2 percent of registered physicians are identified as impaired by alcoholism. Currently there are estimated to be 10,000 alcoholic physicians in the USA. More than 100 physicians commit suicide every year, a number equivalent to the size of an average medical school class. The suicide rate for male physicians is 1.15 times greater than that of the general population, and for female physicians 3 times greater. In one study, 47 percent of physicians were reported to have unsatisfactory marriages, as compared with 32 percent in a control group. *(Scheiber and Doyle, pp 4–7)*

888. **The answer is E (all).** Axis I includes the major psychiatric syndromes. Axis II includes disorders that usually begin in childhood and adolescence, such as developmental and personality disorders. Conditions that are not attributable to a mental disorder but are a focus of attention or treatment (e.g., marital problem, malingering) may be recorded in axis I or axis II depending on the nature. Medical diseases are recorded in axis III. Axis IV records the severity of psychosocial stressors, and axis V records the global assessment of functioning. *(American Psychiatric Association, pp 15–34)*

889. **The answer is A (1,2,3).** In conversion disorder, there is an alteration or loss of a physical function-ing that is an expression of a psychologic conflict. Body dysmorphic disorder (dysmorphophobia) is a preoccupation with an imagined defect of a body part. Hypochondriasis is a preoccupation with the fear of having a serious disease. In addition, somatization disorder (characterized by recurrent multiple somatic complaints not due to a physical disorder), somatoform pain disorder (preoccupation with pain in the absence of adequate physical findings to account for the pain), and somatoform disorder not otherwise specified comprise the *DSM-III-R* somatoform disorders. Malingering is a diagnosis "not attributable to a mental disorder." *(American Psychiatric Association, pp 255–267)*

BIBLIOGRAPHY

American Psychiatric Association. *Diagnostic and Statistical Manual of Mental Disorders* 3rd ed. rev. (*DSM-III-R*). Washington, DC: American Psychiatric Association, 1987.

Bornstein MH, Kessen W, eds. *Psychological Development from Infancy.* Hillsdale, NJ: Lawrence Erlbaum Associates, Inc, 1979.

Caldwell BM, Ricciuti NH, eds. *Review of Child Development Research.* Chicago: University of Chicago Press, 1973; vol. 3.

Campbell D, and Stanley J. *Experimental and Quasi-Experimental Designs for Research.* Skokie, Ill: Rand McNally & Co, 1966.

Colton T. *Statistics in Medicine.* Boston: Little, Brown & Co, 1974.

Committee on Adolescence, American Academy of Pediatrics. Teenage suicide. *Pediatrics.* July 1980; 144–146.

Department of Health and Human Services. *Health.* Washington, DC: Department of Health and Human Services, 1982.

Deykin EY, MacMahon B. The incidence of seizures among children with autistic symptoms. *Am J Psychiatry.* October 1979; 1310–1312.

Feinstein AR. *Clinical Biostatistics.* St. Louis: CV Mosby Co, 1977.

Freud A. *Normality and Pathology in Childhood.* New York: International Universities Press, 1965.

Friedlander BZ. Receptive language development in infancy: Issues and problems. *Merrill-Palmer Q.* January 1970; 7.

Holder A. *Medical Malpractice Law.* 2nd ed. New York: John Wiley & Sons, Inc, 1978.

Kaplan HI, Sadock BJ, eds. *Comprehensive Textbook of Psychiatry/IV.* Baltimore: Williams & Wilkins, 1985.

Kleinbaum D, and Kupper L. *Applied Regression Analysis and Other Multivariable Methods.* North Scituate, Mass: Duxbury Press, 1978.

Leigh H, ed. *Psychiatry in the Practice of Medicine.* Menlo Park, Calif: Addison-Wesley Publishing Co, 1983.

Leigh H, Reiser MF. *The Patient: Biological, Psychological, and Social Dimensions of Medical Practice*. 2nd ed. New York: Plenum Publishing Corp, 1985.

Lewis DO, Shanok SS, Pincus TH, Glaser GH. Violent juvenile delinquents: psychiatric, neurological, psychological, and abuse factors. *J Am Acad Child Psychiatry*. Spring 1979; 307–319.

Lilienfeld A, Lilienfeld D. *Foundations of Epidemiology*. 2nd ed. New York: Oxford University Press, 1980.

MacMahon B, Pugh T. *Epidemiology, Principles and Methods*. Boston: Little, Brown & Co, 1970.

Nagera H. The imaginary companion. *The Psychoanalytic Study of the Child*. 1969; 165–196.

O'Malley JE, Kocher G, Foster D, Slavin L. Psychiatric sequelae of surviving childhood cancer. *Am J Orthopsychiatry*. October 1979; 608–616.

Robins LH. *Deviant Children Grown Up: A Sociological and Psychiatric Study of Sociopathic Personality*. Baltimore: Williams & Wilkins Co, 1966.

Rutter, M, Hersov L, eds. *Child Psychiatry*. Oxford: Blackwell Scientific Publications, 1977.

Rutter M, Tizard J, Whitmore K. *Education, Health, and Behavior*. London: Longman Group, Ltd, 1970

Scheiber SC, Doyle BB, eds. *The Impaired Physician*. New York: Plenum Publishing Corp, 1983.

Simons RC, ed. *Understanding Human Behavior in Health and Illness*. 3rd ed. Baltimore: Williams & Wilkins, 1985.

Thomas AS, Chess S, Birch HG. *Temperament and Behavior Disorders in Children*. New York: New York University Press, 1968.

Weiss G, Hechtman L. The hyperactive child syndrome. *Science*. September 28, 1979; 1348–1354.

Winnicott DW. *Collected Papers*. London: Tavistock Publications, Ltd, 1958.

Subspecialty List: Behavioral Sciences

Question Number and Subspecialty

763. Anxiety/learning theory
764. Individual dynamics
765. Epidemiology
766. Medicine as a career
767. Doctor–Patient Relationship Psychotherapy
768. Psychopathology
769. Geropsychiatry
770. Ethology
771. Hospital community
772. Epidemiology
773. Child psychology
774. Child psychology
775. Child psychology
776. Epidemiology
777. Child psychology/child development
778. Epidemiology
779. Pharmacologic correlates of behavior
780. Biofeedback
781. Psychopharmacology
782. Anxiety
783. Psychopathology
784. Psychopathology
785. Neurobiology
786. Alcoholism
787. Alcoholism
788. Alcoholism
789. Alcoholism
790. Child psychology
791. Sleep
792. Psychophysiology
793. Sleep/neurobiology
794. Sleep/neurobiology
795. Sleep/neurobiology
796. Sleep/neurobiology
797. Sleep/neurobiology
798. Sleep/neurobiology
799. Sleep/neurobiology
800. Sleep/neurobiology
801. Sleep/neurobiology
802. Epidemiology
803. Epidemiology
804. Epidemiology
805. Biostatistics

806. Biostatistics
807. Biostatistics
808. Biostatistics
809. Individual dynamics
810. Individual dynamics
811. Individual dynamics
812. Individual dynamics
813. Individual dynamics
814. Individual dynamics
815. Individual dynamics
816. Neurobiology
817. Neurobiology
818. Neurobiology Psychosis
819. Neurobiology
820. Neurobiology Geropsychiatry
821. Neurobiology
    Psychopharmacology
822. Psychopharmacology
823. Neurobiology
824. Child development
825. Child development
826. Child development
827. Child development
828. Biostatistics
829. Biostatistics
830. Biostatistics
831. Biostatistics
832. Epidemiology
833. Epidemiology
834. Epidemiology
835. Epidemiology
836. Epidemiology
837. Epidemiology
838. Individual dynamics
839. Individual dynamics
840. Individual dynamics
841. Individual dynamics
842. Individual dynamics
843. Individual dynamics
844. Individual dynamics
845. Individual dynamics
846. Pain/psychopharmacology
847. Pain/psychopharmacology
848. Pain/psychopharmacology
849. Pain/psychopharmacology

850. Pain/psychopharmacology
851. Pain/psychopharmacology
852. Pain/psychopharmacology
853. Pain/psychopharmacology
854. Pain/psychopharmacology
855. Depression
856. Anxiety/psychophysiology
857. Child psychology
858. Pain
859. Pain
860. Pain
861. Pain
862. Pain
863. Child psychology
864. Child psychology
865. Child psychology
866. Child psychology
867. Child psychology
868. Child psychology
869. Child psychology
870. Child psychology
871. Child psychology
872. Child psychology/child development
873. Elderly patient/geropsychiatry
874. Assessment
875. Placebo
876. Mental status
877. Ethics and law
878. Human sexuality
879. Social epidemiology
880. Anxiety Neurobiology
881. Substance abuse/psychopharmacology
882. Addiction
883. Addiction
884. Substance abuse
885. Substance abuse
886. Diagnosis/psychopathology
887. Epidemiology/alcoholism
888. Diagnosis
889. Diagnosis/psychopathology

CHAPTER 8

Practice Tests

Carefully read the following instructions before taking the Practice Tests.

1. This examination consists of 311 questions divided into **two test periods.** The first test consists of 143 questions and takes 2 hours. The second test consists of 168 questions and takes 2 hours and 20 minutes.
2. The tests mimic the actual Boards. You should not carry any extra time from one test over to the other. Any remaining time from either test should be used to review your answers in that test only. You should take a break of 1 or 2 hours at least between the two tests.
3. The test items are explained in the Introduction to this book. We urge you to read the entire Introduction prior to taking this practice test.
4. Be sure you have an adequate number of pencils and erasers, a clock, a comfortable setting, and an adequate amount of undisturbed, distraction-free time.
5. Be sure to fill out the answer sheet on page 273 properly (see Introduction).
6. After completion of the entire practice test, check your answers and assess your areas of weakness against the subspeciality list on pages 269–272.

Practice Test I
Questions

DIRECTIONS (Questions 1 through 143): Each of the numbered items or incomplete statements in this section is followed by answers or by completions of the statement. Select the <u>ONE</u> lettered answer or completion that is <u>BEST</u> in each case.

1. The medulla and pons are supplied by all of the following arteries EXCEPT the

    (A) anterior spinal artery
    (B) posterior spinal artery
    (C) branches of the basilar artery
    (D) branches of the vertebral artery
    (E) middle cerebral artery

2. Which of the following fatty acids can be the precursor of prostaglandins in humans?

    (A) oleic
    (B) palmitic
    (C) stearic
    (D) arachidonic
    (E) palmitoleic

3. All of the following are associated with primary hyperparathyroidism EXCEPT

    (A) parathyroid adenoma
    (B) nephrolithiasis
    (C) bone disease
    (D) hyperphosphatemia
    (E) chief cell hyperplasia

4. Hilton's law states that the nerve supply to a joint is derived from the same nerves that supply muscles acting on that joint. Applying this simple theory, which of the following nerves will NOT contribute to the nerve supply of the hip joint?

    (A) obturator
    (B) femoral
    (C) tibial portion of the sciatic
    (D) common peroneal portion of the sciatic
    (E) superior gluteal

5. Vitamin B_{12} is needed for the reduction of the C-2' atom of ribonucleoside triphosphate to produce the corresponding 2'-deoxyribonucleoside. The mineral necessary for the ring system of vitamin B_{12} is

    (A) iron
    (B) cobalt
    (C) calcium
    (D) manganese
    (E) magnesium

6. Squamous cell carcinoma of the lung shows all of the following features EXCEPT

    (A) increasing incidence in women
    (B) most common type of bronchogenic carcinoma
    (C) peripheral location in the lung
    (D) high association with a history of smoking
    (E) greater predilection for men than women

7. The luminal epithelium and glands of the lower respiratory tract are derived from

    (A) foregut endoderm (primitive pharynx)
    (B) midgut endoderm (primitive small intestine)
    (C) cardiogenic mesenchyme
    (D) splanchnic mesenchyme
    (E) neural crest tissue

8. A solution of acetic acid (pK_a 4.75) is titrated with sodium hydroxide until 80 percent of the acetic acid has been converted to sodium acetate. What is the pH of the solution?

    (A) 4.15
    (B) 5.35
    (C) 4.75
    (D) 8.75
    (E) 2.35

9. The occurrence of malignant mesothelioma has been correlated with industrial exposure to

(A) beryllium
(B) silica
(C) coal dust
(D) asbestos
(E) nitrogen dioxide

10. All of the following are important compensatory mechanisms in hemorrhagic shock EXCEPT

(A) tachycardia
(B) venoconstriction
(C) decreased peripheral vascular resistance
(D) absorption of fluid from interstitial space
(E) formation of angiotensin II

11. Which of the following veins DO NOT drain into the right atrium via the coronary sinus?

(A) great cardiac
(B) middle cardiac
(C) anterior cardiac
(D) small cardiac
(E) oblique vein of the left atrium

12. Temporary occlusion of both common carotid arteries is promptly accompanied by

(A) vasodilatation throughout the peripheral circulation
(B) an increase in the number of impulses from the carotid sinus nerve
(C) an increase in venous capacity
(D) an increase in arterial pressure
(E) a decrease in heart rate

13. Under normal metabolic conditions, the energy produced from 1 g of glycogen is approximately

(A) 0.8 kcal
(B) 1.0 kcal
(C) 4.2 kcal
(D) 8.2 kcal
(E) 9.5 kcal

14. A skin biopsy showing the following features, hyperkeratosis, parakeratosis, thickening of the epidermis and club-shaped papillae, and collections of neutrophil leukocytes in clusters in the upper layers of the epidermis, is most characteristic of which of the following conditions?

(A) basal cell carcinoma
(B) malignant melanoma
(C) squamous cell carcinoma
(D) pemphigus vulgaris
(E) psoriasis

15. The scalp receives sensory innervation from all of the following nerves EXCEPT the

(A) auriculotemporal nerve
(B) supraorbital nerve
(C) greater occipital nerve
(D) lesser occipital nerve
(E) temporal branch of the facial nerve

16. Long-term regulation of arterial blood pressure (BP) is primarily a function of

(A) the CNS
(B) the sympathetic nervous system
(C) peripheral baroreceptors
(D) urine output and fluid intake
(E) total peripheral vascular resistance

17. The major amino acid precursor for gluconeogenesis is

(A) alanine
(B) aspartate
(C) cysteine
(D) glutamate
(E) serine

18. Constrictive pericarditis with dense fibrosis and calcification of the pericardium is most likely to be associated with which of the following conditions?

(A) acute rheumatic fever
(B) acute staphylococcal infection
(C) uremia
(D) tuberculosis
(E) lupus erythematosus

19. If in a medical school department it is observed that most of the junior faculty and residents dress and speak like the department's chairperson, this phenomenon may be an example of

(A) sublimation
(B) projection
(C) denial
(D) reaction formation
(E) identification

20. Which of the following statements concerning the function and structure of glands is true?

(A) exocrine glands secrete internally
(B) hormones are ineffective in very small quantities
(C) endocrine glands are ductless
(D) the thyroid gland is an exocrine gland
(E) the thyroid gland is an abdominal gland

21. Atrial fibrillation is a common arrhythmia that accompanies several forms of heart disease. During atrial fibrillation, the atria do not contract sequentially and thus do not contribute to ventricular filling. Which of the following statements best describes this pathophysiologic condition?

    (A) on ECG, the P waves usually are normal in atrial fibrillation
    (B) a drug such as quinidine, which acts in part by prolonging the effective refractory period of conducting tissue, is useful therapy
    (C) the interval between QRS complexes remains constant
    (D) atrial fibrillation is life threatening and usually requires application of strong electric current to place the entire myocardium in refractory period
    (E) since the atria contribute little to ventricular function, the pulse is usually extremely regular in spite of the abnormality

22. Which one of the following statements about the peptide of Val-Ala-Pro-Glu-Gly is true?

    (A) its isoelectric point will be found at a high pH
    (B) it has an overall positive charge at pH 11
    (C) it has an overall positive charge at pH 7
    (D) it has an overall negative charge at pH 7
    (E) it has an overall negative charge at pH 1

23. Glomerular wire-loop lesions are most often found in renal biopsy specimens of patients with

    (A) diabetes mellitus
    (B) systemic lupus erythematosus
    (C) hypertension
    (D) hepatorenal syndrome
    (E) acute tubular necrosis

24. All of the following are common examples of society's sick-role expectations EXCEPT that

    (A) individuals are exempt from normal responsibilities
    (B) individuals are responsible for maintenance of health
    (C) being sick is an undesirable state
    (D) a sick person cannot be expected to get well by "pulling himself together"
    (E) a sick person should seek help from a competent professional

25. Which of the following statements correctly describes the lymphatics?

    (A) the lymphatic circulatory system consists exclusively of lymph nodules, lymph nodes, and aggregates

    (B) lymph tissue is made up of cells (mostly WBCs) separated by a fluid intercellular substance
    (C) the valves in lymphatic vessels are remarkable in that they allow for a reversal of direction of the flow when needed
    (D) the function of the lymphatic system is relatively unknown and unappreciated
    (E) lymph nodes are located only in the upper part of the body (above the waist)

26. Numerous ion channels are involved in the generation of the cardiac action potential. The ion channel most closely associated with the plateau phase of the cardiac action potential is

    (A) voltage-gated sodium channel
    (B) voltage-gated potassium channel
    (C) calcium-gated potassium channels
    (D) voltage-gated calcium channels
    (E) phosphoptidyl inositol-gated calcium channels

27. Which of the following amino acids is purely ketogenic?

    (A) cysteine
    (B) serine
    (C) glycine
    (D) leucine
    (E) alanine

28. Activator of the alternate complement pathway is

    (A) interleukin 1 (IL-1)
    (B) β-interferon
    (C) lipoproteins
    (D) endotoxin
    (E) complement component C1

29. A red infarct would be most likely to occur in the

    (A) heart
    (B) spleen
    (C) kidneys
    (D) lungs
    (E) pancreas

30. Which of the following is LEAST effective as an anti-inflammatory agent?

    (A) indomethacin
    (B) aspirin
    (C) acetaminophen
    (D) phenylbutazone
    (E) tolmetin

31. If a bell rings each time a dog is given food, the dog will soon salivate at the sound of the bell. This phenomenon is called

    (A) operant conditioning
    (B) classical conditioning
    (C) cognitive learning
    (D) shaping
    (E) instinctual behavior

32. All of the following correctly describe the relationship of the heart and great vessels EXCEPT that the

    (A) base is formed by the ventricles
    (B) apex is in the fifth intercostal space
    (C) pulmonary ostium (opening) is under the second left interspace
    (D) aortic ostium largely lies substernally
    (E) coronary sinus opening is a feature of the right atrium

33. Certain tumors produce a substance closely resembling PTH in its biologic activity. The physiologic effects of this substance would include all of the following EXCEPT

    (A) stimulation of bone resorption
    (B) decreased renal phosphate excretion
    (C) increased serum calcium
    (D) increased metabolism of vitamin D to the 1,25-OH form
    (E) increased serum calcitonin levels

34. The steroid compound of greatest potency in the control of plasma sodium ion concentration is

    (A) pregnenolone
    (B) progesterone
    (C) aldosterone
    (D) cortisol
    (E) cortisone

35. The microbicidal oxygen-dependent mechanisms of phagocytes depend on all of the following EXCEPT

    (A) superoxide radical
    (B) singlet oxygen
    (C) ferrous ions
    (D) hydrogen peroxide
    (E) hydroxyl radicals

36. The biology of chemical induction of carcinoma includes all of the following principles EXCEPT

    (A) irreversible dose dependency
    (B) dependency on hormonal promoters
    (C) fixed latency period

    (D) transmission to daughter cells
    (E) enhancement by cell proliferation

37. Propylthiouracil is useful in the treatment of

    (A) derangement toxicosis
    (B) hyperthyroidism
    (C) thyroiditis
    (D) hypoparathyroidism
    (E) hypothyroidism

38. The functions of the limbic system include all of the following EXCEPT

    (A) cognition
    (B) emotion
    (C) reproduction
    (D) nutrition
    (E) aggression

39. The long thoracic nerve arises from

    (A) the medial cord
    (B) the lateral cord
    (C) the posterior cord
    (D) the anterior division of the upper trunk
    (E) none of the above

40. The stimulation in salivary gland acini results in a loss of intracellular and a rise in extracellular potassium ions. The efflux of potassium ions is believed to be primarily due to the action of

    (A) a Na^+-K^+ exchange mechanism
    (B) voltage-dependent nonspecific cation channels
    (C) calcium-activated potassium channels
    (D) Na^+-K^+-Cl^- cotransport
    (E) an ouabain-sensitive pump

41. All of the following bonding reactions are important in the stabilization of the tertiary structure of proteins EXCEPT

    (A) peptide bonds
    (B) hydrogen bonds between peptide groups
    (C) ionic bonds
    (D) hydrophobic interactions
    (E) hydrogen bonds between side chains of amino acids

42. The figure below represents the antibiotic

(A) streptomycin
(B) cephalothin
(C) erythromycin
(D) penicillin
(E) gentamicin

43. Adrenocortical carcinoma is a rare malignant tumor that is

(A) most common among children
(B) a small occult lesion
(C) associated with Cushing's syndrome
(D) of neural crest origin
(E) usually bilateral

44. Within 48 to 72 hr after the last dose of heroin, an addicted individual may experience

(A) anorexia, hypotension, and paralysis of the respiratory muscles
(B) severe irritability, insomnia, anorexia, nausea, and vomiting
(C) yawning, hypothermia, and excruciating pain
(D) mild discomfort with more severe symptoms peaking earlier, 12 to 24 hr after the last dose
(E) mild discomfort with more severe symptoms peaking 4 to 5 days after the last dose

45. All of the following are associated with the use of benzodiazepines EXCEPT

(A) antianxiety effects
(B) addictive effects
(C) anticonvulsant effects
(D) impaired conditioned avoidance learning
(E) additive action with alcohol

46. A patient has injured the common peroneal nerve as it wraps around the neck of the fibula. This injury could affect all of the following muscles EXCEPT the

(A) tibialis posterior
(B) tibialis anterior
(C) extensor digitorum longus
(D) peroneus longus
(E) extensor hallucis longus

47. In the pathways for the synthesis of steroids, a deficiency of the enzymes 21β-hydroxylase or 11 β-hydroxylase may result in abnormally high levels of circulating androgens. A major factor that contributes to this increase is

(A) loss of inhibition of androgen synthesis by corticosteroids
(B) increased synthesis of testosterone within the gonads
(C) decreased conversion of androgens to estrogen
(D) increased release of ACTH
(E) increased release of luteinizing hormone (LH)

48. Which of the following events takes place during the complete biosynthesis of collagen?

(A) biosynthesis is completed within fibroblasts
(B) procollagen is secreted by fibroblasts
(C) triple-helix formation occurs from procollagen
(D) tropocollagen is secreted by fibroblasts
(E) conversion of proline to hydroxyproline occurs after secretion of collagen precursors

49. The virulence of *Streptococcus pneumoniae* is primarily associated with the presence of

(A) cell wall teichoic acid
(B) pneumolysin
(C) polysaccharide capsule
(D) M protein
(E) peptidoglycan

50. Which of the following descriptions of the histology of non-Hodgkin's lymphoma best describes the least aggressive or lowest grade of tumor?

(A) nodular: small cell with cleaved nuclei
(B) diffuse: large cell with noncleaved nuclei
(C) nodular: large cell with cleaved nuclei
(D) diffuse: small cell with noncleaved nuclei
(E) diffuse: immunoblastic

51. The following effects are associated with phenothiazine administration EXCEPT

(A) antiemetic
(B) release of prolactin
(C) prevention of parkinsonism
(D) gynecomastia
(E) antihistaminic

52. All of the following are characteristics of predatory aggression EXCEPT

    (A) always aiming at success
    (B) stalking postures
    (C) frenzied and mutilating attack
    (D) association with feeding
    (E) little autonomic activation

53. Which of the following statements regarding the reproductive anatomy of human males is true?

    (A) the epididymis is subdivided into anterior, median, and posterior lobes
    (B) the testes contain major and minor calcyes
    (C) the tunica albuginea is the innermost layer of the testes
    (D) anorchidism is the musculature of the appendix testis
    (E) the ductus deferens connects the epididymis with the ejaculatory duct

54. One effect of androgens is to promote linear bone growth. This effect is transient because

    (A) androgens cause epiphyseal closure
    (B) androgens slow the synthesis of collagen
    (C) receptors for androgens are down regulated
    (D) androgens increase the excretion rate of calcium and phosphate ions
    (E) androgens stimulate bone resorption

55. All of the following are true concerning the formation of a δ-aminolevulinic acid EXCEPT that it

    (A) requires glycine
    (B) is prerequisite to the formation of porphobilinogen
    (C) requires succinyl-coenzyme A (CoA)
    (D) is catalyzed by δ-aminolevulinate dehydrogenase
    (E) is the rate-limiting step in the formation of heme

56. Retroviruses are unique among all viruses in that

    (A) the mature virus contains a strand of RNA and a strand of DNA
    (B) they can carry out replication of their genomes extracellularly within intact vesicles
    (C) they contain reverse transcriptase in the virion
    (D) they are nonantigenic
    (E) the mature virus contains no nucleic acid

57. The changes seen in the kidney shown in the photograph below may be produced by

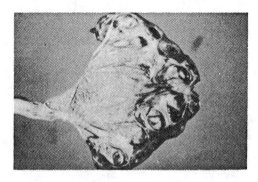

    (A) postrenal obstruction
    (B) renal infarct
    (C) hypertension
    (D) renal cell carcinoma
    (E) abuse of analgesics

58. Bacterial resistance to penicillin usually occurs by

    (A) thickening of the bacterial wall
    (B) changes in the activity of the transpeptidase required for wall formation
    (C) reduced requirement for folic acid
    (D) enzymatic hydrolysis of the β-lactam ring
    (E) decreased affinity of the ribosomal subunit for the drug

59. An attenuated form of anxiety that plays an important role in psychologic defense mechanisms is

    (A) signal anxiety
    (B) actual anxiety
    (C) neurotic anxiety
    (D) panic anxiety
    (E) psychotic anxiety

60. The great cerebral vein (Galen's vein) usually drains directly into the

    (A) transverse sinus
    (B) superior sagittal sinus
    (C) straight sinus
    (D) internal jugular vein
    (E) arachnoid villi

61. In normal adult men, the major source of circulating estradiol is provided by

    (A) secretion from the Leydig's cells in the testes
    (B) secretion from the Sertoli's cells in the testes
    (C) the action of aromatase on circulating androgens
    (D) the action of aromatase on circulating estrone
    (E) release from the inner layers of the adrenal cortex

62. Which of the following is present only in the intrinsic pathway of clotting?

    (A) fibrinogen (factor I)
    (B) accelerin (factor V)
    (C) prothrombin (factor II)
    (D) antihemophilic factor (factor VIII)
    (E) Stuart factor (factor X)

63. All of the following are DNA viruses EXCEPT

    (A) variola
    (B) herpes simplex
    (C) molluscum contagiosum
    (D) papova
    (E) measles

64. Down's syndrome is characterized by the karyotype

    (A) trisomy 13
    (B) trisomy 18
    (C) trisomy 21
    (D) XO
    (E) XXY

65. The most common serious side effect of a single dose of one aspirin tablet is

    (A) infertility
    (B) hepatotoxicity
    (C) nephrotoxicity
    (D) allergic asthma
    (E) hemolytic anemia

66. A physician neglected to discuss with a patient potential complications of proposed surgery. When a colleague pointed this out, the physician claimed that the patient did not want to know it anyway. This may be an example of

    (A) reaction formation
    (B) denial
    (C) organic brain syndrome
    (D) rationalization
    (E) sublimation

67. The circular muscle fibers responsible for closing or reducing the lumen of a viscus, such as the intestine, are collectively termed the

    (A) intercostal muscles
    (B) dilator muscles
    (C) sphincter muscles
    (D) detrusor muscles
    (E) cremaster muscles

68. Tumors of acidophilic cells in the anterior pituitary of adults are most likely to lead to

    (A) dwarfism
    (B) acromegaly
    (C) Cushing's syndrome
    (D) gigantism
    (E) adrenogenital syndrome

69. The blood protein thrombin is known to

    (A) have an enzymatic specificity similar to trypsin
    (B) form clots by complexing with fibrin
    (C) be an oligomeric protein
    (D) require vitamin K in its activated form
    (E) contain γ-carboxyglutamate residues

70. A 3-yr-old child has a temperature of 38.3°C (101°F). On examination, discrete vesiculoulcerative lesions (Koplik's spots) are noted on the mucous membranes of the mouth. The most probable diagnosis is

    (A) rubella
    (B) herpangina
    (C) measles
    (D) herpetic gingivostomatitis
    (E) scarlet fever

71. Which of the following is NOT characteristic of the process of atherosclerosis?

    (A) primarily and initially an intimal disease
    (B) associated with elevated serum cholesterol levels
    (C) monoclonal proliferation of smooth muscle cells in the intima
    (D) associated with increase in serum lipids of the low-density lipoprotein (LDL) class
    (E) associated with increase in serum high-density lipoproteins (HDL)

72. In most individuals, endogenous cortisol plasma concentrations may be described as

    (A) highest in the early morning
    (B) lowest in the late morning and early afternoon
    (C) lowest in the late afternoon
    (D) highest in the late afternoon
    (E) nonvariable throughout the day

73. Which of the following statements correctly characterizes unsuccessful attempts at suicide?

    (A) advanced age is usually a factor
    (B) females are more likely than males to attempt suicide
    (C) subsequent successful suicide attempts are unlikely
    (D) interpersonal difficulties usually are not a factor
    (E) such attempts are infrequent among Catholics

74. The layers of the wall of viscera (from the external to the internal) are the

    (A) adventitia, serous, muscular, submucous, and subserous
    (B) serous, muscular, submucous, and mucous
    (C) serous, adventitia, submucous, mucous, and epithelial
    (D) serous, submucous, muscular, media, and mucous
    (E) serous, adventitia, peritoneal, muscular, and mucous

75. A circadian rhythm in the synthesis and release of melatonin occurs primarily in the

    (A) suprachiasmatic nuclei
    (B) adrenal medulla
    (C) raphe nuclei
    (D) pineal gland
    (E) skin

76. The number of moles of ATP produced by complete mitochondrial oxidation of 1 mol of pyruvate to CO_2 and water is

    (A) 1
    (B) 6
    (C) 12
    (D) 15
    (E) 24

77. The DiGeorge syndrome is characterized by

    (A) a depletion of lymph node lymphocytes in both T- and B-dependent areas

    (B) defective development of the third and fourth pharyngeal pouches
    (C) an absence of isohemagglutinins
    (D) a defect in neutrophil chemotaxis
    (E) a depletion of B-dependent areas in lymph nodes

78. All of the following are signs of local inflammation EXCEPT

    (A) redness
    (B) heat
    (C) numbness
    (D) pain
    (E) swelling

79. In anticoagulant therapy, an increased response would be expected with

    (A) barbiturates
    (B) rifampin
    (C) phenylbutazone
    (D) cholestyramine
    (E) glutethimide

80. Which of the following are considered to be pain receptors?

    (A) Meissner's corpuscles
    (B) Vater-Pacini corpuscles
    (C) basal cells
    (D) rods
    (E) free nerve endings

81. All of the following are primary functions of amniotic fluid contained in the amniotic cavity EXCEPT

    (A) preventing adhesions between the embryo and amnion
    (B) protecting the embryo from physical blows to the mother
    (C) maintaining a relatively constant temperature for the embryo
    (D) providing a major source of nutrition to the embryo
    (E) enabling fetal movements to occur

82. In the absence of hormone replacement therapy, adrenalectomy may result in death within a few days. This is most likely to be caused by the loss of the adrenal hormone

    (A) cortisol
    (B) corticosterone
    (C) aldosterone
    (D) dehydroepiandrosterone
    (E) epinephrine

83. All of the atoms composing urea are contained within

   (A) aspartate and ornithine
   (B) carbamoyl phosphate and citrulline
   (C) ornithine and citrulline
   (D) aspartate
   (E) argininosuccinate

84. Sterilization of surgical instruments that are sensitive to heat can best be accomplished by

   (A) the autoclave
   (B) ionizing radiation
   (C) ethylene oxide
   (D) phenol
   (E) ethyl alcohol

85. The characteristic pathologic lesion of sarcoid is

   (A) fibroblastic proliferation
   (B) noncaseating granuloma
   (C) pyogenic abscess
   (D) mucoid cyst
   (E) hyaline membrane formation

86. Propranolol is beneficial in the treatment of angina because it

   (A) dilates capacitance vessels
   (B) increases coronary blood flow
   (C) increases oxygen delivery
   (D) decreases contractile force
   (E) reduces oxygen requirements

87. Lithium salts are most effective in

   (A) generalized anxiety disorder
   (B) unipolar depression
   (C) panic disorder
   (D) acute mania
   (E) schizophrenia

88. The ischiorectal fossae are correctly described as the

   (A) wings of the uterus
   (B) fimbriae of the ovary and sphincter of the oviducts or uterine tubes
   (C) spaces at either side of the anal canal
   (D) fat-containing spaces that accommodate the broad ligaments of the uterus
   (E) the lateral depressions on each ischial tuberosity as they relate to the rectum

89. The secretion of glucagon from α cells of pancreatic islets is

   (A) inhibited by elevated amino acid concentrations in plasma
   (B) inhibited by elevated cyclic AMP levels
   (C) stimulated by elevated plasma glucose
   (D) stimulated by insulin
   (E) enhanced by sympathetic stimulation

90. In mammals, all of the following can serve as a substrate for the net synthesis of glucose EXCEPT

   (A) glycerol
   (B) β-hydroxybutyric acid
   (C) oxaloacetic acid
   (D) glutamic acid
   (E) propionic acid

91. In a positive viral hemagglutination inhibition test, hemagglutination is inhibited by which of the following substances in the serum?

   (A) antiviral antibody
   (B) latex agglutinins
   (C) Rh antibody
   (D) hemolysin
   (E) virus

92. Malignant melanomas may do all of the following EXCEPT

   (A) metastasize via the lymphatic vessels
   (B) metastasize hematogenously
   (C) arise in sun-exposed areas of skin
   (D) arise in the papillary dermis
   (E) arise de novo

93. In persons suffering from severe anaphylactic shock, the drug of choice for restoring circulation and relaxing bronchial smooth muscle is

   (A) epinephrine
   (B) norepinephrine
   (C) isoproterenol
   (D) phenylephrine
   (E) dopamine

94. All of the following statements concerning suicide are true EXCEPT that

    (A) most people who commit suicide give definite warnings about their intent
    (B) suicide may occur when the patient's mood seems to be lifting
    (C) people who habitually talk of suicide seldom commit suicide
    (D) most people who commit suicide see a physician before the suicidal act
    (E) suicide is more common among professional persons than individuals in lower economic groups

95. The radial nerve supplies the

    (A) teres major
    (B) coracobrachialis
    (C) spraspinatus
    (D) triceps brachii
    (E) serratus anterior

96. The most active form of thyroid hormone in the stimulation of oxygen use is

    (A) thyroxine
    (B) thyroglobulin
    (C) triiodothyronine
    (D) reverse triiodothyronine
    (E) monoiodotyrosine

97. Symptoms of von Gierke's disease include massive enlargement of the liver, severe hypoglycemia, ketosis, hyperlipemia, and hyperuricemia. Biopsy of the tissues of an affected person would show that the liver had a specific deficiency of the enzyme

    (A) glucokinase
    (B) hexokinase
    (C) glucose 6-phosphatase
    (D) phosphofructokinase
    (E) α-1,4-glucosidase

98. In an influenza virus complement-fixation procedure, the indicator system consists of sheep RBCs plus

    (A) ^{51}Cr-labeled sheep RBCs
    (B) antibody to influenza virus
    (C) fluorescent-tagged virus
    (D) antibody to sheep RBCs
    (E) complement

99. The photomicrograph below is from a breast biopsy in a 35-yr-old female. Which of the following most characteristically describes the lesion?

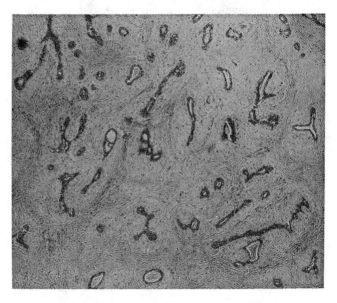

    (A) medullary carcinoma
    (B) fibroadenoma
    (C) Paget's disease
    (D) intraductal carcinoma
    (E) scirrhous carcinoma

100. Atropine, at normal dosages, blocks the effects of acetylcholine by

    (A) inhibiting the synthesis of acetylcholine
    (B) competing at the muscarinic receptor sites
    (C) blocking the release of acetylcholine from storage sites
    (D) enhancing the effects of acetylcholinesterase
    (E) competing at the nicotinic receptor sites

101. All of the following occur during the rapid-eye-movement (REM) sleep EXCEPT

    (A) rapid eye movements
    (B) sleepwalking
    (C) visual dreams
    (D) penile and clitoral erection
    (E) irregular heart rate

102. Which of the following statements concerning the structures of the perineum is true?

    (A) the perineum, defined anatomically, is the entire outlet of the pelvis
    (B) the perineum comprises only the pelvic diaphragm
    (C) the male perineum and female perineum differ because the rectal muscles are fused with the urethral bundles
    (D) the ischial symphysis is the median insertion of the perineal body
    (E) the puborectal muscle is the most lateral bundle of the levator ani

103. Damage to Wernicke's area in the cerebral cortex is associated with

    (A) impaired vocalization
    (B) impaired comprehension of speech
    (C) impaired recognition of visual forms
    (D) dyslexia
    (E) loss of short-term memory

104. The figure shown below demonstrates enzyme kinetics of

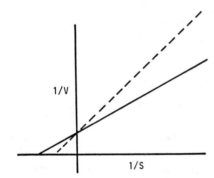

Double-reciprocal plot of enzyme kinetics.

    (A) a competitively inhibited enzyme
    (B) a noncompetitively inhibited enzyme
    (C) an allosteric enzyme with and without effector
    (D) two enzymes, each with a different Vmax
    (E) an irreversibly inhibited enzyme

105. A graft-versus-host reaction may occur

    (A) because the graft is contaminated with gram-negative microorganisms
    (B) only when tumor tissues are grafted
    (C) when immunocompetent lymphoid cells are present in the graft and the recipient is immunosuppressed
    (D) because the graft has histocompatibility antigens not found in the recipient

    (E) when a histocompatible graft is irradiated before engraftment

106. A primary adenocarcinoma of the colon that has invaded the muscle wall but not the serosa, has no local spread, and has invaded local lymph nodes is regarded as stage

    (A) T1,N1,M0
    (B) T2,N0,M1
    (C) T2,N1,M0
    (D) T3,N1,M1
    (E) T4,N1,M1

107. The uptake and elimination of inhalational anesthetics may be affected by all of the following EXCEPT

    (A) pulmonary ventilation
    (B) blood flow
    (C) the extent of liver metabolism
    (D) the solubility of gas in blood
    (E) the solubility of gas in tissue

108. Insight-oriented psychotherapy is an example of which of the following models of doctor–patient relationships?

    (A) activity–passivity
    (B) exploitive
    (C) guidance–cooperation
    (D) mutual participation
    (E) authoritarian

109. The superior lobe of the left lung comprises segments described as

    (A) apical, posterior, and anterior
    (B) apicoposterior and anterior
    (C) apicoanterior and posterior
    (D) superior lingular and lateral
    (E) inferior and superior lingular

110. All of the following statements about the skeletal muscle circulation of experimental animals are true EXCEPT that

    (A) it contributes significantly to the maintenance of systemic arterial blood pressure (BP)
    (B) blood flow within a given group of muscles is relatively homogeneous
    (C) an increase in carotid sinus pressure produces vasodilatation of the vascular bed of most muscles
    (D) contracting muscle can be shown to autoregulate
    (E) stimulation of a pathway from the cortex and hypothalamus may produce vasodilatation

111. All of the following statements concerning mutations are correct EXCEPT that

    (A) substitutions of base pairs may cause mutations
    (B) transition or transversion may cause mutations
    (C) insertion of base pairs may cause mutations
    (D) deletions of base pairs may cause mutations
    (E) most mutations are caused by thymine dimers

112. Tissue grafts in which the same individual acts as both donor and recipient are termed

    (A) allografts
    (B) autografts
    (C) xenografts
    (D) isografts
    (E) homografts

113. The tetrology of Fallot most characteristically includes all of the following EXCEPT

    (A) pulmonary stenosis
    (B) ventricular septal defect
    (C) coarctation of the aorta
    (D) right ventricular hypertrophy
    (E) overriding of the aorta over the septal defect

114. All of the following gaseous anesthetics may cause liver toxicity EXCEPT

    (A) methoxyflurane
    (B) halothane
    (C) enflurane
    (D) isoflurane
    (E) chloroform

115. All of the following factors have been clearly associated with poor adherence to medical regimens EXCEPT

    (A) field dependence
    (B) very old age
    (C) male sex
    (D) socially marginal status
    (E) severe physical illness

116. All of the following are considered parts of the arterial circle of Willis EXCEPT the

    (A) superior cerebellar artery
    (B) internal carotid artery
    (C) anterior cerebral artery
    (D) posterior communicating artery
    (E) posterior cerebral artery

117. Left coronary blood flow is greatest

    (A) near the end of systole
    (B) in early systole
    (C) at the peak aortic systolic pressure
    (D) near the end of diastole
    (E) in early diastole

118. Introns are correctly described as

    (A) noncoding intervening sequences splitting genes for a single protein
    (B) noncoding intervening sequences separating genes for different proteins
    (C) all noncoding sequences of DNA
    (D) untranslated regions of mature mRNA that separate different protein messages
    (E) untranslated regions of mature mRNA that intervene in the message for a single protein

119. Rh_0-specific immune globulin (RhoGAM) therapeutic preparations are correctly described as composed of

    (A) anti-inflammatory agents
    (B) blocking antibodies
    (C) antilymphocyte antibodies
    (D) antiallergen antibodies
    (E) enhancing antibodies

120. Cells that exhibit neoplastic transformations may show all of the following changes EXCEPT

    (A) increased sensitivity to contact inhibition of growth
    (B) decreased sensitivity to density-dependent inhibition
    (C) loss of anchoring ability for growth
    (D) infinite potential for replication and survival
    (E) the ability to produce malignant transformations in synergistic hosts

121. All of the following may cause hypokalemia EXCEPT

    (A) carbenicillin
    (B) furosemide
    (C) triamterene
    (D) amphotericin B
    (E) glycyrrhizic acid

122. A patient complains of pain in the chest and nausea. A thorough medical workup does not reveal any organic pathologic condition. It is learned that the patient's mother, who died recently, had exactly these symptoms. This patient's symptoms may be caused by

(A) generalized anxiety disorder
(B) pathologic grief reaction
(C) posttraumatic stress disorder
(D) major depression
(E) none of the above

123. The sensorimotor strip of cerebral cortex representing the right foot would derive its primary blood supply from which of the following arteries?

(A) left middle cerebral artery
(B) right middle cerebral artery
(C) left anterior cerebral artery
(D) right anterior cerebral artery
(E) right posterior cerebral artery

124. In the normal heart, the major source of energy for oxidative metabolism is

(A) glucose
(B) lactate
(C) fatty acids
(D) pyruvate
(E) amino acids

125. Addition of a competitive inhibitor to an enzymatic reaction will result in which of the following changes to a Lineweaver–Burk plot of that reaction?

(A) increase in the slope
(B) increase in the slope and decrease in the Y intercept
(C) decrease in the slope
(D) decrease in the slope and increase in the Y intercept
(E) decrease in both the slope and the Y intercept

126. Antibody against autologous IgG would be synthesized in

(A) central lymphoid organs
(B) peripheral lymphoid organs
(C) thymic tissue
(D) macrophages
(E) phagosomes

127. In order to heal properly, wounds require all of the following EXCEPT

(A) fibroblast secretion of tropocollagen
(B) cross-linkage of collagen
(C) fibroblast synthesis of elastic fibers

(D) the presence of collagenase
(E) the hydroxylation of collagen

128. The most serious result of acute acetaminophen intoxication is

(A) hypoglycemic coma
(B) methemoglobinemia
(C) respiratory depression
(D) renal tubular necrosis
(E) hepatic necrosis

129. The single best approach that physicians may use in dealing with a chronically angry patient is to

(A) express their own emotions freely
(B) let the patient use catharsis
(C) be neutral and objective
(D) consult a psychiatrist
(E) use sarcasm to defuse the anger

130. A lesion involving the superior cervical ganglion would mostly affect the

(A) accommodation reaction
(B) convergence reaction
(C) pupillary constriction reflex
(D) pupillary dilatation reflex
(E) corneal reflex

131. All of the following statements regarding systemic hemodynamics are true EXCEPT that the

(A) greatest cross-sectional area is within the capillaries rather than small veins
(B) greatest percentage of blood volume is in the small veins and the least is in the arterioles
(C) greatest drop in pressure occurs in the arterioles rather than the large arteries
(D) compliance of the venous circulation is less than the arterial circulation
(E) velocity of blood flow is lowest in the capillaries

132. Which of the following has its highest concentration in erythrocyte plasma membranes?

(A) cholesterol
(B) plasmalogens
(C) gangliosides
(D) a lipid containing glycerol, two fatty acids, and serine phosphate
(E) phosphatidyl ethanolamine

133. The sketch below represents the organism that may cause

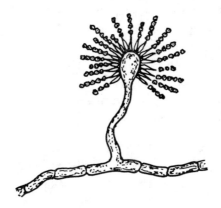

(A) phycomycosis
(B) tinea barbae
(C) tinea corporis
(D) tinea pedis
(E) aspergillosis

134. The most important component in the formation of the hemostatic plug is

(A) red blood cells
(B) fibrin
(C) lymphocytes
(D) platelets
(E) collagen

135. The phenothiazine antipsychotic that is LEAST likely to have extrapyramidal side effects is

(A) chlorpromazine
(B) trifluoperazine
(C) thioridazine
(D) haloperidol
(E) prochlorperazine

136. All of the following are often associated with decreased sexual activity EXCEPT

(A) mania
(B) depression
(C) chronic schizophrenia
(D) diabetes mellitus
(E) multiple sclerosis

137. Retinal detachments usually occur at the plane between

(A) choroid and pigmented epithelium
(B) pigmented epithelium and visual cells
(C) bipolar and ganglion cells
(D) ganglion and amacrine cells
(E) visual and horizontal cells

138. In a healthy individual with normal cardiovascular function cardiac output is controlled ultimately by

(A) the heart
(B) the sympathetic nervous system
(C) the central nervous system
(D) the peripheral circulation
(E) none of the above

139. Under normal conditions, the brain relies primarily on glucose as an energy source. Of the total calories consumed by the body, this accounts for

(A) 5 percent
(B) 20 percent
(C) 50 percent
(D) 60 percent
(E) 75 percent

140. A patient is suffering from eruptions and multiple draining sinuses with copious suppuration. The lesions are located in the cervicofacial region. Microscopic examination of material taken from the lesions reveals small sulfur granules. This patient is most likely suffering from

(A) amebiasis
(B) mucormycosis
(C) histoplasmosis
(D) candidiasis
(E) actinomycosis

141. The lesion shown below is characteristic of

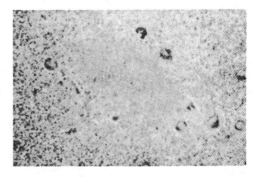

(A) an abscess
(B) a granuloma
(C) a keloid
(D) an infarct
(E) a thrombus

142. Which of the following oral hypoglycemic agents has the longest duration of action?

    (A) tolazamide

    (B) tolbutamide

    (C) acetohexamide

    (D) chlorpropamide

    (E) isopropamide

143. If a diagnostic test is positive in 98 of 100 patients with a particular disease and is negative in 90 of 100 controls without the disease, which of the following statements is true?

    (A) specificity is 98 percent and sensitivity is 90 percent

    (B) specificity is 90 percent and sensitivity is 98 percent

    (C) positive predictive accuracy is 98 percent

    (D) negative predictive accuracy is 98 percent

    (E) none of the above

Practice Test II
Questions

DIRECTIONS (Questions 144 through 189): Each group of items in this section consists of lettered headings followed by a set of numbered words or phrases. For each numbered word or phrase, select the <u>ONE</u> lettered heading that is most closely associated with it. <u>Each lettered heading may be selected once, more than once, or not at all.</u>

Questions 144 through 147

For each hormone listed below, select the metabolic derangement that would most likely result from its deficiency.

    (A) osteoporosis
    (B) ketoacidosis
    (C) sodium wasting
    (D) somnolence
    (E) hypoglycemia

144. Aldostrone

145. Cortisol

146. Insulin

147. Thyroid hormone

Questions 148 through 150

The Lineweaver-Burk plot below is based on an enzyme-catalyzed reaction in the absence of an inhibitor, the presence of a competitive inhibitor, and the presence of a noncompetitive inhibitor. For each description below, indicate the lettered point in the graph with which it is associated.

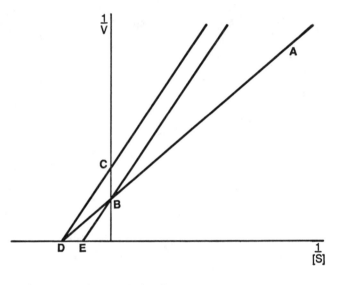

148. K_m of the uninhibited enzyme

149. Vmax of the competitively inhibited enzyme

150. The point that contains all the necessary information to determine the substrate concentration at which half the active sites will be occupied in the presence of the noncompetitive inhibitor.

Questions 151 through 153

For each agent listed below, choose the nucleic acid that best describes it.

 (A) double-stranded RNA
 (B) double-stranded DNA
 (C) single-stranded RNA
 (D) single-stranded DNA
 (E) contains no nucleic acid

151. Adenovirus

152. Prion

153. Coxsackievirus

Questions 154 through 157

For each antihypertensive agent, select the side effect with which it is most commonly associated.

 (A) bradycardia
 (B) tachycardia
 (C) first-dose syncope
 (D) depression
 (E) sedation

154. Hydralazine

155. Propranolol

156. Prazosin

157. Methyldopa

Questions 158 through 161

For each age listed below, select the developmental stage described by Erikson with which it is most likely to be associated.

 (A) identity vs role diffusion
 (B) initiative vs guilt
 (C) industry vs inferiority
 (D) basic trust vs mistrust
 (E) autonomy vs shame, doubt

158. First year

159 Fifth year

160. Tenth year

161. Fifteenth year

Questions 162 through 165

For each ganglion listed below, choose the nerve that carries the preganglionic fibers.

 (A) vagus nerve
 (B) facial nerve
 (C) oculomotor nerve
 (D) glossopharyngeal nerve
 (E) hypoglossal nerve

162. Ciliary

163. Pterygopalatine

164. Otic

165. Submandibular

Questions 166 through 168

For each phase of the cardiac cycle listed below, choose the portion of the electrocardiogram with which it is most closely associated.

 (A) P wave
 (B) QRS complex
 (C) ST segment
 (D) T wave
 (E) QT interval

166. Ventricular repolarization

167. Atrial contraction

168. Plateau phase of cardiac action potential

Questions 169 through 171

 (A) a substitution mutation changes only one specific amino acid of the protein coded
 (B) a codon codes for one specific amino acid
 (C) deletions or insertions cause frame-shifts starting at the codon for the amino acid affected
 (D) the sum of purines in double-stranded DNA is equal to the sum of pyrimidines
 (E) most of the 64 possible base triplets have been shown to code for amino acids

169. Proof that the genetic code is degenerate

170. Proof that the genetic code is nonoverlapping

171. Proof that the sequence of bases in DNA is read sequentially from a fixed starting point

Questions 172 through 174

   (A) *Neisseria meningitidis*
   (B) *Brucella abortus*
   (C) *Treponema pallidum*
   (D) *Borrelia burgdorferi*
   (E) *Legionella pneumophila*

172. Nebulizers filled with tap water have been implicated as sources of infection

173. Lyme disease

174. Cannot be cultured on artificial media

Questions 175 through 178

For each of the findings described below, choose the disease with which it is usually associated.

   (A) Marfan's syndrome
   (B) Pompe's disease
   (C) Tay-Sachs disease
   (D) Niemann-Pick disease
   (E) Lesch-Nyhan syndrome

175. Connective tissue disorder with skeletal, ocular, and cardiovascular abnormalities

176. Accumulation of GM_2 ganglioside in the nervous system

177. Spingomyelin buildup in reticuloendothelial cells

178. Cardiac and neurologic glycogen storage disease

Questions 179 through 184

For each of the following agents, select the pharmacologic effect with which it is associated.

   (A) blockade of muscarinic receptors
   (B) selective blockade of β_1-adrenergic receptors
   (C) inhibition of breakdown of cholinergic neurotransmitters
   (D) stimulation of α_1-adrenergic receptors
   (E) blockade of preganglionic nicotinic receptors

179. D-Tubocurarine

180. Physostigmine

181. Phenylephrine

182. Atropine

183. Metroprolol

184. Norepinephrine

Questions 185 through 189

For each age listed below, select the vocalization or language likely to be heard at that age.

   (A) cooing and vowel sounds
   (B) consonant sounds
   (C) conjunctions
   (D) pronouns
   (E) babbling

185. 3 mo

186. 5 mo

187. 6 mo

188. 24 mo

189. 36 mo

DIRECTIONS (Questions 190 through 230): Each group of items in this section consists of lettered headings followed by a set of numbered words or phrases. For each numbered word or phrase, select

   A if the item is associated with (A) only,
   B if the item is associated with (B) only,
   C if the item is associated with both (A) and (B),
   D if the item is associated with neither (A) nor (B).

Questions 190 through 194

   (A) inhibition of bacterial cell wall peptidoglycan synthesis
   (B) inhibition of protein synthesis at the level of the 30S bacterial ribosome
   (C) both
   (D) neither

190. Gentamicin

191. Penicillin

192. Cephalosporins

193. Sulfonamides

194. Tobramycin

Questions 195 through 197

   (A) facial nerve
   (B) vagus
   (C) both
   (D) neither

195. Carries taste fibers

196. It is predominantly afferent

197. Innervates the stapedius muscle

Questions 198 and 199

(A) P wave
(B) QRS complex
(C) both
(D) neither

198. Depolarization waves

199. Repolarization waves

Questions 200 through 202

(A) proteoglycans
(B) glycosaminoglycans
(C) both
(D) neither

200. Contain disaccharide repeating units

201. Contain core proteins

202. Contain several different polysaccharides

Questions 203 and 204

(A) antigens
(B) haptens
(C) both
(D) neither

203. React with homologous antibodies

204. Induce the production of specific antibodies

Questions 205 and 206

(A) intracerebral hemorrhage
(B) subdural hemorrhage
(C) both
(D) neither

205. Trauma to the head

206. Severe hypertension

Questions 207 and 208

(A) clonidine
(B) propranolol
(C) both
(D) neither

207. Abrupt withdrawal may be associated with hypertension

208. May produce postural hypotension

Questions 209 through 215

(A) operant (instrumental) conditioning
(B) classical conditioning
(C) both
(D) neither

209. Reward

210. Does not occur with the autonomic nervous system

211. Unconditioned response

212. Shaping

213. Phobias may result from this

214. Never occurs in humans

215. Stimulus generalization

Questions 216 through 218

(A) neural crest
(B) neural tube (neuroepithelium)
(C) both
(D) neither

216. Anterior (ventral) horn motor neurons

217. Postganglionic sympathetic neurons

218. Dorsal root neurons

Questions 219 through 221

(A) loss of consciousness
(B) clonic muscle contractions
(C) both
(D) neither

219. Petit mal seizures

220. Grand mal seizures

221. Psychomotor seizures

Questions 222 through 224

(A) eukaryotic mRNA
(B) bacterial mRNA
(C) both
(D) neither

222. Undergoes little modification after transcription

223. A poly A tail is added after transcription

224. Contains numerous methylated base or ribose units that are posttranslational modifications

Questions 225 and 226

    (A) toxoid
    (B) exotoxin
    (C) both
    (D) neither

225. Immunogenic

226. Toxic

Questions 227 and 228

    (A) reactive follicular hyperplasia (RFH)
    (B) nodular lymphoma (NL)
    (C) both
    (D) neither

227. Preservation of nodal architecture

228. Even distribution of follicles or nodules throughout the cortex and medulla of the node

Questions 229 and 230

    (A) myelosuppression is an important side effect
    (B) relatively high degree of specificity in its actions on T cells
    (C) both
    (D) neither

229. Cyclosporine

230. Azathioprine

DIRECTIONS (Questions 231 through 311): For each of the items in this section, ONE or MORE of the numbered options is correct. Choose the answer

    A if only 1, 2, and 3 are correct,
    B if only 1 and 3 are correct,
    C if only 2 and 4 are correct,
    D if only 4 is correct,
    E if all are correct.

231. Organisms that produce potent exotoxins that have a pathogenic function include

    (1) *Brucella abortus*
    (2) *Corynebacterium diphtheriae*
    (3) *Mycobacterium tuberculosis*
    (4) *Clostridium botulinum*

232. Important viral factors involved in viral disease production include the

    (1) immunologic status of the host
    (2) cytopathic effect of the virus on target cells
    (3) nutritional status of the host
    (4) alterations of the host's cell membranes

233. A carbon skeleton for the biosynthesis of amino acids in humans is supplied by

    (1) pyruvate
    (2) oxaloacetate
    (3) 3-phosphoglycerate
    (4) α-ketoglutarate

234. The protein coat (capsid) of true viruses is known to

    (1) serve as an antigen in serologic tests
    (2) function to maintain infectivity of nucleic acid in the extracellular state
    (3) serve as an antigen in vaccines
    (4) aid in the penetration of the virion into susceptible cells

235. Amino acids whose side chains contribute to the charge of a protein at pH 7 include

    (1) cysteine
    (2) glycine
    (3) tyrosine
    (4) lysine

236. A 6-yr-old farm boy develops restlessness, hallucinations, and convulsions and dies 2 days later. At autopsy, the only significant finding is eosinophilic inclusions in neurons. These findings are consistent with

    (1) rabies
    (2) polio
    (3) herpes simplex encephalitis
    (4) western equine encephalitis

237. The reagent cyanogen bromide cleaves

    (1) peptide bonds on the α-carboxyl side of arginine residues
    (2) peptide bonds on the α-carboxyl side of lysine residues
    (3) disulfide bridges
    (4) peptide bonds between the α-carboxyl of methionine and the α-amino group of the adjacent amino acid

238. Antibody-mediated antiviral immunity may operate through which of the following mechanisms?

    (1) complement-independent neutralization
    (2) complement-dependent neutralization
    (3) opsonization
    (4) lysis of infected host cells

239. Carcinoma of the colon and rectum is characteristically

    (1) common in North American whites
    (2) most frequently seen in patients over the age of 50 yr
    (3) uncommon in black Africans and Japanese in Japan
    (4) frequently seen in people on high-fiber diets

240. The risk factors for suicide include

    (1) living alone
    (2) previous attempts at suicide
    (3) presence of pain
    (4) male sex

241. The enzyme succinyl-CoA-acetoacetate transferase (3-ketoacid CoA transferase) is found in

    (1) skeletal muscle
    (2) erythrocytes
    (3) the brain
    (4) the liver

242. A virus causes diseases by

    (1) rendering vital target cells nonfunctional
    (2) disrupting the mucosa to allow bacteria to enter and produce a superimposed infection and disease
    (3) stimulating the host to produce immune substances that are deleterious to the host
    (4) altering the growth properties of the cell

243. In the photomicrograph of a cytologic preparation shown below, malignant cells may be characterized by features such as

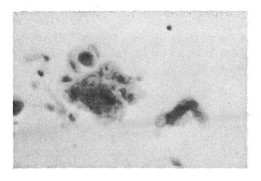

    (1) increased nucleus/cytoplasm ratio
    (2) increased cell size
    (3) pleomorphism of cell shape
    (4) absence of nucleoli

244. Depression may be associated with which of the following?

    (1) cancer of the pancreas
    (2) antihypertensive drugs
    (3) hypothyroidism
    (4) cocaine abuse

245. The embryonic development of the neural tube and derivatives is correctly described by which of the following statements?

    (1) the neural tube is derived from the mesodermal germ layer of the embryo
    (2) the wall of the neural tube is initially a pseudostratified columnar epithelium from which neurons, but no glial cells, are derived
    (3) myelination in the spinal cord is complete by the ninth month in utero
    (4) in newborns, the caudal end of the spinal cord is at approximately the level of the third lumbar vertebra

246. Sodium reabsorption is correctly described as

    (1) occurring in the proximal tubules via an active transport system
    (2) increased by aldosterone in both proximal and distal tubules
    (3) in part coupled with active transport of K^+ into the distal tubular epithelium
    (4) increased with volume expansion

247. Compounds derived from the amino acid tyrosine include

    (1) melanin
    (2) epinephrine
    (3) levodopa
    (4) histamine

248. Influenza viruses are correctly described as

    (1) being of three antigenic types (A, B, and C)
    (2) having a segmented genome
    (3) typed according to the ribonucleoprotein in the virion
    (4) having RNA as their genetic information

SUMMARY OF DIRECTIONS				
A	**B**	**C**	**D**	**E**
1, 2, 3 only	1, 3 only	2, 4 only	4 only	All are correct

249. Emboli are clots or plugs that are

(1) of gas, fat, or amniotic fluid origin

(2) causes of hemorrhagic infarction

(3) carried intravascularly by blood to distant sites

(4) usually of intravascular thrombotic origin

250. Which of the following statements may describe an acute grief reaction?

(1) it seldom is associated with depressive syndrome

(2) waves of somatic distress are common

(3) antidepressant therapy often may be required

(4) hallucinations and illusions may occur

251. The ventral posterior lateral nucleus of the thalamus is correctly described as

(1) receiving fibers conveying impulses associated with pain and temperature from the face

(2) a nonspecific thalamic relay nucleus

(3) projecting to the supplementary motor cortex

(4) processing sensory information from pain, touch, and proprioceptive pathways

252. The course of a premature ventricular systole is correctly described by which of the following statements?

(1) the premature contraction is associated with a diminished development of tension in the left ventricle

(2) a second contraction occurs in an interval shorter than normal

(3) peak left ventricular pressure in the following beat is greater than in previous contractions

(4) peak left ventricular pressure is usually less than normal for several beats after the first postextrasystolic beat

253. The compound tetrahydrofolate, as it occurs in humans, is correctly described as

(1) carrying activated one-carbon units

(2) serving as a donor of one-carbon units in biosynthetic reactions

(3) serving as a receptor of one-carbon units in degradative reactions

(4) not carrying the one-carbon unit CO_2

254. Receptors for C3b are present in the membranes of

(1) macrophages

(2) B lymphocytes

(3) neutrophils

(4) T lymphocytes

255. Which of the following types of change seen in cell injury is LEAST associated with abnormalities of the nucleus?

(1) pyknosis

(2) karyolysis

(3) karyorrhexis

(4) swelling of rough endoplasmic reticulum

256. Depressive syndrome may be characterized by

(1) suicidal thoughts

(2) apathy

(3) anorexia

(4) anhedonia

257. The hypothalamus is correctly described as

(1) projecting to brain stem nuclei

(2) receiving afferent fibers via the medial forebrain bundle

(3) involved in the regulation and modulation of autonomic activity

(4) situated in the walls and floor of the third ventricle

258. The tympanic reflex is associated with

(1) relaxation of the tensor tympani

(2) inward movement of the maleus

(3) inward movement of the foot plate of the stapes

(4) decreased sound transmission

259. Which of the following enzymes can be found in the liver but not in skeletal muscle?

(1) glucose 6-phosphatase

(2) glucokinase

(3) pyruvate carboxylase

(4) fructose 1,6-diphosphatase

260. A preparation of pooled human IgM injected into a rabbit may stimulate production of antibodies reactive with

(1) λ light chain

(2) μ chain

(3) κ light chain

(4) J chain

261. Stings by bees, wasps, or hornets may produce skin responses that may be described as

    (1) acute necrosis
    (2) chronic lymphoid infiltration
    (3) subacute inflammation
    (4) granulomatous necrosis

262. Obsessional neurosis may be characterized by

    (1) undoing
    (2) anal sadistic tendencies
    (3) rigid superego
    (4) isolation

263. Complete destruction of the dorsal cochlear nucleus would

    (1) result in complete unilateral deafness
    (2) decrease the number of fibers in the ipsilateral lateral lemniscus
    (3) produce partial deafness in the contralateral ear
    (4) result in a hearing deficit on the affected side

264. The figure below represents two ventricular function curves of a dog's heart. Curve A is plotted at rest, and curve B is plotted during an experimental protocol. Which of the following protocols would be most likely to cause a shift from curve A to curve B?

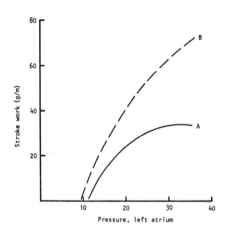

    (1) infusion of norepinephrine
    (2) reducing the temperature of the heart
    (3) sympathetic stimulation of the heart
    (4) injection of a calcium-blocking agent, such as verapamil

265. Which of the following characteristics are indicative of regions of the eukaryotic genome that are actively transcribed?

    (1) sensitivity to digestion by DNase I
    (2) presence of the nonhistone proteins HMG 14 and HMG 17

    (3) reduced levels of 5-methylcytosine
    (4) elevated levels of the core histones

266. Hypervariable regions of IgG molecules exist on

    (1) H chain
    (2) L chain
    (3) Fab fragments
    (4) Fc fragments

267. The features of drug-induced vasculitis include

    (1) lesions that are limited to the skin
    (2) an association with the use of phenylbutazone
    (3) an underlying panniculitis in the subcutaneous tissue
    (4) both leukocytoclastic and lymphocytic forms

268. Captopril inhibits

    (1) angiotensin-converting enzyme
    (2) formation of angiotensin I
    (3) degration of bradykinin
    (4) aldosterone metabolism

269. Psychologic defense mechanisms may be described as

    (1) accentuated during hospitalization
    (2) associated with hormonal states
    (3) adaptive in illness
    (4) consciously mobilized

270. The organ of Corti is

    (1) attached to the bony modiolus at the same site as the tectorial membrane
    (2) located in the cochlear duct
    (3) surrounded by perilymph
    (4) activated by pressure waves in the scala tympani

271. The hormone cholecystikinin (CCK) provides a potent stimulus for emptying of the gallbladder. Each of the following statements regarding CCK are correct EXCEPT

    (1) CCK is released by endocrine cells of the small intestine
    (2) CCK alone strongly stimulates pancreatic secretion of enzymes and juice
    (3) CCK competitively inhibits gastrin-stimulated acid secretion
    (4) CCK is released in response to the presence of monosaccharides in the duodenum

SUMMARY OF DIRECTIONS				
A	**B**	**C**	**D**	**E**
1, 2, 3 only	1, 3 only	2, 4 only	4 only	All are correct

272. Both bacterial and eukaryotic nuclear DNA are

    (1) associated with histones
    (2) linear molecules
    (3) approximately the same size
    (4) replicated in a semiconservative manner

273. Rickettsiae are considered to be bacteria because they

    (1) contain both RNA and DNA
    (2) have a peptidoglycan-containing cell wall
    (3) divide by binary fission
    (4) are facultative parasites of living cells

274. The underdeveloped lungs of immature or premature infants cannot adequately perform their ventilatory functions because

    (1) alveolar capillaries are removed from the air spaces
    (2) alveolar development only begins at about 7 mo gestation
    (3) the alveolar septa are relatively thick
    (4) the diaphragm is incompletely formed

275. Digoxin

    (1) has a high therapeutic index
    (2) is a positive inotrope
    (3) has a relatively short half-time for elimination compared to time required for therapeutic effect
    (4) has both direct and indirect electrophysiologic effects

276. Factors that influence how a patient perceives a symptom include

    (1) the frequency of the symptom in a given population
    (2) the familiarity of the symptoms
    (3) the predictability of the outcome of the illness
    (4) the degree of threat associated with the illness

277. In the cerebral cortex, pyramidal cells are found in which of the following layers?

    (1) V
    (2) III
    (3) II
    (4) I

278. A prolonged deficiency of vitamin A may lead to eye changes, such as

    (1) nyctalopia
    (2) degeneration of cones
    (3) degeneration of rods
    (4) degeneration of retinal cells other than receptors

279. An unesterified glycerol hydroxyl group is produced after hydrolysis of a phospholipid by

    (1) phospholipase A_1
    (2) phospholipase A_2
    (3) phospholipase C
    (4) phospholipase D

280. Which of the following may occur when bacteria are treated with lysozyme?

    (1) the linkage between N-acetylmuramic acid and N-acetylglucosamine is hydrolyzed
    (2) the cell becomes osmotically fragile
    (3) protoplasts are produced
    (4) spheroplasts are produced

281. Which of the following may be implicated as carcinogens?

    (1) vinyl chloride
    (2) aflatoxin B
    (3) 2-naphthylamine
    (4) betel nut chewing

282. A patient is discharged from the hospital with a plasma level of digoxin near 1.0 ng/mL and instructions to continue appropriate maintenance therapy. Several weeks later, the same patient is readmitted with toxic symptoms associated with digoxin and a plasma level > 4.0 ng/ml. Possible explanations for this observation include

    (1) sudden improvement in cardiac function with increased renal perfusion so that renal clearance increased
    (2) inappropriate patient compliance such that patient took digoxin more frequently than suggested
    (3) impairment of hepatic function in the presence of unrelated disease
    (4) decrease in volume of distribution of digoxin in the presence of concurrent therapy with quinidine

283. Which of the following factors will increase the likelihood of a person's seeking medical help?

    (1) high level of stress
    (2) upper socioeconomic class
    (3) anxiety concerning the symptom
    (4) unpleasant experiences with physicians

284. The pharyngeal pouches are correctly described by which of the following statements?

    (1) pouches 2 and 3 communicate with the cervical sinus early in development
    (2) pouch 3 gives rise to the thymus on the right side and the inferior parathyroid gland on the left
    (3) pouch 1 lies in front of the oropharyngeal (buccopharyngeal) membrane
    (4) pouch 1 endoderm contributes to the lining of the adult middle ear cavity

285. The endocochlear potential is correctly described as

    (1) produced by deformation of the basilar membrane
    (2) the potential difference between endolymph and perilymph
    (3) the generator potential of the hair cells
    (4) dependent on ion pump activity in the stria vascularis

286. The carbon atoms of fatty acids synthesized in humans can be derived from

    (1) citrate
    (2) carbohydrates
    (3) proteins
    (4) steroids

287. Rabies virus

    (1) is contained in the saliva of infected dogs
    (2) glycoprotein spikes serve as host cell adhesions
    (3) infects the CNS
    (4) cannot be recovered from the salivary glands of infected carnivores

288. Acute rejection of a renal transplant is characterized by

    (1) an interstitial infiltrate composed of mononuclear cells
    (2) its occurrence within minutes of transplantation
    (3) necrotizing arteritis with a neutrophilic infiltrate
    (4) its failure to respond to immunosuppressive therapy

289. Correct statements regarding the nature of drug–receptor interactions include

    (1) a drug effect is inversely proportional to drug–receptor complex
    (2) potency, not efficacy, is an important characteristic of a drug for clinical purposes
    (3) antagonists are drugs that occupy receptors but bring about less than the maximum response
    (4) the affinity of drugs for receptors can vary independent of their ability to bring about a response

290. The basic elements of informed consent include

    (1) a reasonable explanation of the procedures
    (2) advising patients that they are free to withdraw consent at any time
    (3) a description of potential risks and benefits
    (4) a discussion of potential alternatives

291. Efferent fibers from the cerebellar nuclei leave the cerebellum via the

    (1) brachium conjunctivum
    (2) brachium pontis
    (3) restiform body
    (4) middle cerebellar peduncle

292. During strenuous exercise, cardiac output may increase fourfold with little change in right atrial pressure. The cardiovascular adjustments that underlie this phenomenon are known to

    (1) primarily be the result of an improved cardiac function curve due to the release of epinephrine
    (2) include increased total peripheral vascular resistance due to sympathetic stimulation
    (3) result from dilatation of small veins, thereby increasing venous return
    (4) partly result from increased cardiac function and decreased venous capacitance secondary to sympathetic stimulation

293. Bile salts are required for

    (1) transport of fatty acids across the mitochondrial membrane
    (2) facilitating the action of pancreatic lipase
    (3) buffering of intestinal acids
    (4) intestinal absorption of fatty acids, monoglycerides, and diglycerides

SUMMARY OF DIRECTIONS				
A	**B**	**C**	**D**	**E**
1, 2, 3 only	1, 3 only	2, 4 only	4 only	All are correct

294. True statements concerning the varicella-herpes zoster virus include

    (1) it has a tropism for nerve cells

    (2) it replicates in the cytoplasm

    (3) it can be activated to give manifestations in a dermatome distribution

    (4) infections can be diagnosed by the presence of large cytomegalic cells

295. The lesion shown below is known to cause

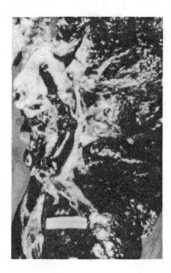

    (1) sudden death

    (2) pulmonary infarction

    (3) hemorrhagic necrosis

    (4) left-sided heart failure

296. Adverse effects of aminoglycoside antibiotics in humans include

    (1) nephrotoxicity

    (2) hepatitis

    (3) ototoxicity

    (4) congestive heart failure

297. Anxiety may correctly be described by which of the following statements?

    (1) it usually reduces the sympathetic tone

    (2) it may improve performance

    (3) it is often unconscious

    (4) it may be a conditioned response

298. Each branchial arch contains

    (1) an aortic arch vessel

    (2) neural crest cells

    (3) a cartilaginous plate

    (4) a cranial nerve or major branch of a cranial nerve

299. According to the Henderson-Hasselbalch equation, pH = pK + log (ionized/un-ionized). The pK of phenobarbital is 7.2. Which of the following therapies would increase renal clearance of phenobarbital in an intoxicated, comatose patient on a ventilator?

    (1) IV infusion of sodium bicarbonate

    (2) IV injection of vasopressin

    (3) IV infusion of mannitol

    (4) lowering the ventilatory rate

300. Hormones that have antagonistic effects to each other include

    (1) serotonin and histamine

    (2) calcitonin and parathyroid hormone

    (3) glucagon and insulin

    (4) epinephrine and norepinephrine

301. Acquired immunodeficiency syndrome (AIDS) leads to

    (1) *Pneumocystis carinii* infections

    (2) Kaposi's sarcoma

    (3) reduction of CD-4+ T cells

    (4) non-Hodgkin's B cell lymphomas

302. The cellular process of apoptosis is best described as

    (1) shrinkage necrosis

    (2) by-product of coagulative necrosis

    (3) individual cell deletion

    (4) gummatous necrosis

303. Cholestyramine adversely affects the absorption of

    (1) lipid-soluble vitamins

    (2) anticoagulants

    (3) digitalis glycosides

    (4) phenobarbital

304. Based on a prospective study of cigarette smoking and the development of lung cancer in physicians, heavy smokers were found to have an annual mortality rate of 2.27 per 1,000 from lung cancer, whereas nonsmokers had an annual death rate of 0.07 per 1,000 from lung cancer. On the basis of this study, we can state that

(1) the relative risk of death from lung cancer for smokers is 32 times as great as for nonsmokers

(2) the attributable risk of smoking for lung cancer is 2.20

(3) smoking accounts for 97 percent of the total risk of death from lung cancer in this population

(4) the population attributable risk of lung cancer resulting from smoking for this population is 2.27/2.20

305. Which of the following enzymatic activities are associated with the DNA polymerase III holoenzyme of *Escherichia coli?*

(1) 5′ to 3′ polymerase

(2) 3′ to 5′ polymerase

(3) 3′ to 5′ exonuclease

(4) 5′ to 3′ exonculease

306. The proximal renal tubules are correctly described as

(1) forming the major part of the tubular mass renal parenchyma

(2) consisting of epithelial cells with an extensive brush border

(3) responsible for approximately 65 percent of all resorptive and secretory processes

(4) responsible for almost complete resorption of glucose, protein, and amino acids

307. γ-Carboxylation of prothrombin is inhibited by which of the following anticoagulants?

(1) heparin

(2) dicumarol

(3) acetic acid

(4) warfarin

308. The ability to survive the host immune response by producing new antigenic variants is characteristic of

(1) *Haemophilus influenzae*

(2) *Trypanosoma gambiense*

(3) *Streptococcus pyogenes*

(4) *Borrelia recurrentis*

309. Diffuse pulmonary interstitial fibrosis can be caused by

(1) busulfan

(2) *Thermopolyspora polyspora*

(3) silica

(4) sarcoidosis

310. Which of the following statements may be true regarding antiseptics and disinfectants?

(1) benzoyl peroxide slowly releases oxygen and is therefore bactericidal against anaerobic and microaerophilic bacteria

(2) the activity of ethyl alcohol is most effective at concentrations of 50 to 70 percent by weight

(3) iodine is a valuable agent in the treatment of wounds and abrasions because of its low toxicity compared with its germicidal potency

(4) the mechanism of action for phenol and phenol derivatives is via protein precipitation

311. Epidemiologic studies, such as the Isle of Wight study, that have examined the association between reading difficulties and psychiatric disorders have shown that

(1) 25 percent of children with specific reading retardation show antisocial behavior

(2) 30 percent of children with a conduct disorder have reading retardation

(3) 4 percent of children in the general population have reading retardation

(4) the association between reading difficulties and conduct disorders is much stronger than the association with emotional disturbance

Answers and Explanations

1. **The answer is E.** The medulla oblongata and the pons (varolii) are supplied by the anterior spinal arteries, posterior spinal artery, and branches of the vertebral and basilar arteries. The middle cerebral is the only artery of those listed in the question that does not supply the medulla and pons. A minor source of arterial blood to the medulla and pons can sometimes include both the superior and anterior inferior cerebellar arteries. *(Carpenter, pp 724–730)*

2. **The answer is D.** Except for arachidonic, all of the fatty acids listed in the question are nonessential and cannot be precursors for the synthesis of essential fatty acids in humans. Prostaglandins are synthesized from arachidonic acid (*cis*-5,8,11,14-eicosatetraenoic acid) or other 20-carbon fatty acids that have at least three double bonds. Prostaglandins are 20-carbon fatty acids that contain a 5-carbon ring. They are hormonelike in their action, but unlike hormones, they often directly modulate the activities of the cells in which they are synthesized. *(Stryer pp 991–992)*

3. **The answer is D.** Primary hyperparathyroidism is a group of diseases characterized by overproduction of parathormone in a setting of no previous parathyroid hypersecretion. It occurs in 2.5 per 1,000 people. The overproduction of parathormone causes bone destruction with increased calcium release and elevated calcium levels in the blood. Subsequently, the kidneys are overloaded with calcium, with leakage of both calcium and phosphorus in the urine. Eventually, there is renal stone formation. This disease is also associated with peptic ulcers, pancreatitis, hypertension, CNS disturbances, and multiple endocrine neoplasia types I and II. The bone disease consists of bone destruction and new bone formation and the development of cysts and fibrosis. The renal disease includes stone formation, polyuria, polydipsia, and renal failure. Laboratory analysis of serum shows hypercalcemia with hypophosphatemia and elevated levels of parathor-

mone. Primary hyperparathyroidism may be caused by adenomas, chief cell or water clear cell hyperplasias, or carcinomas. Parathyroid adenomas are the major cause in most patient series of primary hyperparathyroidism. *(Rubin and Farber, pp 1146–1149)*

4. **The answer is D.** The hip joint is supplied by the following nerves: the obturator and its accessory, the femoral, the superior gluteal, and the tibial portion of the sciatic nerve to the musculus quadratus femoris. The common peroneal portion of the sciatic nerve does not supply the hip joint. *(Gardner et al, p 217)*

5. **The answer is B.** Vitamin B_{12}, or cobalamin, is unique in that its corrin ring requires a cobalt atom in order to function. Cobalamin enzymes are involved in hydrogen rearrangement reactions, as in the synthesis of deoxyribonucleosides from ribonucleosides or as in the conversion of methylmalonyl coenzyme A (CoA) into succinyl CoA. The methylation of homocysteine by N^5-methyltetrahydrofolate to form methionine also requires the involvement of cobalamin as a methylated intermediate. Deficiencies of vitamin B_{12} or cobalt result in anemic symptoms. Pernicious anemia is a disease in which vitamin B_{12} is not absorbed because of a lack of a protein called intrinsic factor. This protein is normally synthesized by the gut epithelium and is required for vitamin B_{12} absorption. *(Stryer, pp 506–509)*

6. **The answer is C.** Squamous cell carcinoma is the most common type of bronchogenic carcinoma, accounting for 60 percent of all reported cases. It is found in males more often than in females and is the form of lung cancer most closely correlated with a history of smoking. This type of tumor is thought to arise from bronchial mucosa and is thus central in location. Its increasing incidence in women is thought to be secondary to the increasing number of women smoking cigarettes in the past 20 yr. *(Robbins et al, pp 750–754)*

7. **The answer is A.** The lower portions of the respiratory system develop as a diverticulum of the foregut, and thus the epithelium lining the airways and forming the glands would be derived from foregut endoderm. The smooth muscle, cartilage, and fibrous connective tissues are derived from splanchnic mesenchyme. The midgut endoderm gives rise to the small intestine, cecum, appendix, and most of the transverse colon. The cardiogenic mesenchyme forms the endocardial heart tubes. Neural crest cells give rise to the spinal ganglia and those of the autonomic nervous system. *(Moore, pp 61, 216–224, 239, 303)*

8. **The answer is B.** Acetic acid is a weak acid, as indicated by its pK_a, and dissociates into a hydrogen ion and its conjugate base, acetate (i.e., $CH_3-COOH \rightarrow H^+ + CH_3-COO^-$). A solution of a weak acid and its salt is referred to as a buffer. The pH of any buffer solution can be determined by use of the Henderson-Hasselbalch equation.

$$pH = pK_a + \log A^-/HA$$

When the acetic acid has been converted into 80 percent acetate, the ratio A^-/HA is 4, and substituting the values provided in the problem into the Henderson-Hasselbalch equation yields:

$$pH = 4.75 + \log 4 = 5.35$$

(Stryer, pp 41–42)

9. **The answer is D.** Mesothelioma is the most common malignant tumor of the pleura. It is a highly invasive lesion and has been linked to asbestos fibers—especially in persons in the shipbuilding and insulation industries. A history of smoking also increases the risk of developing a mesothelioma. Histologically, the tumor may be either sarcomatous (composed of mesenchymal stromal cells), carcinomatous (resembling tubular or papillary structures), or a combination of these two types. These tumors are highly malignant, and most patients die within 1 yr of diagnosis. *(Robbins et al, pp 760–761)*

10. **The answer is C.** Although metabolic acidosis may occur and [H$^+$] increase, the initial compensatory response to hemorrhage results in a large increase in total peripheral vascular resistance. The loss of blood volume initially decreases cardiac output, but baroreceptor-mediated sympathetic drive causes vasoconstriction. Thus, vascular resistance increases, heart rate increases, and blood pressure returns toward normal. Slightly later, the kidneys may secrete renin, and the production of angiotensin II via converting enzyme activity ultimately ensues. Fluid also will shift from the interstitial compartments to the vascular space, help-

ing to restore cardiac output. Other humoral agents, including epinephrine, vasopressin, and glucocorticoids, may also be released to further compensate for the cardiovascular effects of hemorrhage. *(Guyton, pp 327–328)*

11. **The answer is C.** The heart is drained partly by veins that empty into the coronary sinus and partly by small veins that empty directly into the chambers of the heart. The direct veins include the anterior cardiac veins and the minimae cardiac veins. The coronary sinus ends in the right atrium and receives the great cardiac, middle cardiac, small cardiac, and the oblique vein of the left atrium. *(Gardner et al, p 323)*

12. **The answer is D.** Temporary occlusion of both common carotid arteries will decrease vascular pressure within the carotid sinus area. This important peripheral baroreceptor responds to changes in pressure and is an important reflex in maintaining relatively constant arterial pressure on a short-term basis. A decrease in pressure will depress the number of impulses that travel from the carotid sinus nerve. Since these impulses normally inhibit the central vasoconstrictor area and excite the vagal center, a decrease in impulses will reflexively cause arterial pressure to rise and heart rate and contractility to increase. The entire circulation will be stimulated to constrict, and thus there will be a reduction in venous capacitance. *(Guyton, pp 249–251)*

13. **The answer is C.** The normal yield from the complete oxidation of glycogen is about 4.2 kcal/g. Approximately the same amount of energy is derived from the combustion of proteins. In contrast, oxidation of fatty acids derived from triacylglyceride stores is much greater, about 9.5 kcal/g. Despite the fact that glycogen is an important and easily mobilized energy store, fats are the major energy reservoir. *(Stryer, p 471)*

14. **The answer is E.** The condition of psoriasis is characteristically a scaly hyperkeratotic lesion of the skin, with the characteristic features described as parakeratosis, which is abnormal keratin maturation with nucleated material in the stratum corneum and with resultant thickness of the epidermis with club-shaped papillae extending into the dermal collagen. From time to time in various stages of the disease, collections of neutrophil leukocytes in the form of microabscessess can be seen in the upper layers of the epidermis. These are sometimes referred to as Pautrier's microabscesses. The condition is clearly distinguishable microscopically from other thickening of the epidermis, which may be mistaken clinically for basal cell carcinoma or even melanoma or squamous cell carcinoma. The condition of pemphigus vulgaris is a bullous or vesicular

type of lesion that may have produced crusting on the surface and may be clinically similar but is microscopically quite distinct. Psoriasis is thought to be related to an abnormality of cell proliferation and control, resulting from some forms of injury, but its real etiology is still largely unknown. *(Rubin and Farber, pp 1209–1214)*

15. The answer is E. The sensory innervation of the scalp is provided by the supratrochlear and supraorbital branches of the ophthalmic nerve, the zygomaticotemporal branch of the maxillary nerve, the auriculotemporal branch of the mandibular nerve, the lesser occipital nerve of the cervical plexus, and the greater occipital and third occipital nerves (dorsal rami) of the cervical spinal nerves. The temporal branch of the facial nerve (cranial nerve VII) does not supply the scalp. *(Gardner et al, pp 659–660)*

16. The answer is D. Although short-term regulation of arterial BP is primarily affected by the integrated responses of peripheral baroreceptors and the central and sympathetic nervous systems, the primary determinant of regulation of BP in the long run is the relationship of urine output to fluid intake. This system is normally capable of returning BP to normal levels (infinite gain), which is different from the short-term nervous regulation. By adjusting extracellular fluid and blood volumes, renal–body fluid mechanisms alter venous return. Individual beds then adjust their resistance because of the interplay of local and neuronal factors, and thus arterial pressure is slowly readjusted to control levels. The total peripheral vascular resistance is thus altered by those mechanisms rather than being the variable that directly determines BP. *(Guyton, pp 246–247)*

17. The answer is A. The primary precursors for gluconeogenesis in liver are lactate and alanine, which are produced in muscle during intense activity. Alanine is formed from pyruvate by transamination in a reaction catalyzed by alanine aminotransferase. Alanine is converted back to pyruvate in liver and employed in the synthesis of glucose. *(Stryer, pp 444–445, 496)*

18. The answer is D. Constrictive pericarditis is a condition in which the normally thin and delicate pericardium is replaced by dense fibrous tissue with, in some circumstances, calcification within the fibrous tissue, resulting in a rigid, constricting pericardium that causes eventually malfunction of the myocardium and congestive failure. Although there are many reasons why the pericardium may cause an obstructive function to the heart, many of the others result from the acute accumulation of fluid or fluid and fibrin as seen in some cases of acute rheumatic fever or acute staphylococcal in-

fections. In uremia and in lupus erythematosus, there may be hemorrhagic or even fibrinous pericarditis, but it rarely extends long enough to produce the complete constrictive form of the disease with dense fibrosis that is so typically seen in tuberculosis. In fact, tuberculosis is by far the most common cause of this otherwise relatively rare disorder. *(Rubin and Farber, p 536)*

19. The answer is E. Identification is the psychologic defense mechanism by which an individual becomes like an admired (or otherwise psychologically important) person. Identification is an important phenomenon in personality development. *(Leigh and Reiser, pp 77–98)*

20. The answer is C. Hormones are chemical substances secreted by glands and are usually effective in very minute amounts. Glands show marked differences in their structure, function, and pattern of development. Exocrine glands secrete outwardly via a duct. Endocrine glands are ductless, since their secretions or hormones are poured directly in the venous drainage. The thyroid gland is a pure endocrine gland rather than an amphicrine, an adjective meaning "both secretions" (endocrine plus exocrine) and reserved for describing mixed types of glands, such as the pancreas. The thyroid gland is a cervical and not an abdominal gland. *(Gardner et al, p 43)*

21. The answer is B. Atrial fibrillation is a common arrhythmia that accompanies several forms of chronic heart disease. It probably represents some form of reentry phenomenon in which part of the tissue may be excited at an inappropriately early part of the cardiac cycle. Since the atria do not contract, there are no P waves. Activation of conducting tissue in the atrioventricular node becomes variable in time from cycle to cycle, and thus the QRS complex interval becomes less constant. The strength of ventricular contraction is related to the timing of filling, and thus failure of the atria to effectively contract alters ventricular filling. This produces an extremely irregular pulse. Direct current shock is an effective mechanism to return the heart to normal rhythm and reverse atrial fibrillation. However, atrial fibrillation per se is not a life-threatening event, and placing the entire myocardium into refractory period frequently is not the appropriate course of action. A number of drugs are available to prolong the effective refractory period of selective parts of the heart, and these drugs would represent an effective manner in which to revert atrial fibrillation to normal atrial contraction. *(Berne and Levy, pp 49–51)*

22. The answer is D. None of the amino acids composing the peptide Val-Ala-Pro-Glu-Gly have any charged side chains except for glutamate, which bears a charged carboxyl group. Thus, we only have to consider the amino and carboxyl groups of the C- and N-terminals along with the glutamic acid carboxyl group. At neutral pH, the carboxyl groups will be dissociated, since their pKs are always at a low pH. Likewise, the positively charged N-terminal amino group will not be dissociated, since its pK is always at a high pH. Thus, at pH 7, the peptide will contain two negative charges and one positive charge for an overall negative charge. Increasing the pH will only increase the negativity of the peptide, since the amino group will become more dissociated and less charged as its pK is approached. The isoelectric point of the peptide will be found at pH lower than 7. *(Lehninger, pp 71–76; Stryer pp 17, 42)*

23. **The answer is B.** Wire-loop lesions in glomeruli in renal biopsy specimens, though not pathognomonic, are generally associated with renal involvement by systemic lupus erythematosus. The formation of the wire loops is caused by subendothelial electron-dense deposits that produce thickened, refractile capillary walls. Small subepithelial deposits, or spikes, may also be present and produce extension of the deposits through the basement membrane. Wire-loop lesions also may be seen in glomerular lesions of patients with cryoglobulinemia. Diabetes mellitus, hypertension, and acute tubular necrosis may be associated with histologic changes in the renal glomeruli or tubules or both. These entities are not typically associated with wire-loop lesions, however. In the hepatorenal syndrome, renal dysfunction appears to be functional rather than associated with anatomic renal changes. *(Rubin and Farber, pp 864–867)*

24. **The answer is B.** Society's sick-role expectations, as described by Parsons, include exemption from normal social role expectations, the recognition that the individual is not responsible for being sick and that he or she cannot be expected to get well simply by wanting to get well, being sick is an undesirable state, and the individual should try to get well, and that the sick person should seek competent help to get well. The idea that an individual is responsible for the maintenance of his or her health is contrary to the second expectation described above. *(Leigh and Reiser, pp 17–24)*

25. **The answer is B.** The function and structure of the lymphatics are well known and appreciated. The lymphatics consist of the lymphatic vessels and collecting ducts, lymph nodules, lymph nodes, and aggregates. Lymph tissue is primarily made up of WBCs separated by a fluid intercellular substance. Reversal of flow in the lymphatic vessels may be caused by the dilatation of the vessel where it faces an obstruction, consequently rendering incompetent the corresponding valves. Lymph nodes are located throughout the body, both above and below the waist. *(Gardner et al, pp 40–41)*

26. **The answer is D.** The prolonged depolarization of the plateau phase of the cardiac action potential is attributable to slowly inactivating voltage-gated calcium channels. *(Guyton, p 113)*

27. **The answer is D.** Alanine, cysteine, glycine, and serine are all converted to pyruvate during amino acid degradation. Thus, each of these amino acids can give rise to glucose via conversion of pyruvate to oxaloacetate and then phosphoenolpyruvate. In addition, ketone body formation can proceed by conversion of pyruvate to acetyl-CoA. In contrast, leucine can only be converted to potential ketone body precursors. The degradation of leucine leads to the formation of acetyl-CoA and acetoacetate. *(Stryer, pp 503–511)*

28. **The answer is D.** The classic complement pathway is usually activated by the antigen-antibody union then involving complement components C1q, C4, C2, and C3–C9. The alternate complement pathway proceeds through C3–C9, and it can be activated by aggregated immunoglobulins IgA, IgG_4, IgE, lipopolysaccharides, and endotoxins but not IL-1, β-interferon, lipoproteins, or the complement component C1. IL-1 activates T cells. β-Interferon is an antiviral protein, and the complement component C1 binds to the antigen-antibody complex and initiates the cascade of the classic complement pathway. *(Jawetz et al, p 186; Roitt, pp 14, 94; Joklik et al, p 175)*

29. **The answer is D.** Red infarcts are localized areas of ischemic necrosis resulting from a vascular interruption. These infarcts usually occur secondary to venous occlusion, with necrosis of the tissue due to ischemia accompanied by congestion and hemorrhage. Red infarcts occur in loose tissues that have a double circulation and are easily congested. The lungs are classically affected. As with arterial interruption, there is necrosis. At the same time, large amounts of hemorrhagic blood accumulate in the pulmonary parenchyma, so the infarct remains red. The intestines and brain are other organs that may have red infarcts. The heart, spleen, and kidneys classically have pale infarcts because they are solid tissues. Infarcts may occur with arterial occlusions, but there is no seepage or reflux of blood, since there is no dual blood supply, and the tissue is solid. *(Robbins et al, pp 108–111)*

30. **The answer is C.** Acetaminophen is an effective analgesic and antipyretic agent but has only weak anti-inflammatory activity because of weak peripheral prostaglandin inhibitory properties. Indomethacin, aspirin, phenylbutazone, and tolmetin have prominent anti-inflammatory properties and

hence may be useful in the treatment of patients with acute gout, rheumatoid arthritis, and other diseases associated with inflammation. (Gilman et al, pp 692–695)

31. **The answer is B.** Temporal pairing of a neutral stimulus with a stimulus that produces an inherent response (food in the case described in the question) characterizes classical conditioning. Operant conditioning involves reward and punishment. (Leigh and Reiser, pp 41–76)

32. **The answer is A.** The base of the heart, an organ compared to a pyramid, is formed by the atria rather than the ventricles. The apical region of the heart frequently is rounded, but the apex itself is often difficult to discern. The opening of the coronary sinus is in the right atrium near the valve of the inferior vena cava. The pulmonary ostium is located at approximately the second or third costal cartilage on the left side. The aortic valve is located on the posterior border of the left side of the sternum at the level of the third intercostal space. (Gardner et al, pp 309–312)

33. **The answer is B.** A PTH-like effect would be expected to stimulate bone resorption, vitamin D conversion, and elevate serum calcium levels. Serum calcitonin would consequently be expected to rise. A PTH-like effect on the kidneys would increase calcium absorption while markedly increasing phosphate excretion. (Guyton, pp 937–946)

34. **The answer is C.** Aldosterone is the major mineralocorticoid hormone. It acts by enhancing renal reabsorption of sodium ions and excretion of potassium ions. Cortisol and cortisone are the primary glucocorticoids that promote glycogen synthesis and gluconeogenesis and increase fat and protein degradation. Progesterone is required for implantation of a fertilized ovum in the uterus and maintenance of pregnancy. Pregnenolone is a common precursor in the biosynthesis of all the above hormones (Stryer, pp 565–568)

35. **The answer is C.** Killing of microbes by phagocytes is regulated by both oxygen-dependent and oxygen-independent mechanisms. The oxygen-dependent mechanisms involve the participation of superoxide anion, hydrogen peroxide, singlet oxygen, and hydroxyl radicals, all of which are powerful microbicidal agents. Ferrous ions are not part of the oxygen-dependent microbicidal mechanisms of phagocytes. (Roitt, p 4)

36. **The answer is C.** Chemical carcinogenesis is the induction of cancer by chemical agents. Although the mechanisms are still poorly understood, chemical carcinogenesis is dose dependent. As the dose is increased, over time the risk of developing cancer also is increased. This dose relationship is irreversible and additive. A variable latency period, from the time of insult to the time of cancer induction, may range from several months to years. When the cells with malignant induction divide, they transmit the carcinogenic effects to their daughter cells, so malignant clones arise. Chemical promoters, which are often hormonal, interact with the chemical carcinogens to decrease the latency period and increase the number of tumor cells. All cells undergoing active proliferation are more susceptible to carcinogenic induction. Susceptibility to chemical carcinogenesis is largely genetically determined, varying greatly among cell and tissue strains. (Robbins et al, pp 237–241)

37. **The answer is B.** Propylthiouracil inhibits the synthesis of thyroid hormones and thus is effective in treating hyperthyroidism. Although the complete mechanism of action is not fully understood, it is believed that propylthiouracil interferes with the incorporation of iodine into tyrosyl residues of thyroglobulin and inhibits the coupling of the iodotyrosyl residues to form iodothyronines. However, propylthiouracil does not inactivate existing thyroxine and triiodothyronine, nor does it interfere with the effectiveness of exogenous thyroid hormones. (Gilman et al, pp 1401–1406)

38. **The answer is A.** The limbic system is concerned with basic instinctual and emotive behaviors and memory. Higher functions, such as thinking (cognition), are performed by the cerebral cortex. (Leigh and Reiser, pp 41–76)

39. **The answer is E.** The long thoracic nerve usually arises by three roots. It descends behind the brachial plexus and the first part of the axillary artery. It supplies many branches to the musculus serratus anterior. All of the other choices listed in the question are parts of the brachial plexus and its divisions. (Gardner et al, p 101)

40. **The answer is C.** The stimulation of afferent nerves to salivary gland acini results in the secretion of a solution that resembles plasma. This is accompanied by a loss of cellular potassium ions, which is brought about by a rise in the intracellular concentration of calcium ions. In experiments in which single ionic channels have been recorded directly, it has been demonstrated that the basolateral plasma membranes of salivary gland acinar cells contain calcium-activated potassium channels. It is believed that these account for the efflux of potassium following stimulation. Na^+-K^+-Cl^- cotransport and the ouabain-sensitive Na^+-K^+ pump may each contribute to the reuptake of potassium ions by these cells. (Petersen and Maruyama)

41. The answer is A. Although peptide bonds define the primary structure (the sequence of amino acids) and, hence, supply the information necessary to specify the three-dimensional structure of a protein, they play no active role in stabilizing the tertiary structure of proteins. Four major types of weak bonds are important in tertiary structure—hydrogen bonds between R groups of the amino acids composing the protein, hydrogen bonds between the peptide groupings of α-helical and β-pleated sheet regions, ionic bonds between positively and negatively charged R groups, and hydrophobic interactions between nonpolar R groups. Study has revealed that hydrophobic interactions are the most important forces involved in maintaining the tertiary structure of proteins. *(Stryer, pp 28–30)*

42. The answer is D. The penicillin binucleate core structure is a cyclized dipeptide formed by condensation of L-cysteine and D-valine. Several different side chains are found at the R portion of the figure that accompanies the question. These impart important biologic characteristics to the molecule, such as acid stability, resistance to β-lactamase, broadened spectrum, and so forth. *(Joklik et al, pp 129–131)*

43. The answer is C. Adrenocortical carcinoma is a rare malignant tumor of the adrenal cortex. It almost never affects children. These tumors are consistently large, bulky, and unilateral, with extension into the soft tissues and retroperitoneum apparent at the time of diagnosis. They often show necrosis and hemorrhage, invade vascular and lymphatic structures, and frequently metastasize. The tumor is considered to be an adenocarcinoma and ranges in structure from well differentiated to anaplastic. About half of the tumors are functional and secrete steroids, especially cortisol. Clinically, affected patients may have symptoms of Cushing's syndrome—hypoglycemia, virilization, feminization, or a combination of these. These tumors are thought to arise from the adrenal cortical cells and are not of neural crest origin. *(Rubin and Farber, pp 1150–1154)*

44. The answer is B. Eight to 12 hr after the last dose of heroin, an addicted individual may experience nonpurposive symptoms, such as lacrimation, rhinorrhea, yawning, and sweating. After 12 to 14 hr, the sufferer may fall into a restless sleep. The syndrome progresses, and symptoms such as restlessness, gooseflesh, anorexia, tremor, and dilated pupils appear. At 48 to 72 hr, nonpurposive symptoms reach their peak, and the addicted person experiences increasing irritability, insomnia, anorexia, violent yawning, sneezing, lacrimation, coryza, weakness, depression, nausea, vomiting, intestinal spasm, diarrhea, increased heart rate and blood pressure, chilliness alternating with flushing and

excessive sweating, and myalgias and arthralgias. *(Gilman et al, pp 541–544)*

45. The answer is D. Benzodiazepines are antianxiety agents. They are habit-forming and have additive sedative action with alcohol. Patients who use these drugs should be cautioned to drive carefully, especially after drinking alcohol. Antipsychotic drugs, such as phenothiazines, impair conditioned avoidance learning in animals. *(Leigh and Reiser, pp 401–418)*

46. The answer is A. The common (fibular) peroneal nerve supplies the short head of the musculus (m) biceps, the m tibialis anterior, the m peroneus (fibularis) longus, the m extensor digitorum longus, and the m extensor hallucis longus. The m tibialis posterior is supplied by the tibial nerve. *(Gardner et al, pp 224–230)*

47. The answer is D. Inhibition or loss of the 21 β-hydroxylase or 11 β-hydroxylase enzyme in the pathways for the synthesis of steroids results primarily in a deficiency of glucocorticoids in the adrenal cortex. Because glucocorticoids normally act to inhibit the release of ACTH, the secretion of ACTH from the pituitary is enhanced. Deficiencies in these enzymes do not, however, prevent the synthesis of androgens in the adrenal cortex, and their release from this organ becomes enhanced by the elevated ACTH levels. Such deficiencies also result in adrenal hyperplasia. *(Ganong, pp 308–309)*

48. The answer is B. Fibroblasts synthesize procollagen intracellularly. Procollagen is a triple helix containing glycosylated residues and hydroxylated proline. Once procollagen is secreted, it must be hydrolyzed by extracellular peptidases to form tropocollagen. The peptidases cleave the nonhelical peptides of the N-terminal and C-terminal ends. Tropocollagen spontaneously associates into collagen fibers in the extracellular space. *(Stryer, pp 261–270)*

49. The answer is C. The importance of the capsule in the virulence of the pneumococcus is apparent from the observations that only encapsulated strains are virulent, and vaccine efficacy is type specific (the organisms are divided into more than 80 types on the basis of antigenic differences in the capsular carbohydrate composition). Cell wall teichoic acids and peptidoglycan are found in rough pneumococci (and most other bacteria as well) and are not intimately involved in the pathogenesis of disease. M protein is the potent antiphagocytic cell wall component of group A streptococci. *(Joklik et al, pp 368–372)*

50. The answer is A. There have been many classifications of the histologic appearance of non-

Hodgkin's lymphoma. In more recent times, it has become apparent that a particular classification that recognizes certain types of differentiation of the lymph node into nodular, diffuse, and cleaved nuclei or noncleaved of the cells can be related to the grade of aggressiveness of the tumor and, therefore, can be used as both a clinical and a histologic classification. The least aggressive of the lymphomas would be those that still retain the nodular pattern and in which the cells are small, with cleaved nuclei resembling the central germinal center cells from which they arose. Although nodular large, cleaved cell would be the next in degree of aggressiveness and would be probably classified as intermediate, all of the others are diffuse with varying degrees of cellular cleaving and are usually in the intermediate to high grade of aggressiveness. *(Rubin and Farber, pp 1094–1104)*

51. **The answer is C.** Phenothiazines antagonize dopaminergic neurotransmission and chronically can cause a variety of extrapyramidal symptoms, including parkinsonism, akathisia, and tardive dyskinesia. On withdrawal of drug treatment, parkinsonism usually abates, but akathisia and tardive dyskinesia can sometimes worsen temporarily. *(Gilman et al, p 402)*

52. **The answer is C.** Predatory aggression is a type of behavior that is usually associated with feeding and does not involve anger at the object of aggression. Frenzied, mutilating aggression is characteristic of the anger–fear response in affective aggression rather than in a predatory aggression. *(Hine et al, pp 261–280)*

53. **The answer is E.** The epididymis consists of a central portion (body), an upper enlarged extremity (head), and a lower pointed extremity (tail). The testes do not contain calyces. The tunica albuginea is the outer covering of the testes. Anisorchidia is the normal asymmetry between the testes (the left is larger and lower). The ductus deferens, formerly called the vas deferens, is a long tube that carries the spermatozoa from the tail of epididymis (reservoir of spermatozoa) to the ejaculatory ducts. *(Gardner et al, pp 475–481)*

54. **The answer is A.** Androgens stimulate the synthesis of proteins, and this effect accounts for much of the increase in rate of growth that occurs during puberty. Within long bones, androgens also eventually cause the epiphyses to fuse with the shaft of the bone. When this takes place, no further linear bone growth occurs. Other effects of androgens include some increase in the amount of retention of ions, such as calcium and phosphate. *(Ganong, pp 346–348)*

55. **The answer is D.** The rate-limiting step in the synthesis of heme is the condensation of glycine and succinyl-CoA to form δ-aminolevulinate. The mitochondrial enzyme δ-aminolevulinate synthetase catalyzes this reaction. δ-Aminolevulinate dehydrogenase catalyzes the condensation of two molecules of δ-aminolevulinate to porphobilinogen. Four molecules of porphobilinogen condense to form a linear tetrapyrrole, which undergoes a series of reactions to produce protoporphyrin IX. Chelation of iron by this molecule yields heme. *(Lehninger, pp 718–719; Stryer, pp 594–595)*

56. **The answer is C.** The Retroviridae are characterized by the presence of a reverse transcriptase (RNA-dependent DNA polymerase) in the virion. This family contains oncornaviruses that cause leukemias, sarcomas, lymphomas, and mammary carcinomas in animals as well as a few nononcogenic species, such as the lentivirus that causes visna in sheep. They are RNA viruses that are able to insert their genome into the DNA of the host cell through the action of the transcriptase. In this form they are nonantigenic, as they are hidden in the genetics of the host cell. Once the virus is expressed again and mature particles are produced, the virus will take on the antigenic characteristics of its capsid proteins. *(Joklik et al, pp 685–686, 736–743)*

57. **The answer is A.** The photograph that accompanies the question demonstrates severe hydronephrosis of the kidney. Hydronephrosis refers to dilatation of the renal pelvis and calices associated with progressive atrophy of the kidney due to obstruction of the flow of urine from the kidney. The obstruction may be located at any site along the urinary outflow tract and may be partial or total, unilateral or bilateral. Since glomerular filtration may continue for some time after the development of the obstruction, the renal pelvis and calices become dilated by the continued urine production. The resultant back-pressure produces atrophy of the renal parenchyma with obliteration of the pyramids. The degree of hydronephrosis depends on the extent and rapidity of the obstructive process. *(Robbins et al, pp 1051–1052)*

58. **The answer is D.** Resistant bacteria produce penicillinase, which hydrolyzes the β-lactam ring to form penicilloic acid, a molecule with no antibacterial activity. Penicillinase is produced by a number of clinically important bacteria, most notably *Staphylococcus*. In infections with these organisms, therapy often is based on penicillinase-resistant penicillins. *(Gilman et al, p 1115)*

59. **The answer is A.** An individual usually is not consciously aware of signal anxiety, a type of anxiety that serves as a signal of an impending danger intrapsychically. Panic anxiety, neurotic anxiety, and

psychotic anxiety are severe forms of anxiety and are pathologic. *(Leigh and Reiser, pp 41–76)*

60. The answer is C. The venous drainage of the brain includes (1) the superior cerebral veins, (2) the superficial middle cerebral vein, (3) the inferior cerebral veins, (4) the basal vein, and (5) the single great cerebral vein. The last is formed between the splenium and the pineal body and receives several tributaries, which include the basal veins. It drains into the straight sinus or rectus sinus of the dura mater. *(Gardner et al, pp 612–614)*

61. The answer is C. Aromatase is the enzyme that controls the conversion of testosterone to estradiol. It also catalyzes the formation of estrone from androstenedione. The major proportion of circulating estradiol in adult men is formed directly by aromatization of these circulating androgens. Lesser amounts may be secreted by both the Leydig's cells and the Sertoli's cells in the testes and by the adrenal cortex. *(Ganong, pp 374–375)*

62. The answer is D. The activation of factor X is the final reaction of both the extrinsic and intrinsic pathways of clotting. Activated factor X proteolytically cleaves prothrombin to thrombin, which in turn cleaves fibrinogen to fibrin. Accelerin stimulates the activation of factor X, and fibrin-stabilizing factor (factor XIII) stabilizes the clot by cross-linking fibrin. All of these factors are part of the common pathway. The defect in hemophilia is a deficiency in factor VIII, or antihemophilic factor. This factor acts at the last step of the intrinsic pathway. Factor VIII acts in concert with factor IX, a proteolytic enzyme, to activate factor X. *(Stryer, pp 248–251)*

63. The answer is E. There are five genera of DNA animal viruses. The HAPPPy mnemonic device (**H**erpes, **A**deno, **P**apova, **P**arvo, and **P**ox) enumerates these. All others are RNA viruses. Variola is a poxvirus, as is molluscum contagiosum; measles is caused by a paramyxovirus. *(Joklik et al, pp 640–642)*

64. The answer is C. Down's syndrome is the most common chromosome abnormality, occurring in 1 of 800 live births. It is characterized by a trisomy 21 karyotype with an extra G group chromosome (chromosome 21), making 47 total chromosomes. In the majority of cases, the parents are phenotypically and genetically normal, and Down's syndrome is secondary to a meiotic error in the ovum. The risk of having a Down's syndrome child is proportional to increasing maternal age. The clinical features of Down's syndrome include fat facies, epicanthic folds, oblique palpebral fissures, and severe mental retardation. The majority of affected individuals die early from cardiac or infec-

tious complications. Thirty percent have a ventricular septal defect.

Trisomy 13 is also called Patau's syndrome, and affected children have microcephaly and severe mental retardation, with absence of a portion of the forebrain. These children die soon after birth. Trisomy 18, or Edwards' syndrome, is also a very severe genetic defect, and the average life span is 10 wk. Affected children have severe mental retardation and cardiac anomalies, including a ventricular septal defect. The chromosome abnormality is an extra chromosome 18 due to a meiotic error. Patients with an XO karyotype have Turner's syndrome and are phenotypically females. Only 3 percent of affected fetuses survive to birth. Fetuses that survive birth have severe edema of the hands, feet, and neck. They have a webbed neck, short stature, and congenital heart disease. At puberty, there is failure to develop normal secondary sex characteristics, so their genitalia remain immature. The ovaries are atrophic and infertile, with primary amenorrhea. Klinefelter's syndrome, or testicular dysgenesis, is characterized by an XXY karyotype. It occurs in 1 of 600 live births. Affected individuals usually are diagnosed after puberty and have eunuchoid habitus, long legs, and small atrophic testes and penis. Secondary male characteristics fail to develop. These men are infertile and often have a low IQ. *(Robbins et al, pp 123–134)*

65. The answer is D. In patients with endogenous asthma and nasal polyps, a single dose of aspirin may cause bronchoconstriction and vasomotor collapse. Analgesic nephropthy, hepatotoxicity, and infertility are rare side effects, which occur most often during protracted or high-dose therapy. Hemolytic anemia may occur as an uncommon side effect in patients with glucose 6-phosphate dehydrogenase deficiency. *(Gilman et al, pp 686–688)*

66. The answer is D. Rationalization is a defense mechanism in which the person gives a post hoc plausible explanation for an unacceptable action. *(Leigh and Reiser, pp 77–98)*

67. The answer is C. A pylorus is a muscular mechanism made up of two components: a dilator for opening and a sphincter to close or reduce the lumen or the orifice of a hollow viscus. As a rule, the dilator component consists of longitudinal muscle bundles or fibers, and each sphincter has circular, oblique, or spiral bundles or fibers. *(Gardner et al, p 383)*

68. The answer is B. Acidophilic cells of the anterior pituitary are those cells that stain with acidic dyes. The major peptide hormones found in cells of this type are growth hormones and prolactin. Tumors of acidophilic cells may lead to excessive secretion of growth hormone, which, in children, produces gigantism and, in adults, results in acromegaly. Acromegaly is associated with changes in facial features and enlargement of the hands and feet. Dwarfism may be the result of deficiencies in growth hormone or of growth factors. Cushing's syndrome is caused by excess secretion of glucocorticoids and may result from tumors of ACTH-containing cells in the pituitary. In contrast to the growth hormone-containing cells, the cells that synthesize ACTH may be chromophobic or basophilic. Adrenogenital syndrome results from excessive secretion of androgens. (Ganong, pp 204–205)

69. **The answer is A.** The proteolytic blood enzyme thrombin has a specificity for arginine–glycine bonds similar to trypsin. Thrombin is synthesized as prothrombin, which contains γ-carboxyglutamate residues deriving from vitamin K-dependent, posttranslational modification of glutamate. In order to be activated, prothrombin is proteolytically cleaved by factor X_a after being anchored to platelet membranes in a calcium-γ-carboxyglutamate-dependent reaction. The γ-carboxyglutamate end of the prothrombin molecule is removed, leaving an active thrombin. Fibrinogen is converted to fibrin by the proteolytic cleavage of four arginine–glycine bonds. The A and B fibrinopeptides released spontaneously associate to form a clot of insoluble fibrin fibers. (Stryer, pp 250–251)

70. **The answer is C.** Koplik's spots on the buccal mucosa are characteristic of infection with morbilli (measles) virus. Microscopic examination of these lesions would reveal giant cells containing viral nucleocapsids. Macroscopically, these lesions will appear as small, erythematous macules with white centers. Rubeola (red measles) is an acute febrile disease characterized by fever, maculopapular rash, and respiratory symptoms. A cell culture-produced attenuated vaccine is available. There is only one antigenic variety of measles virus, so the vaccine is monovalent. It should not be given until after 12 mo of age to allow maternal antibody, which could interfere with the infection established by the vaccine strain, to dissipate from the infant's circulation. (Joklik et al, pp 826–837)

71. **The answer is E.** Atherosclerosis is a complex condition that is primarily and initially an intimal disease. It has now been long established and associated with an elevated serum cholesterol, but the lipoproteins are considered to be of equal importance in that a high level of LDL in association with elevated cholesterol is a very poor prognostic sign in the potential of an individual to develop severe atheroma and its complications. High levels of HDL appear to balance out the negative effect of cholesterol and are, therefore, considered good prognostic signs. (Rubin and Farber, pp 459–461)

72. **The answer is A.** The rate of cortisol secretion in normal persons is approximately 20 mg/day and is subject to fluctuations occurring throughout the day. Endogenous glucocorticoid concentrations in plasma follow a diurnal cycle, with peak concentrations occurring during early morning hours, a gradual decline in mid- to late afternoon, and the lowest concentrations occurring at night. This diurnal variation is not observed in patients with Cushing's disease. (Wyngaarden and Smith, p 89)

73. **The answer is B.** Persons who unsuccessfully attempt suicide tend to be young and female, unlike persons who complete suicide. Suicidal attempt often occurs at times of interpersonal difficulties and is not infrequent among Catholics. (Leigh and Reiser, pp 99–141)

74. **The answer is B.** Viscera may be either solid or hollow. The wall of hollow viscera consists of several concentric layers. A typical viscus, from the innermost to the outermost portion, has mucous, submucous, muscular, and serous or adventitious layers. (Gardner et al, pp 42, 383)

75. **The answer is D.** The major site of melatonin synthesis is within parenchymal cells of the pineal gland. It is formed by N-acetylation of 5-hydroxytryptamine followed by methylation. The rate of its synthesis is phase locked to the light–dark cycle, being high in the dark and very markedly diminished in the light portions of the cycle. Its synthesis and release are primarily regulated by sympathetic nerves whose activity appears to be entrained to the light–dark cycle via the suprachiasmatic nuclei. Sympathetic input regulates the N-acetyltransferase reaction within the pineal cells by controlling intracellular cyclic AMP levels. (Ganong, pp 394–395)

76. **The answer is D.** Conversion of pyruvate to acetyl-CoA results in the production of 1 mol of NADH. Oxidation of the resultant acetyl-CoA to CO_2 and water via the citric acid cycle yields 3 mol of NADH, 1 mol of $FADH_2$ and 1 mol of guanosine triphosphate (GTP). Oxidation of each mol of NADH during electron transport yields 3 mol of ATP, whereas oxidation of $FADH_2$ results in the formation of 2 mol of ATP. Therefore, beginning with pyruvate, the yield is 12 mol of ATP from 4 mol of NADH, 2 mol of ATP from 1 mol of $FADH_2$, and 1 mol of ATP equivalent (GTP) from substrate level phosphorylation, giving a total of 15 mol of ATP. (Stryer, pp 373–374, 377–379)

77. **The answer is B.** The DiGeorge syndrome is a form of glandular aplasia due to defective embryonic development of the third and fourth pharyngeal pouches, which give rise to the thymus, parathyroid, and thyroid glands. This anomaly results

in a depletion of thymic-dependent areas in lymphoid tissues. In Bruton's hypogammaglobulinemia, B-dependent areas are depleted. Hence, antibody formation is severely restricted. In severe combined immunodeficiency disease, both B cell and T cell functions are absent, and the affected individual is completely without any immune capability. Job's disease, or lazy leukocyte syndrome, is characterized by a defect in the chemotactic response of neutrophils. *(Joklik et al, pp 230–234)*

78. The answer is C. Celsus and Virchow defined clinical signs of acute inflammation that included redness, heat, swelling, pain, and loss of function. The heat and redness are related to dilatation of the vasculature. The swelling is a result of exudation of fluid, proteins, and cells into the interstitial tissue. Pain is thought to be secondary to prostaglandin secretions. Virchow describes loss of function as a result of the combined effects of the other factors of the inflammatory response. Numbness, which implies neurologic involvement, is not characteristic of the local acute inflammatory response. *(Robbins et al, pp 41–44)*

79. The answer is C. Phenylbutazone impairs platelet aggregation and displaces anticoagulant drugs from their binding with blood proteins. Barbiturates, glutethimide, and rifampin all induce microsomal enzymes systems in the liver that increase drug metabolism and thus reduce the response. Cholestyramine, a plasma cholesterol-lowering agent, binds anticoagulants in the intestine, reducing their absorption. *(Craig and Stitzel, p 425)*

80. The answer is E. Pain receptors are considered to be free nerve endings. Meissner's and Vater-Pacini corpuscles are thought to be involved with touch and proprioception. Rods are retinal light-sensitive cells. *(Leigh and Reiser, pp 209–240)*

81. The answer is D. The amniotic fluid is derived from maternal tissue fluid and excretions from the embryo. When contained within the amnion, it serves as a hydraulic cushion for the embryo. Although it contains dissolved substances, it does not provide a major nutrient source for the embryo. The major source for nutrients, gases, and so forth is the fetal blood returning from the placenta, where substances from the maternal blood have passed through the placental membrane to become constituents of the fetal blood. Fetal metabolic waste products are passed through the placental membrane and become incorporated in the maternal circulation. *(Moore, p 128)*

82. The answer is C. Aldosterone is synthesized and secreted by cells of the adrenal cortex. A primary role for mineralocorticoids, such as aldosterone, is to stimulate the renal reabsorption of sodium ions.

After adrenalectomy, the excretion of sodium ions in the urine is significantly increased and plasma sodium ion concentrations fall. At the same time, plasma potassium concentrations increase. If mineralocorticoids are not administered, blood pressure and the volume of the plasma decrease and death ensues. Although the loss of glucocorticoids, such as cortisol and corticosterone, may also become lethal in certain circumstances, such as fasting, their loss in adrenalectomy is not as critical as is the loss of aldosterone. Neither the loss of the androgen dehydroepiandrosterone, secreted by the adrenal cortex, nor the loss of catecholamines, such as epinephrine, secreted by the adrenal medulla, produce similar life-threatening changes in body functions. *(Ganong, p 320)*

83. The answer is E. The atoms composing the CO_2 and ammonia (NH_4^+) that form the carbamoyl group of carbomoyl phosphate are ultimately incorporated into urea. Likewise, the atoms forming the amino group of aspartate constitute the remainder of the urea molecule. Thus, of the molecules listed in the question, only argininosuccinate contains all of the atoms destined to become urea. *(Stryer, pp 500–502)*

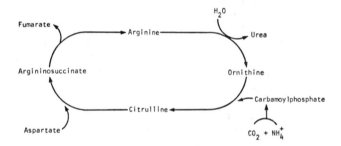

84. The answer is C. For sterilization of surgical instruments sensitive to heat, the method of choice is ethylene oxide. The autoclave uses high temperatures for sterilization. Both phenol and ethyl alcohol are used for disinfection, but neither can be relied on to kill spores. Ethylene oxide is effective against all types of bacteria, including the tubercle bacilli and spores. It is a gas and can be used for the sterilization of fragile and heat-labile materials and other items packaged in cloth or paper containers. Sterilization is complete in 4 to 12 hr, which must be followed by 12 to 24 hr of aeration to allow dissipation of the dissolved gas. Ionizing radiation would not penetrate many surgical instruments evenly and hence would not sterilize effectively. *(Joklik et al, pp 166–167)*

85. The answer is B. Sarcoid is a multisystem disease of unknown cause. It affects all organ systems, and young women are most often the victims. The characteristic lesions are noncaseating epithelioid granulomas that contain multinucleated giant cells.

Schaumann's bodies or crystalline inclusion bodies may be identified. The lung and thoracic lymph nodes are the most commonly involved sites, and pulmonary involvement may be quite serious, causing severe restrictive lung disease. Besides tissue biopsy as a method of diagnosing sarcoid, the Kveim test is the most commonly used clinical diagnostic procedure: Antigenic tissue suspensions from patients with sarcoid are injected into the skin, and positive reactions show papules 4 to 6 wk later. Biopsy specimens of the papules show noncaseating granulomas. The findings are rarely unequivocally positive, and the reliability of this test is being questioned. Patients with sarcoid usually have a progressive downhill course over years, and steroid therapy can only ameliorate their disease. (Robbins et al, pp 390–392)

86. **The answer is E.** Propranolol is useful in treating angina by decreasing myocardial oxygen consumption during rest and exercise. Propranolol decreases cardiac demand for oxygen because of its negative chronotropic effect (especially during exercise), its negative inotropic effect, and its minor depression of arterial pressure. (Gilman et al, p 821)

87. **The answer is D.** Lithium salts are particularly effective in treating acute mania. They also may be effective in preventing recurrences of unipolar depression, but not to the extent of their use in treatment of mania. Lithium is not particularly effective in panic disorders, anxiety disorder, or schizophrenia. (Leigh and Reiser, pp 401–418)

88. **The answer is C.** The ischiorectal fossae are spaces at either side of the anal canal and were formerly considered the terminal or aboral portion of the rectum. The wings of the uterus correspond to the broad ligaments. The fimbriae of the ovary and sphincters of the uterine tube are tubal parts. There is no special fat-containing space to accommodate the broad ligaments and no lateral depression or ischial tuberosity exists that is related to the rectum. (Gardner et al, p 507)

89. **The answer is E.** Activity in the sympathetic afferent nerves to the pancreas results in the enhanced secretion of glucagon from the α cells within the pancreatic islets. The stimulation of sympathetic afferents also inhibits insulin secretion from the β cells. The increase in glucagon secretion is a β-adrenergic response that uses a cyclic AMP second messenger mechanism. Thus, agents that elevate cyclic AMP promote glucagon secretion. An inhibitory α-adrenergic receptor also is present, but the β-adrenergic response usually is dominant on sympathetic stimulation. The secretion of glucagon is enhanced also by elevated amino acid concentrations in plasma and is inhibited by glucose and insulin. (Ganong, p 237)

90. **The answer is B.** In mammals, unlike plants, there is no mechanism for synthesizing net glucose from acetyl-CoA or substances whose metabolism will lead only to the production of acetyl-CoA. The ketone body β-hydroxybutyrate can only be metabolized to acetoacetyl-CoA and, ultimately, to acetyl-CoA. In contrast, glycerol can enter the gluconeogenic or glycolytic pathways at the level of dihydroxyacetone phosphate. Propionate, the end product of β oxidation of odd-chain fatty acids, and the amino acid glutamate can be converted to the citric acid cycle intermediates succinyl-CoA and α-ketoglutarate, respectively. These intermediates, as well as the citric acid cycle intermediate oxaloacetate, can all be converted to phosphoenolpyruvate for use in gluconeogenesis. (Stryer, pp 438–442)

91. **The answer is A.** In a positive viral hemagglutination test, the virus is the hemagglutinating particle. Antibody specific to the viral hemagglutinin will block this activity and inhibit hemagglutination. The assay is similar to a neutralization test, with the erythrocyte taking the place of a susceptible nucleated host cell. Many different viruses possess hemagglutinating activity. Hence, this assay can be used to identify serum antibodies that are reactive with numerous different viral agents. The limiting ingredient is the availability of the viruses. (Joklik et al, p 663)

92. **The answer is D.** Malignant melanoma is a neoplasm of melanocytes that usually occurs in patients 40 to 60 yr old. It most often arises in the skin but may originate in other mucosal surfaces. These tumors may arise either de novo, from preexisting benign nevi, or in rare cases in familial groups. Lentigo maligna, one subtype, tends to arise in sun-exposed areas of the skin. Clinically, these tumors are raised lesions with irregular notched borders and may be red, white, or black or have black and brown foci. Malignant melanoma arises from melanocyte cells in the epidermis. These malignant cells form clusters or nodules and spread laterally within the epidermis or vertically into the dermis. Tumor in the papillary dermis only occurs as a result of direct tumor spread or recurrence. Tumor cells are frequently pigmented with melanin granules and have large eosinophilic nucleoli. Malignant melanomas frequently metastasize, either by lymphatic vessels to regional lymph nodes or hematogenously to the skin, lungs, and liver. Nodular melanoma has the worst prognosis and is the most likely form to metastasize. (Rubin and Farber, pp 1243–1254)

93. **The answer is A.** Epinephrine is the drug of choice for treating severe anaphylactic shock, since it has both α and β effects. The α and β effects constrict the smaller arterioles and precapillary

sphincters, thereby markedly reducing cutaneous blood flow. Veins and larger arteries also respond to epinephrine. The β effects of epinephrine cause relaxation of the bronchial smooth muscle and induce a powerful bronchodilatation, which is most evident when the bronchial muscle is contracted, as in anaphylactic shock. Neither norepinephrine nor dopamine would be the drug of choice, since neither has action on the β₂ receptors and, therefore, would not cause the bronchodilatation needed for treating anaphylactic shock. Isoproterenol has a powerful action on all β receptors but almost no action on the α receptors, so vasodilatation instead of vasoconstriction would be produced. Phenylephrine would be a poor drug of choice for analphylactic shock, since it has little effect on the β receptors and causes no bronchodilatation. *(Gilman et al, pp 145–164)*

94. The answer is C. Suicide and suicidal attempt occur more frequently among people who seem to think of suicide or consider it as an option. Most people who commit suicide have seen a physician or given warnings of their intent. Suicide may occur when a patient's mood seems to be lifting. At this time, these persons may either gain more energy or experience a sense of resolution as the option of suicide has been decided. *(Leigh and Reiser, pp 99–141)*

95. The answer is D. The radial nerve, from the brachial plexus, innervates the triceps brachii. The musculus (m) teres major is supplied by the lower scapular nerve, the m coracobrachialis is innervated by the musculocutaneous nerve, the m supraspinatus is supplied by the suprascapular nerve, and the m serratus anterior is supplied by the long thoracic nerve. *(Gardner et al, p 116)*

96. The answer is C. The thyroid gland synthesizes and secretes thyroxine (3,5,3',5',-tetraiodothyronine, T₄) and 3,5,3'-triiodothyronine (T₃) as well as lesser amounts of reverse triiodothyronine (3,3',5'-triiodothyronine, RT₃) and monoiodotyrosine. Of these, T₃ is most active in stimulating oxygen consumption in the body, being three to five times as potent as T₄, although it is secreted in smaller amounts. RT₃ and monoiodotyrosine are not active. Thyroglobulin is a glycoprotein of the thyroid gland that plays a major role in the synthesis of the thyroid hormones and that may be released into the circulation. It is not, however, believed to play a role in the actions of the thyroid hormones. *(Ganong, pp 268–269)*

97. The answer is C. Of the enzymes listed in the question, only glucokinase and glucose 6-phosphatase are found in the liver and not in most other tissues. A deficiency in glucokinase would lead to increased blood sugar levels, not hypoglycemia.

This would occur because of the liver's decreased ability to phosphorylate free glucose for use. In contrast, a defect in glucose 6-phosphatase would cause the symptoms observed in von Gierke's disease. This endoplasmic reticulum enzyme catalyzes the dephosphorylation of glucose 6-phosphate, allowing glucose to be released into the blood when levels are low. A lesion at this point would result in massive storage of glycogen in liver. *(Stryer, pp 465–466)*

98. The answer is D. Complement-fixation procedures are performed in two stages. The test system consists of antigen and antibody (one of which is unknown) plus complement. The indicator system consists of sheep erythrocytes and hemolysin (an antisheep-RBC serum), which will sensitize the cells to the lytic action of complement. If complement is fixed in the test system, it is effectively bound (or consumed) in the antigen-antibody complexes there and is not free to participate in the lysis of the sensitized erythrocytes present in the indicator system. *(Stites et al, pp 361–362)*

99. The answer is B. The photomicrograph shows the characteristic appearance of hyperplastic ducts surrounded by what appears to be fibrous tissue and also smooth muscle. The pattern is a uniform one, in which the ducts are evenly distributed in this background of muscle and fibrous tissue. This is characteristic of so-called fibroadenoma of the breast, which tends to occur in younger females and is usually discrete and of a rubbery consistency. It is, however, very important that this be distinguished from the other forms of lumps in the breast, such as the various forms of carcinoma. Intraductal carcinoma and Paget's disease usually are both clinically and pathologically easily distinguishable from this lesion. The fibroadenoma is an entirely benign condition. *(Kissane, p 1550)*

100. The answer is B. The major action of atropine is to competitively antagonize the muscarinic action of acetylcholine at postganglionic parasympathetic neuroeffecter junctions. Atropine and scopolamine are, therefore, known as antimuscarinic agents. Because of the relatively small effect at the nicotinic receptor sites at autonomic ganglia, atropine produces a partial block only at relatively high doses. An example of an agent that prevents the release of acetylcholine is botulin toxin, whereas hemicholinium exerts its anticholinergic action by interference with acetylcholine synthesis. *(Gilman et al, p 132)*

101. The answer is B. In REM sleep, there is autonomic activation and a suppression of skeletal muscle activity. Thus, sleepwalking does not occur during REM but rather in the slow wave phase of sleep (stages 4 and 3). *(Leigh and Reiser, pp 241–269)*

102. **The answer is A.** From an anatomic standpoint, the perineum comprises the entire outlet of the pelvis, whereas the obstetric standpoint defines it as only the space between the vaginal and the anal orifice. The pelvic diaphragm is above the perineum. The rectal muscles are not fused with the urethral muscles and are the same in both sexes. There is no ischial symphysis. The urogenital triangle is not found in the female perineum. *(Gardner et al, pp 502–503)*

103. **The answer is B.** Wernicke's area, which is located at the posterior end of the superior temporal gyrus, is believed to play an important role in the understanding of language, either written or spoken. Patients with lesions in this area have a form of fluid aphasia in which the ability to vocalize is not impaired but the subject matter of speech is not intelligible. Moreover, the ability to understand either speech or writing is impaired. This is in contrast to lesions of Broca's area, in which understanding is preserved but the ability to vocalize speech is impaired. Deficits in the processing of visual information, dyslexia, or disorders of short-term memory may each result from cerebral lesions but are not specifically associated with Wernicke's area. *(Ganong, pp 228–229)*

104. **The answer is A.** The double-reciprocal Lineweaver-Burk plot that accompanies the question illustrates a competitively inhibited enzyme. In competitive inhibition, the intercept on the y axis, which is equal to 1/Vmax, does not change. This points out that at significantly high substrate concentration, the inhibition can be overcome. In noncompetitive inhibition, the Vmax, and hence the y-axis intercept, does change. Noncompetitive inhibition cannot be overcome by increasing the substrate concentration. Allosteric enzymes do not obey Michaelis-Menten kinetics and cannot be plotted as straight lines on double-reciprocal curves. Likewise, irreversibly inhibited enzymes cannot be treated by Michaelis-Menten kinetics. *(Stryer, pp 189–191, 193–195)*

105. **The answer is C.** The graft-versus-host reaction occurs when immunocompetent lymphoid cells are transferred to a histoincompatible recipient who is unable to reject them. The donor cells then mount an immune response against the foreign histocompatibility antigens of the recipient and attempt to reject them. This usually occurs in bone marrow transplantation performed as a therapeutic modality in patients with certain leukemias or other blood diseases, such as aplastic anemia. *(Joklik et al, pp 220–221)*

106. **The answer is C.** Staging of a cancer requires clinical and pathologic judgment regarding the extent of spread of the lesion. It does not depend on the tumor's microscopic appearance. T is used to grade the size and extent of the primary tumor. N indicates the presence of lymph node metastases, and M indicates distal metastases. T0 indicates a carcinoma in situ or tumor confined to the mucosa. T1 is a superficial invasive tumor without extension into the underlying muscle wall or deeper connective tissue. T2 indicates muscle wall extension, and T3 shows full-thickness involvement of the organ by tumor. A T4 lesion has local extension and spread and is larger. An N0 tumor shows no lymph node involvement, whereas N1 has positive lymph node metastases. M0 tumors show no distant metastases, and M1 indicates distant tumor. The tumor described in the question invades the muscle wall but does not extend through the wall or into adjacent organs or tissue, so it is classified as T2. The lymph nodes are involved, thus N1, but there are no other metastases, so it is M0. Thus it is regarded as a T2,N1,M0 tumor. *(Robbins et al, pp 229–230)*

107. **The answer is C.** The uptake and elimination of gaseous anesthetics are influenced by pulmonary ventilation, blood flow to tissues, and the solubility of the agent in tissue as well as in blood. Increased pulmonary ventilation increases the exchange of the agent across alveolar membranes, thus increasing the transfer of gas to blood when the alveolar gas tension is high relative to the blood. Conversely, if air ventilated to the lungs has a lower alveolar tension relative to blood, the rate of removal of gas from blood will increase. The solubility of an agent in blood and tissue is important. Agents that are highly soluble raise the blood or tissue tension of an agent slowly. High blood flow to tissues accelerates the delivery or removal of an agent from that tissue. The extent of liver metabolism does not influence the uptake and elimination of inhalational anesthetics. However, metabolism may be a determinant of toxicity. *(Gilman et al, pp 262–266)*

108. **The answer is D.** The three basic models of the doctor–patient relationship are activity–passivity, guidance–cooperation, and mutual participation models. Activity–passivity model is the traditional model, in which the patient is a passive recipient of treatment. Guidance–cooperation model implies patient cooperation with the treatment regimen. Mutual participation implies a model of doctor–patient relationship in which the physician aids the patient in self-help. *(Simons, pp 19–26)*

109. **The answer is B.** The two lobes of the left lung are separated by the oblique fissure. The superior lobe lies above and in front of this fissure. The superior lobes of the right and left lungs have a different number of bronchopulmonary segments or segments of ventilation. The right has three (apical, posterior, and anterior), and the left has only two because of fusion (apicoposterior and anterior). *(Gardner et al, p 295–299)*

110. The answer is B. Skeletal muscle constitutes the major mass of the body, and thus alterations in its resistance will greatly affect systemic BP (i.e., product of cardiac output times resistance). For instance, when carotid sinus pressure is elevated, a reflex is elicited that inhibits activity in the vasoconstrictor regions of the brain and causes vasodilatation in the skeletal muscle bed and others. A separate sympathetic colinergic pathway has been described as arising from areas in the cortex and hypothalamus and producing vasodilatation in skeletal muscle. This reflex may induce vasodilatation in anticipation of exercise. In addition to these extrinsic neuronal regulatory mechanisms, local metabolic factors contribute to the regulation of muscle blood flow. This is especially true in stimulated or exercising muscle. For instance, metabolically active muscle can be shown to autoregulate, that is, increase its resistance as perfusion pressure rises to maintain constant blood flow and, conversely, decrease resistance when pressure decreases. Skeletal muscle is very heterogeneous. Within the same muscle group, blood flow is high to red muscle and relatively low to white muscle. Precapillary sphincter contraction and relaxation further confound local flow patterns via intermittent activity and perhaps by shunting of blood to nonnutrient pathways. *(Berne and Levy, pp 227–231)*

111. The answer is E. Mutations are caused by changes in the base sequence of DNA. Substitution of one base pair for another is the most common type of mutation. A transition substitution refers to the replacement of one purine by another purine or one pyrimidine by another. Transversions refer to replacement of either a purine or a pyrimidine with either a pyrimidine or a purine, respectively. Frame-shift mutations (insertions or deletions) are less common than substitutions. The formation of thymine dimers is not the most common cause of mutations. In fact, most cells have repair mechanisms for dealing with DNA so affected. *(Stryer, pp 635–638)*

112. The answer is B. Isografts are tissue exchanges between genetically identical individuals (inbred animals or identical twins). Allografts (also called homografts) are exchanges between genetically nonidentical individuals of the same species. Xenografts (heterografts) cross species boundaries. *(Joklik et al, p 253)*

113. The answer is C. The classic description of Fallot's tetralogy, a congenital heart disease, includes pulmonary stenosis, ventricular septal defect, and overriding of the aorta over the septal defect and,

as a result of these abnormalities, right ventricular hypertrophy.

Coarctation of the aorta is a totally separate congenital anomaly and may occur in both infants and adults depending on its relationship to the ducts and on whether or not the ductus arteriosus closes. It is not a characteristic part of the tetralogy of Fallot, although theoretically the two could occur in the same individual. *(Kissane, pp 663–683)*

114. The answer is D. Liver toxicity is an uncommon but significant adverse reaction associated with the use of halogenated anesthetics. The mechanism of injury with halothane, methoxyflurane, and enflurane appears to involve hypersensitivity or hepatotoxic metabolites or both. The potential for hepatotoxicity appears to correlate with the degree of liver metabolism. Halothane, methoxyflurane, and enflurane undergo liver biotransformation. All of these agents have been reported to cause liver damage. Isoflurane undergoes little biotransformation in vivo. This agent does not appear to be hepatotoxic. *(Lewis et al)*

115. The answer is C. There is controversy concerning the factors influencing adherence to medical regimens. Among the demographic factors, female sex has clearly been associated with poor adherence. Field dependence has been associated with poor adherence among individuals suffering from alcoholism. Severe physical illness, contrary to what one would suspect, also has been associated with poor adherence. *(Simons, pp 38–47)*

116. The answer is A. The superior cerebellar artery does not participate in the formation of the cerebral arterial circle of Willis. The other vessels listed in the question are all contributors to the formation of the anastomosis between the internal carotid and vertebral arteries. *(Heimer, pp 56–59)*

117. The answer is E. When cardiac muscle contracts, it squeezes blood vessels that course through it, and this extravascular compression has a significant effect on coronary blood flow. In early systole, there is an actual reversal of blood flow, and although coronary blood flow increases during systole, it is not until the ventricle relaxes that maximal left coronary artery blood flows are obtained. Since aortic pressure is maximal during systole, it is obvious that choice **C** in the question is incorrect. Peak flows are obtained in early diastole, when the ventricle is relaxed and aortic pressure has not declined to its diastolic level. *(Berne and Levy, pp 213–219)*

118. The answer is A. Although in bacteria a continuous sequence of triplet codons encode for each protein, genes may be discontinuous in eukaryotic cells. Noncoding intervening sequences of DNA that split genes in eukaryotes are called introns. Mature mRNA translated from such DNA does not contain the intron message. However, newly synthesized mRNA may contain intron message. These intervening sequences in the primary transcripts are specifically excised and ligated so that the mature mRNA contains no intron message. The coding sequences of split genes are called exons. *(Stryer, pp 110–113)*

119. The answer is B. Erythroblastosis fetalis can occur when an Rh_0-positive child is being carried by an Rh_0-negative mother. If the mother makes antibodies against the $Rh_0(D)$ antigen, these may cross the placenta and destroy fetal erythrocytes. The induction of this immune response can be blocked if an antibody specific for the Rh_0 antigen is injected into the mother at the time of her first exposure to the fetal RBCs, which usually occurs at parturition. Rh_0 immune globulin (RhoGAM) is a human γ-globulin preparation rich in antibodies specific for the Rh_0 antigen. It is used to prevent the sensitization of the mother, which will then protect a subsequent antigenically incompatible fetus from this disease. *(Joklik et al, pp 250–251)*

120. The answer is A. Neoplastic transformation is a phenotypic change in cells that characterizes the malignant state and is passed on to progeny. These transformed cells show anaplasia and transplantability. They also show decreased sensitivity to contact inhibition and to density-dependent inhibition for growth. Thus, these tumor cells are more mobile and do not cease to grow when in contact with other cells or when more than a monolayer of confluent cells is present. Instead, they continue to replicate and pile up. Unlike normal cells, these tumor cells also can grow and divide on fluid media and have lost the need for anchorage to grow. Malignant transformed cells have an infinite ability to replicate and survive under appropriate conditions. These transformed cells are capable of tumorigenesis, so they are able to produce a neoplasm when placed within a synergistic host. *(Robbins et al, pp 230–236)*

121. The answer is C. Hypokalemia is a frequent complication of therapy with loop diuretics (e.g., furosemide) as well as thiazide-type agents. These agents cause an increase in the amount of sodium delivered to distal sites of the nephron, where sodium is exchanged for potassium. Diuretics, such as triamterene and spironolactone, are potassium-sparing in that they produce a weak diuresis and cause potassium retention. Amphotericin B causes hypokalemia by producing renal tubular acidosis (type IV). Large doses of certain penicillins (e.g., carbenicillin) may produce hypokalemia by acting in the nephron as nonreabsorbable anions, which

are paired with potassium for urinary excretion. Glycyrrhizic acid, a flavoring agent in certain foods and medications, may cause hypokalemia through its aldosterone-like effects. *(Lindeman and Papper)*

122. The answer is B. Pathologic grief reactions include distorted reactions in which there may be acquisition of symptoms belonging to a deceased loved one. Posttraumatic stress disorder involves unusual and catastrophic disasters, not simple bereavement. *(Leigh and Reiser, pp 99–141)*

123. The answer is C. The sensorimotor cortex related to the right foot is located in the left cerebral hemisphere. The representation of the body in the sensorimotor cortex is such that the area related to the foot is situated on the medial aspect of the hemisphere. This region is in the vascular territory of the anterior cerebral artery. *(Heimer, pp 357–373)*

124. The answer is C. Although the heart is versatile in its use of substrates, more than 60 percent of myocardial oxygen consumption is derived from free fatty acids. Glucose and lactate are the major carbohydrate sources but make up only 30 to 35 percent of the sources for myocardial energy. In the normal heart, pyruvate uptake is very low, and oxidation of amino acids provides little to myocardial energy expenditure. In general, the heart uses the substrate in greatest supply. For example, ketone bodies may be used in diabetic acidosis. However, under normal conditions, free fatty acids are the major substrate. *(Berne and Levy, p 221)*

125. The answer is A. A Lineweaver–Burk analysis of enzyme kinetics in the presence and absence of an inhibitor allows the characterization of the type of inhibition. The analysis is based on a transformation of the Michaelis–Menten equation, which produces a straight line when the reciprocal of the velocity is plotted against the reciprocal of substrate concentration (i.e., $1/v$ vs $1/[S]$). The intercept on the Y axis is equal to $1/Vmax$, and the slope is equal to $K_m/Vmax$. Addition of a competitive inhibitor to an enzymatic reaction results in a higher value for K_m but no change in Vmax. This means that in a Lineweaver-Burk analysis, the slope will increase, but the Y intercept will remain unchanged. *(Stryer, pp 189–191, 193–195)*

126. The answer is B. Antibodies are synthesized in peripheral lymphoid tissues, such as the spleen and lymph nodes. The central lymphoid tissues are the thymus (responsible for T cell development) and the bursa of Fabricius (in birds) or certain gut-associated lymphoid tissues (in mammals), which are thought to be responsible for B cell development. Macrophages are important accessory cells in the induction of an immune response and are a prerequisite for most humoral immune responses. They process the antigen in some way and present it to T and B cells, which collaborate in the production of antibody molecules. In all probability, the antigen does not go through the normal phagocytic process (i.e., engulfment into a phagosome, lysosomal fusion with the phagosome to form a phagolysosome, the development of this inclusion to a digestive vacuole, and so forth) but rather is mildly degraded or modified and is reinserted into the membrane of the phagocytic cell. *(Davis et al, pp 386–389)*

127. **The answer is D.** The rapidity with which wounds heal is primarily related to fibroblast proliferation and secretion of collagen. Collagen is the major component contributing to the tensile strength of the wound. It is produced by fibroblasts as tropocollagen. Collagen is composed of a triple helix of three α chains, which are hydroxylated and have lysine oxidations. These modifications allow cross-linkages between the chains, and these cross-links are the most important factor contributing to the stability and strength of collagen and scar tissue. Fibroblasts also synthesize elastic fibers, which aid in the repair of wounds. Collagenase is an enzyme that cleaves collagen and digests it, retarding healing. It is rarely found in uncomplicated, healing wounds. *(Robbins et al, pp 76–80)*

128. **The answer is E.** Dose-dependent, potentially fatal hepatic necrosis is the most serious consequence of acute acetaminophen poisoning. Renal failure and hypoglycemia also may occur. Methemoglobinemia and respiratory depression are manifestations of phenacetin poisoning. Although acetaminophen is a metabolite of phenacetin, symptoms of their toxicities are very different. *(Gilman et al, p 694)*

129. **The answer is C.** In dealing with a chronically angry patient, physicians should be as neutral and objective as possible. It may be helpful for the physician to recognize that these patients arouse anger, but an angry reaction will only increase the patient's angry behavior. Sarcasm used by a physician in this situation tends to increase the patient's anger. *(Simons, pp 101–120)*

130. **The answer is D.** The accommodation reflex, convergence reflex, and pupillary constriction in response to increased levels of light all have their efferent limbs within the oculomotor nerve (cranial nerve III). Pupillary dilatation occurs in response to lowered levels of light or to a reaction (fight, flight, or frolic) mediated via the sympathetic division of the autonomic nervous system. The major sympathetic ganglion, which contains the majority of the postganglionic sympathetic neurons subserving the head, is the superior cervical ganglion. Loss of this ganglion would not affect oculomotor nerve–mediated reflexes but would limit the sympathetic reflexes, which include dilatation of the pupil pro-

duced by the dilator pupillae muscle of the iris. The corneal reflex—bilateral blinking in response to touching the edge of the cornea—is a polysynaptic reflex with the afferent limb in the trigeminal nerve and its efferent limb in the facial nerve. *(Heimer, pp 242–243, 309–320)*

131. **The answer is D.** Although the capillaries are the smallest vessels, by virtue of their large number and parallel existence, their effective cross-sectional area is very large. Since velocity is inversely related to cross-sectional area, the velocity in the capillaries is very low. This large surface area and low velocity promote exchange of substances between blood and tissue. Resistance to blood flow primarily occurs in arterioles with smooth muscle, and thus this is the site of the largest pressure drop. Blood volume is greatest in small veins by nature of their high compliance. *(Berne and Levy, pp 2–3)*

132. **The answer is A.** The lipid composition of erythrocytes, as well as most mammalian plasma membranes, is approximately half cholesterol and half phospholipid. Of the phospholipids, most is either phosphatidyl choline or spingomyelin, with phosphatidyl ethanolamine also contributing a lesser, but considerable, amount. Gangliosides and phosphatidyl serine also are present but constitute smaller percentages of the lipid. Plasmalogens are phospholipids containing a long-chain unsaturated alcohol in ester linkage at the l′ position. They are especially abundant in the membranes of nerve and muscle cells. *(Stryer, pp 284–287)*

133. **The answer is E.** The organism represented in the sketch that accompanies the question is septate (note the divisions, or cross-walls) in the hypha. This observation rules out any of the phycomycetes, since these organisms are coenocytic. The position of the conidiospores in strings arising from the columnella is characteristic of the genus *Aspergillus*. The dermatophytes that are the causative agents of the tinea infections usually have single conidiospores and are characterized by their macroconidial forms. *(Joklik et al, pp 940–941)*

134. **The answer is D.** The simplest form of a blood clot at a site of injury is a hemostatic plug. It is composed of an aggregation of platelets with a web of fibrin, which prevents leakage of blood into the extravascular spaces. Platelets are the most important component in the formation of this plug. When the blood vessel is injured, cells and plasma start to leak out, but platelets are immediately attracted to the site of injury. They accumulate, pile up, and stop the leakage. They also release tissue thromboplastin, which activates the intrinsic blood coagulation pathway, causing the fibrin mesh to form. The fibrin tightens the plug and traps other cells, strengthening the platelet plug and forming a more

permanent plug. RBCs and lymphocytes are seen in hemostatic plugs as they are trapped from the circulating blood by the aggregation of platelets and fibrin. They act as filler material in the plug and have no other defined role in the formation of hemostatic plugs. Collagen is important in the initiation of hemostasis, as when blood vessels are damaged. The collagen fibrils in the subendothelial wall of the vessel are exposed to the circulation and are the substance that the platelets initially stick to when they form a hemostatic plug. (*Robbins et al, pp 91–95*)

135. **The answer is C.** Extrapyramidal reactions are most likely to occur with piperazine-type phenothiazines, including trifluoperazine and prochlorperazine, as well as the butyrophenone haloperidol. Thioridazine, a piperidine-type phenothiazine, is least likely to cause extrapyramidal reactions. Prochlorperazine is mainly used as an antiemetic. (*Gilman et al, pp 402–407*)

136. **The answer is A.** Common causes of sexual dysfunction include many types of neuropathy and chronic illnesses. Diabetic neuropathy is probably the most common organic cause of sexual dysfunction. Depression and anxiety are common functional causes of sexual dysfunction. Chronic schizophrenia is often associated with decreased sexual function. Mania, however, is often associated with increased sexuality. (*Simons, pp 316–401*)

137. **The answer is B.** Most retinal detachments occur at the potential cleft between the rod and cone cells and the pigmented epithelium of the retina. This potential cleft represents the point of contact between the inner and outer layers of the embryonic optic cup. The inner layer of the optic cup differentiates into the neural retina. The outer layer becomes the retina pigmented epithelium and fuses with the connective tissue of the choroid. (*Heimer, p 36*)

138. **The answer is D.** The normal heart is capable of pumping all of the blood that is returned to it over a wide range of volumes. By virtue of the Frank-Starling law of the heart, in normal persons the heart is capable of pumping 13 to 15 L/min without excessive backing up of pressure. Accordingly, it is the summation of all peripheral blood flows that return to the heart that ultimately regulates cardiac output. Thus, local metabolic factors and their integrated responses with neurohumoral regulation of specific beds determine venous return, which is identical to cardiac output in the closed circulatory system. Changes in cardiac function or activity in the central or peripheral nervous system contribute to this regulation indirectly. (*Guyton, p 273*)

139. **The answer is B.** Under normal metabolic conditions, the brain oxidizes about 140 g of glucose each day. This amounts to approximately 80 percent of the total glucose consumed each day and about 20 percent of the total O_2 consumed by the body. During starvation, the rate of glucose use by the brain is decreased and that of ketone bodies is increased, such that in late starvation, about 40 g of glucose (from gluconeogenesis) and 100 g of ketone bodies are daily consumed by the brain. (*Lehninger, p 838; Stryer, pp 551–553*)

140. **The answer is E.** Cervicofacial actinomycosis (lumpy jaw) is an endogenous infection that is usually preceded by a tooth extraction or some other traumatic injury to the mouth. The lesion commonly drains to the cheek or submandibular area. The presence of sulfur granules is of great diagnostic importance. These are actually small (approximately 1 mm in diameter) colonies of the organism in a calcium phosphate matrix. They consist of a central filamentous mass of branching bacilli surrounded by radially oriented, club-shaped structures. (*Joklik et al, pp 451–454*)

141. **The answer is B.** The lesion shown in the question is a granuloma, which is a small, circumscribed collection of inflammatory cells. These cells primarily consist of modified macrophages called epithelioid cells. There is an outer rim of lymphocytes. There are also multinucleated giant cells of the Langhans type. Other cells, such as plasma cells, eosinophils, and neutrophils, may be seen in granulomas, but the epithelioid cells are the single diagnostic feature. The center of a granuloma may be necrotic, like that pictured in the question, or it may be a solid mass of epithelioid cells. Granulomas are a form of response to chronic irritants associated with either infectious or noninfectious causes. An abscess is seen in acute inflammatory processes and is a circumscribed collection of pus secondary to liquefactive tissue necrosis. It is accompanied by a neutrophilic response. A keloid is an abnormal formation of collagenous connective tissue in a scar, forming a dense, bulging tumor. It is accompanied by minimal cell response. An infarct is an area of ischemic necrosis of tissue secondary to circulatory obstruction, producing an area with coagulation necrosis and neutrophilic cell response. A thrombus is a clot in a blood vessel formed intravascularly, causing vascular obstruction. They are composed of fibrin, platelets, RBCs, and WBCs. (*Robbins et al, pp 61–65*)

142. **The answer is D.** In general, the duration of action of the oral hypoglycemic agents correlates with their half-lives. Several compounds (acetohexamide, tolazamide) have active metabolites that may contribute to hypoglycemic activity. Tolbut-

amide, the shortest-acting agent, has a duration of action of 6 to 12 hr (half-life of 7 hr). Tolazamide produces hypoglycemic activity for 12 to 16 hr or more (half-life of 7 hr). Acetohexamide, although its half-life is 6 hr, has a duration of 12 to 18 hr or more because its metabolite is more active than the parent compound. Chlorpropamide has the longest half-life (35 hr) and longest duration of action (24 to 72 hr). Isopropamide is not an oral hypoglycemic but is an antimuscarinic compound. *(Katcher et al, p 1376)*

143. The answer is B. Sensitivity is defined as the extent to which patients with a particular disease or characteristic are accurately classified as having the disease, according to the diagnostic test. In this question, 98 percent of patients with the disease are accurately classified on the basis of the test result, so the sensitivity of the test is 98 percent. Specificity is defined as the extent to which patients who do not have the disease are correctly classified. In this question, 90 percent of the patients without disease had negative results and would have been correctly classified, so that specificity of the test is 90 percent. Positive and negative predictive accuracy refers to the accuracy of positive and negative results when the test is applied to a particular population, and these values will depend on the prevalence of the disease in the population. *(MacMahon and Pugh, pp 261–263)*

PRACTICE TEST II

144–147. The answers are 144-C, 145-E, 146-B, 147-D. Aldosterone is required for appropriate renal retention of salt and water. Its absence is accompanied by a salt-wasting diuresis. Cortisol is necessary for maintaining serum glucose levels between meals, and hypoglycemia results from its absence. In the absence of insulin, fatty acids are metabolized to ketones in the liver, resulting ultimately in ketoacidosis. The absence of thyroid hormone results in a number of symptoms, including extreme somnolence. *(Guyton, pp 427–428,907,920,927–928)*

148–150. The answers are 148-D, 149-B, 150-D. The kinetic parameters K_m and Vmax can be determined by plotting reaction rate as a function of varying substrate concentrations in the form of a Lineweaver-Burk plot. Vmax is determined from the y-intercept and K_m is calculated from the x-intercept. In addition, such plots allow the characterization of competitive and noncompetitive inhibitors. The K_m of an enzyme is increased in the presence of a competitive inhibitor, but the Vmax remains unchanged, whereas, in the presence of a noncompetitive inhibitor, K_m remains unaltered,

but Vmax is decreased. Therefore, the lines for the uninhibited and competitively inhibited reactions will intersect on the y axis, and the lines for the uninhibited and noncompetitively inhibited enzyme will intersect on the x axis. K_m may be defined as the substrate concentration at which one half of the enzyme's active site will be occupied. Thus, the answers to questions 148 and 150 are both D. *(Stryer, pp 190–191,193–197)*

151–153. The answers are 151-B, 152-E, 153-C. The following generalities may assist in determining the characteristics of viral nucleic acids: Most DNA animal viruses are double-stranded; therefore, herpesviruses, adenoviruses, papovaviruses, and poxviruses are all double-stranded DNA, and parvoviruses are single-stranded DNA. The rest of the animal viruses are RNA, and most of these are single stranded (the exception here being the reoviruses). Prions are *proteinacious virions* with no nucleic acid content. *(Joklik et al, pp 643–646,810–814,875)*

154–157. The answers are 154-B, 155-A, 156-C, 157-E. The antihypertensive action of hydralazine is primarily arteriolar venodilatation, which results in reflex tachycardia. This tachycardia may precipitate or aggravate myocardial ischemia. Propranolol is a nonselective β-adrenergic blocking agent. Blockade of cardiac β_1 receptors results in slowing of the heart rate. Prazosin dilates arterioles and venules. This may cause inadequate blood return to the right side of the heart as well as hypotension, which can result in syncopal episodes, particularly after the first dose. This phenomenon can be minimized by administering a small dose initially, preferably at bedtime. Methyldopa routinely causes sedation. This usually dissipates with continued use but uncommonly may persist enough to interfere with daily living activities, particularly mental work. *(Gilman et al, pp 788–796)*

158–161. The answers are 158-D, 159-B, 160-C, 161-A. Erikson propounded what he called the epigenetic principle, in which each "part" in proper sequence has a critical time of ascendancy until all the related parts have arisen to form a functioning whole. The sequence of parts is as follows: basic trust (first year), autonomy (second year), initiative (third to fifth year), industry (sixth year to adolescence), identity (adolescence), intimacy (young adulthood), generativity (adulthood), and integrity (mature age). Failure to consolidate these crises may give rise to later psychopathology. *(Erikson, pp 101–172)*

162–165. The answers are 162-C, 163-B, 164-D, 165-B. The parasympathetic fibers in the oculomotor nerve are the axons of cells in the oculomotor nucleus that synapse in the ciliary ganglion. The postganglionic fibers pass to the short ciliary nerves and supply the ciliary muscle and the spinchter pupillae. Parasympathetic fibers by way of the greater petrosal nerve from the facial nerve synapse in the pterygopalatine ganglion and then send postganglionic parasympathetic fibers to the lacrimal gland. Preganglionic fibers derived from the chorda tympani of the facial nerve synapse in the submandibular ganglion. The postganglionic fibers pass to the submandibular and sublingual glands. Preganglionic fibers from the lesser petrosal of the glossopharyngeal nerve synapse in the otic ganglion. The postganglionic fibers pass to the parotid gland. *(Gardner et al, pp 642,676,679,685)*

166–168.   The answers are 166-D, 167-A, 168-C. The depolarization observed in the P wave signals the onset of atrial contraction, whereas the QRS complex is associated with the initiation of ventricular contraction. The sustained depolarization of the plateau phase is represented by the ST interval (which is not normally associated with any voltage deflection). Finally, the T wave is associated with the onset of ventricular repolarization. *(Guyton, p 178)*

169–171.   The answers are 169-E, 170-A, 171-C. The genetic code defines the relationship between the sequence of bases in DNA and the corresponding sequence of amino acids in proteins. Three bases form a codon that codes for an amino acid. Since it has been demonstrated that most of the 64 possible arrangements of bases into codons do code for specific amino acids and since there are only about 20 amino acids, the code is degenerate. If a single base pair is substituted, only one amino acid is changed (provided that a degenerate codon for the same amino acid is not substituted). This demonstrates that the code is not overlapping. Finally, deletions or additions of a single base pair cause a shift of the reading frame subsequent to the point of change. Consequently, all amino acids in the coded protein subsequent to that point will be altered. This demonstrates a sequential reading of bases from a fixed starting point. *(Stryer, pp 99–101)*

172–174.   The answers are 172-E, 173-D, 174-C. Legionellosis, or legionnaire's disease, was first detected in 1976 when an outbreak of deadly pneumonia occurred in over 200 persons attending an American Legion convention. Epidemiologic investigations showed that the disease was caused by a gram-negative rod that was named *Legionella pneumophila.* The organism was spread from water reservoirs contaminating air-conditioning units, nebulizers filled with water, or evaporative condensers. Active cases or carriers constitute the sources of infection for *N. meningitidis. B. abortus*

causes brucellosis, and contaminated unpasteurized milk or contaminated dairy products serve as sources of infection. *T. pallidum,* the causative agent of syphilis, is transmitted venereally. *B. burgdorferi* causes Lyme disease, and wild animals or birds serve as the source of infection. This recently discovered disease is transmitted by tick bites. Lyme disease is characterized by unique skin lesions, known as erythema chronicum migrans (ECM). A unique property of *T. pallidum* is that it cannot be cultured on artificial media. *(Joklik et al, pp 382,516,557,566,589)*

175–178.   The answers are 175-A, 176-C, 177-D, 178-B. Marfan's syndrome is a rare, usually autosomal dominant disease characterized by abnormally formed connective tissue. Affected patients are very tall and have long extremities and tapering fingers and toes with hyperextensive joints. They have bilateral dislocation of the ocular lens, cystic medial necrosis of the aorta, and floppy mitral valve leaflets. The underlying connective tissue defect is still unknown. Patients usually survive to 40 yr of age.

Tay-Sachs disease is an autosomal recessive disease resulting from absence of hexosaminidase A. This GM_2 ganglioside accumulates in neurons of the central and autonomic nervous systems, retina, heart, liver, and spleen. The buildup of the ganglioside in the neurons causes their destruction, with gliosis and lipid deposits in the brain. Affected persons are normal at birth. By age 6 mo, there is progressive motor and mental deterioration, and death occurs by age 3 yr.

Niemann-Pick disease is an autosomal recessive disease characterized by a deficiency in sphingomyelinase, causing a buildup of sphingomyelin and cholesterol in reticuloendothelial cells and parenchymal cells in tissues. These abnormal cells are lipid laden, foamy, and large. Affected individuals suffer neurologic deterioration and organomegaly and usually die by the age of 3 yr.

Pompe's disease is glycogen storage disease type II, which is autosomal recessive. It is caused by absence of the enzyme α-glucosidase in lysosomes, which causes defective glycogenolysis resulting in abnormal buildup of glycogen. The heart and nervous system show the most severe involvement, and patients die of congestive heart failure by 2 yr of age.

Lesch-Nyhan syndrome is an X-linked disorder caused by a defect of the enzyme hypoxanthine guanine phosphoribosyltransferase, which is involved in purine metabolism. Affected persons suffer from hyperuricemia, gout, pyelonephritis, and renal stones. Neurologic deficits are the most prominent abnormality and include severe mental retardation, spastic cerebral palsy, and self-mutilating behavior. *(Robbins et al, pp 136–156)*

179–184. The answers are 179-E, 180-C, 181-D, 182-A, 183-B, 184-D. Neurohumoral transmission may be classified into two basic types—cholinergic and adrenergic transmission. Cholinergic transmission involves the stimulation of either nicotinic or muscarinic receptors by acetylcholine. Postsynaptic nicotinic receptors may be blocked by D-tubocurarine. Blockade of these receptors at motor end-plates results in muscle paralysis. Muscarinic receptors of postganglionic parasympathetic fibers also are stimulated by acetylcholine. However, these receptors are blocked by atropine and not by D-tubocurarine. The activity of cholinergic neurotransmitters (e.g., acetylcholine) is rapidly terminated by acetylcholinesterase. This enzyme may be inhibited reversibly by anticholinesterases, such as physostigmine.

Adrenergic neurotransmission occurs through stimulation of α or β receptors. Norepinephrine (noradrenalin) is a potent stimulant of postsynaptic α and β receptors. Phenylephrine selectively stimulates only postsynaptic α_1 receptors, β receptors may be classified as either β_1 (e.g., heart) or β_2 (e.g., bronchial muscle) receptors, β_1 receptors may be selectively blocked by metoprolol. *(Gilman et al, p 92)*

185–189. The answers are 185-A, 186-B, 187-E, 188-D, 189-C. As crying diminishes during infant development, cooing and vowel sounds (e.g., "oo") increase. Words appear at about 1 yr, between a range of 8 and 18 mo of age. Vocabulary increases to as many as 50 words by 18 mo and 200 words by age 2 yr. The sequence of appearance of different classes of words is as follows: nouns, verbs, adjectives, and adverbs. Pronouns appear by age 2 yr, and conjunctions after the age of 2½ yr. *(Lennenberg, pp 128–130)*

190–194. The answers are 190-B, 191-A, 192-A, 193-D, 194-B. All β-lactam antibiotics, including the penicillins and cephalosporins, kill susceptible bacteria by inhibiting transpeptidation, the final step of peptidoglycan synthesis. The aminoglycoside antibiotics (e.g., gentamicin, kanamycin, amikacin, and tobramycin), after being actively transported to intracellular sites, kill susceptible bacteria by inhibiting protein synthesis primarily at the level of the 30S ribosome. This results in misreading of the genetic code. Sulfonamides, such as sulfisoxazole, are competitive antagonists of para-aminobenzoic acid, which is required for synthesis of folic acid. *(Gilman et al, pp 1096,1116,1152)*

195–197. The answers are 195-C, 196-B, 197-A. The facial nerve contains taste fibers for the anterior two thirds of the tongue. The vagus carries taste fibers for the base of the tongue (epiglottic region). The vagus nerve is predominantly afferent, and the facial nerve supplies the stapedius muscle. *(Gardner et al, pp 626–627,706)*

198–199. The answers are 198-C, 199-D. The P wave is the electrical result of atrial depolarization before contraction. The QRS is the electrical result of ventricular depolarization before contraction. The T wave is primarily due to repolarization in the ventricles. *(Guyton, pp 177–178)*

200–202. The answers are 200-C, 201-A, 202-A. In addition to containing collagen and elastin, connective tissues are rich in ground substance composed of proteoglycans and glycosaminoglycans. Glycosaminoglycans (acid mucopolysaccharides) are the polysaccharide chains of proteoglycans. They are disaccharide repeating units containing a derivative of an amino sugar. Major glycosaminoglycans include hyaluronate, chondroitin sulfate, keratin sulfate, heparin, and heparin sulfate. Proteolgycans are glycoproteins having an extremely high content of carbohydrate (about 95 percent) and an extremely high molecular weight. Their core proteins are linked to glycosaminoglycans. Proteoglycans are polyanionic biomolecules that bind water and cations, thereby forming the ground substance of connective tissues. *(Stryer, pp 275–277)*

203–204. The answers are 203-C, 204-A. Haptens react specifically with the appropriate antibodies, although they cannot by themselves induce the production of homologous antibodies. There are two types of haptens—simple and complex. Simple haptens can neither induce the formation of antibodies nor visibly react with them by themselves. Reactions can only be visualized if the hapten is complexed with another molecule, which will give it a valence sufficient to react visibly. An alternate method of visualizing the reaction between a simple hapten and its specific antibody is by an inhibition test in which the simple hapten reacts with the antibody and interferes with its subsequent reaction with a form of the hapten that can be seen. Complex haptens have the ability to react visibly with the antibody (they are multivalent and can build a lattice of sufficient size to be seen), but they are not immunogenic by themselves. Both types of haptens gain immunogenicity when they are coupled with appropriate molecules, such as large proteins, called carrier molecules. These carriers make possible the induction of an immune response by imparting to the hapten sufficient size or chemical complexity to allow it to interact with the cells taking part in the collaboration process involved in the immune response. *(Joklik et al, pp 180,192–193)*

205–206. The answers are 205-C, 206-A. Trauma to the head can cause both intracerebral hemorrhage and subdural hemorrhage. Subdural hemorrhage is seen more frequently with more trivial head injuries, whereas intracerebral hemorrhage usually requires a severe blow to the head, often associated with a fracture of the skull. It is usually associated, therefore, with searing stress through the cerebral substance forming rupture of the vessels. A subdural hemorrhage may be slow and accumulative following a trivial injury and easily missed. Severe hypertension may cause rupture of small vessels in the brain, with the classic intracerebral hemorrhage resulting in stroke. Subdural hemorrhage is not associated with hypertension and results usually from trauma. (Rubin and Farber, pp 1436–1439)

207–208. The answers are 207-C, 208-B. Clonidine and propranolol are two effective antihypertensive agents. Although the mechanisms underlying their respective reduction in systemic blood pressure are unclear, clonidine appears to act as a central α_2-adrenergic agonist, and propranolol's effect is via β receptor antagonism. This latter drug's effect may involve antagonism of β_1 receptors of heart, kidney, or brain. Regardless of their differences in mechanism of action, abrupt withdrawal of each agent is associated with rebound hypertension. Clonidine is without significant effects on postural hypotension, since most cardiovascular reflexes remain intact. Propranolol is frequently associated with profound decreases in blood pressure on standing, since effective cardiovascular blockade has occurred. (Gilman et al, pp 790–794)

209–215. The answers are 209-A, 210-D, 211-B, 212-A, 213-C, 214-D, 215-B. Operant or instrumental conditioning rewards a desirable behavior through reinforcers (which may be an actual reward or the removal of a noxious stimulus). In classical conditioning, a neutral stimulus is repeatedly paired with a stimulus that naturally results in a response (unconditioned stimulus and unconditioned response). Eventually, the neutral stimulus alone elicits the response (the neutral stimulus has become the conditioned stimulus). In classical conditioning, stimulus generalization may occur; i.e., a stimulus similar to the conditioned stimulus may produce the conditioned response. Shaping of a behavior by gradation is an operant conditioning characteristic. Phobias may result from classical conditioning (e.g., by being trapped in an elevator, elevators may become a conditioned stimulus causing fear response) and from operant conditioning (by avoiding the phobic stimulus, the patient is rewarded by not having fear reactions). Both types of conditioning obviously occur in human beings. At one time, operant conditioning, being a more advanced form of learning, was thought to be possible only through the voluntary nervous system, but more recent studies have shown that the autonomic nervous system is capable of operant conditioning

(e.g., heart rate, blood pressure). (Leigh and Reiser, pp 41–76; Simons, pp 607–618)

216–238. The answers are 216-B, 217-A, 218-A. Neural ectoderm (neuroepithelium) forming the neural tube and its derivatives (i.e., brain and spinal cord) gives rise to all neurons having their cell bodies (soma or perikaryon) located within the CNS. It also gives rise to the oligodendroglia and astroglia. Neural crest tissue gives rise to the cells of the spinal and cranial nerve sensory ganglia, the postganglionic autonomic neurons, melanocytes, and several other types of cells. (Moore, pp 375–383)

219–221. The answers are 219-A, 220-C, 221-D. Petit mal seizures, which typically occur in children, are characterized by a repetitive spike and wave pattern occurring at a frequency of about 3/sec in the EEG. The abnormal neuronal discharge that this pattern represents is believed to be generated at a subcortical locus. Such seizures are associated with a transient loss of consciousness without convulsions. Petit mal seizures may become less frequent and then disappear with maturity.

Grand mal seizures are characterized by loss of consciousness together with generalized convulsions. This form of seizure may be caused by the activity of an abnormally discharging focus of neurons that progressively recruits neighboring neurons into a synchronous discharge. This spreads into the motor cortex and to subcortical areas, producing a tonic to clonic pattern of muscle contractions and the loss of consciousness. The EEG displays a characteristic sequence of rapid spikes and spikes followed by slow waves during the seizure. Grand mal convulsions frequently are preceded by a subjective aura, which represents the onset of seizure activity before it has entered motor areas.

Psychomotor seizures are caused by abnormal neuronal discharges in a focus within the temporal lobe. Complex symptoms may include stereotyped behaviors and abnormal emotional reactions without loss of consciousness or abnormal muscle contractions. (Ganong, p 167)

222–224. The answers are 222-B, 223-A, 224-D. Except for bacterial mRNA, which undergoes little or no posttranslational modification, most RNA molecules are either cleaved or otherwise chemically altered after transcription. Eukaryotic mRNAs are greatly modified from the primary transcripts originally generated. In addition to being extensively spliced and cleaved from heterogeneous nuclear RNA, most eukaryotic mRNAs have modified caps (methylated G nucleotide) at their 5'-end and long poly A tails at their 3' ends. However, methylation of bases or methylation of ribose units does not occur in mRNA to any great extent. tRNA of bacterial cells contains methylated bases, and tRNA of eukaryotic cells contains methylated ribose units. *(Stryer, pp 704–721)*

225–226. The answers are 225-C, 226-B. An immunogenic substance is one that, on injection into a proper individual or animal, is capable of eliciting an antibody response with which it reacts specifically. Both exotoxins and toxoids are immunogenic. Toxoids are exotoxins that have been treated with formaldehyde or other chemicals so that they have lost the toxic properties possessed by the exotoxins from which they were derived. Toxoids are used for vaccination against diphtheria, tetanus, clostridial infections, and other diseases. *(Joklik et al, p 295)*

227–228. The answers are 227-A, 228-B. In the microscopic evaluation of lymph nodes, RFH can at times be difficult to differentiate from NL. Several histologic architectural features can be helpful in the decision-making process. In RFH, the nodal architecture is preserved, the follicles are more prominent in the cortex than in the medulla, there is marked variation in the size and shape of the follicles, which are sharply demarcated, and there is only moderate, if any, infiltration of the capsule and pericapsular fat by inflammatory cells. NL, on the other hand, produces effacement of the normal nodal architecture, has follicles or nodules distributed more or less evenly throughout the cortex and medulla of the lymph node, shows slight to moderate variation in the size and shape of the follicles, which are not well demarcated, and demonstrates prominent infiltration of the capsule and pericapsular fat by the neoplastic process. *(Kissane, pp 1288–1289,1301–1304)*

229–230. The answers are 229-B, 230-A. Azathioprine is the most commonly used agent for immunosuppression therapy. However, a new drug, cyclosporine, is being used increasingly, especially in transplantation procedures. This increased use of cyclosporine is in part due to its enhanced specificity and lower toxicity compared to other conventional cytotoxic agents. Cyclosporine appears to inhibit the production and acquisition of responsiveness to interleukins in T cells, thereby inhibiting the proliferative response of T cells to many antigens. Cyclosporine does not produce either leukopenia or thrombocytopenia as do other agents, including azathioprine. The major adverse effect of cyclosporine is renal toxicity. Azathioprine is a purine antimetabolite that is phase specific to cells involved in nucleic acid synthesis. It is converted to thioinosinic acid, which inhibits the synthesis of inosinic acid, resulting in inhibition of DNA. Bone marrow depression is the major side effect of azathioprine. Although it is still commonly used, especially with corticosteroids for inhibition of transplant rejection and some other autoimmune

disorders, it is nonetheless relatively nonspecific and toxic. *(Craig and Stitzel, pp 840–844)*

231. The answer is C (2,4). Diphtheria toxin is a general cell poison that blocks protein synthesis by ADP-ribosylating elongation factor 2. The median lethal dose per kilogram of body weight (LD_{50}kg) is 0.3 μg for guinea pigs. Botulinum toxin is a potent neurotoxin that blocks the exocytosis of acetylcholine-containing vesicles. The LD_{50}kg for guinea pigs is approximately 1 ng. *B. abortus* and *M. tuberculosis* do not excrete any potent toxic products during infection. *(Joklik et al, pp 70, 335, 423–432, 513–517)*

232. The answer is C (2,4). Viruses cause disease by disturbing cell function, either by a direct cytolytic event or by induced alterations in cell functions or synthetic capabilities or both. Viruses are able to cause disease more easily in individuals who are nutritionally or immunologically deficient. Host cell membrane changes that are important in disease production include loss of contact inhibition, which may lead to a malignant transformation, and changes in permeability or antigenic composition, which could lead to loss of cytoplasmic content due to leakage or immunologic destruction of the infected cell. *(Davis et al, pp 1033–1034)*

233. The answer is E (all). Except for tyrosine, which is synthesized from the essential amino acid phenylalanine, all of the basic nonessential amino acids found in humans can be synthesized from either pyruvate, oxaloacetate, 3-phosphoglycerate, or α-ketoglutarate. Glutamate is derived from the incorporation of ammonium ion into α-ketoglutarate by the action of glutamate dehydrogenase. In turn, glutamine synthetase catalyzes ammonium ion amidation of glutamate to form glutamine. Alternatively, glutamate can be synthesized into proline. Pyruvate and oxaloacetate are transaminated by glutamate to form alanine and aspartate, respectively. Aspartate can be amidated by ammonium ion to form asparagine. Serine can be synthesized from 3-phosphoglycerate in a sequence of reactions involving oxidation, glutamate transamination, and phosphate hydrolysis. Serine is the precursor of glycine and cysteine. In glycine formation, the side chain β-carbon of serine is transferred to tetrahydrofolate to yield glycine and methylenetetrahydrofolate. Glycine can also be formed from NH_4^+, CO_2, and methylenetetrahydrofolate via catalysis by glycine synthase. Formation of cysteine from serine involves substitution of a sulfur atom derived from methionine for the side chain O_2 atom. *(Lehninger, pp 694–699; Stryer, pp 487–491)*

234. The answer is E (all). The capsid proteins of viruses are external components of the virion and as such are in a position to interact with the immunologic apparatus of the host. Thus, they are the inducers of antibody synthesis both in an infection and in the vaccines that are employed to prevent viral diseases. They also function to protect the viral nucleic acids from nucleases present in the plasma and in phagocytic vacuoles. One of the viral capsid proteins is responsible for adsorption of the virus to susceptible cells, and it, or perhaps other capsid components, may also function in penetration of the virus into the cell. *(Joklik et al, pp 115,631)*

235. **The answer is D (4).** Cysteine and tyrosine are amino acids with uncharged, polar side chains. Cysteine contains a thiol group, and tyrosine possesses a phenolic hydroxyl group. Glycine, the simplest amino acid, has no side chain. Lysine bears an unbranched, four-carbon aliphatic chain ending in an ε-amino group. At physiologic pH, this side chain amino group is positively charged. *(Stryer, pp 16–21)*

236. **The answer is B (1,3).** The symptoms shown by the patient described in the question could have been caused by any of the agents listed. The pathologic process observed in the CNS is similar in all of these. The detection of inclusion bodies is a valuable aid in diagnosis. The rabies inclusion body (Negri body) occurs in the cytoplasm of the infected nerve cell, whereas the inclusion body of herpes simplex (Lipshütz body) has an intranuclear location. Polioviruses do not produce inclusion bodies of diagnostic significance; neither do the togaviruses. *(Hoeprich, pp 864, 1093)*

237. **The answer is D (4).** Cyanogen bromide is one of several chemical reagents that cleave proteins at specific points. Cyanogen bromide splits polypeptides only on the carboxyl side of methionine residues. Trypsin hydrolyzes peptide bonds on the carboxyl side of arginine and lysine residues. Disulfide bonds may be split by a variety of reducing agents, of which β-mercaptoethanol is one. *(Stryer, pp 55–56)*

238. **The answer is E (all).** Viruses can be neutralized by antibody alone if the antibody is directed against a viral component important in adsorption, penetration, or uncoating. Antibody-coated viruses in the circulation or in the tissues are phagocytized and destroyed. This opsonization by antibody is due to the fact that phagocytic cells have a membrane receptor for the Fc portion of certain immunoglobulin molecules, and this antibody–receptor complex serves to hold the viral particle close to the phagocytic cell until it can be engulfed. Complement can augment this neutralization, and it also can inactivate virions directly by covering their surfaces and, in some instances, lysing the virus even in the absence of specific antiviral antibody. If infected host cells are lysed, the site of viral replication is destroyed, and the infection can be brought under control. *(Davis et al, pp 1023–1024)*

239. **The answer is A (1,2,3).** Carcinoma of the colon and rectum is one of the major cancers in the western world and is frequently seen in North American whites, usually over the age of 50. It is a disease that is relatively rare in black Africans and in Japanese living in Japan, although there is some indication that Japanese living in the USA and changing their diets also may have an increased incidence of this disease. There is some evidence that the incidence may be increasing with urbanization in Africa.

The key to the disease appears to be related to the level of fiber in the diets, which is high in Africa and Japan and low in modern western diets, to a large extent. *(Hutt and Burkitt, pp 27–30)*

240. **The answer is E (all).** Males are more likely to complete suicide, although more females attempt suicide. Living alone, previous attempts at suicide, and the presence of pain have been shown to be associated with increased likelihood of suicide. History of depression, family history of depression or suicide, alcohol use, and ready availability of means of suicide also are important risk factors. *(Leigh and Reiser, pp 99–141)*

241. **The answer is B (1,3).** The enzyme 3-ketoacid CoA transferase is required to transfer CoA from succinyl-CoA to acetoacetate to form acetoacetyl-CoA. This reaction precedes the thiolysis of the acetoacetyl-CoA to two molecules of acetyl-CoA, which may then be used for energy production in the citric acid cycle. Ketone bodies may be oxidized in the mitochondria of all tissues containing these enzymes. This includes virtually all tissues except liver, where ketone bodies are manufactured, and cells lacking mitochondria, such as erythrocytes. *(Stryer, pp 478–480)*

242. **The answer is E (all).** Viruses can damage the host and produce disease by all of the mechanisms listed in the question. Cells can be rendered nonfunctional by direct cytopathic effects, depression of synthesis of cellular macromolecules, and alterations of lysosomes or cell membranes. Viral transformation of normal cells to hyperplastic or malignant cells is also a mechanism of disease production. *(Joklik et al, pp 773–778)*

243. **The answer is A (1,2,3).** Malignant cells may show a variety of anaplastic changes. They show irregularities in size and shape of the cell, with extreme variation and overall increase in cell size. The nucleus has an increased amount of DNA and is hyperchromatic. The nuclei are larger than expected for the cell size, with an elevated nucleus/cytoplasm ratio approaching 1:1 instead of the normal 1:4. The nuclei may show coarsely clumped, irregularly dispersed chromatin, and one or more prominent nucleoli. Some tumors may create tumor giant cells that are multinucleated conglomerations of malignant cells. *(Robbins et al, pp 218–220)*

244. **The answer is E (all).** Depression is commonly associated with malignancies, especially visceral malignancies, such as cancer of the tail of the pancreas, as well as with various endocrinopathies, such as hypothyroidism. Many antihypertensive drugs cause depression, especially reserpine and propranolol. Cocaine abuse often is associated with depression, especially with cocaine crash, which commonly occurs following the high. *(Leigh and Reiser, pp 99–141; American Psychiatric Association, pp 177–179)*

245. **The answer is D (4).** The neural tube is formed from neural ectoderm. The cells of the tube are initially pseudostratified in configuration but change with future differentiation of the tissue. The neurons with cell bodies located within the CNS are derived from the neural tube as well as all of the glial cells except the microglia. Although myelination begins before birth, it is not completed until approximately a year after birth. The spinal cord is the same length as the vertebral column initially. However, the cord does not lengthen as rapidly as the column. At birth, the cord ends at about the level of the third lumbar vertebra and ultimately ends at about the level of the intervertebral disk between the second and third lumbar vertebrae in adults. *(Moore, pp 375–380, 383, 384)*

246. **The answer is B (1,3).** Na⁺ reabsorption involves active processes in both proximal and distal tubules. Reabsorption is increased at the distal tubules by the mineralocorticoid aldosterone. Coupling with active transport of K⁺ into the distal tubule cell is well documented. Expansion of extracellar fluid leads to an increase in excretion of Na⁺ secondary to an unknown natriuretic hormone or physical factors depressing reabsorption. *(Guyton, pp 419–420)*

247. **The answer is A (1,2,3).** The catecholamines dopamine, norepinephrine and epinephrine all are sequentially derived from levodopa, which is synthesized from tyrosine by a one-step ring hydroxylation catalyzed by tyrosine hydroxylase. Levodopa also serves as the precursor of the pigment melanin. Norepinephrine is the neurotransmitter at sympathetic innervations of smooth muscle junctions. Likewise, dopamine is synthesized in sympathetic nerve terminals, whereas epinephrine is produced by the adrenal medulla and acts as a circulating hormone. Remarkable success has been achieved in treating the symptoms of Parkinson's disease using levodopa. In contrast to the catecholamines, the vasodilator histamine is formed

from histidine by decarboxylation. *(Stryer, pp 1025–1026)*

248. **The answer is E (all).** All of the statements in the question correctly describe influenza virus. Three serotypes of influenza viruses are known to occur in nature. These are divided into types A, B, and C on the basis of differences in their ribonucleoprotein antigens. Within the types, there are antigenic differences based on changes in the nature of the hemagglutinin and neuraminidase spikes that protrude from the envelope. It is changes in these subtypes that cause the emergence of epidemics and pandemics of influenza, and these changes are also the reason that vaccine prophylaxis of the disease is so difficult. Each pandemic is caused by a new antigenic subtype. Hence, there has not been sufficient time to produce the large quantities of vaccine that would be needed to protect the world's population. Thus, the vaccine is usually reserved for medical personnel and the aged (who are particularly at risk of fatal influenzal disease). It is thought that the segmented genome of the virus may play a role in the antigenic changes that the organism undergoes. *(Joklik et al, pp 642, 662, 821–823)*

249. **The answer is E (all).** Emboli are detached intravascular fragments of material that are carried by the blood to distant sites. These emboli are then lodged in vessels that are too small, causing partial or total obstruction. These masses may be solid, liquid, or gaseous and may include air, nitrogen, fragments of bone, marrow, atherosclerotic plaque, tumor, or foreign bodies. Ninety-nine percent of all emboli are of thrombotic origin. Pulmonary emboli are the most common form of emboli. The majority arise in thrombosed veins of the legs. When released, they cause pulmonary obstruction with hypoxia and right-sided heart failure. Pulmonary emboli rarely cause infarction. Systemic emboli arise in the arterial system, usually in the left ventricle or left atrium, and travel to blood vessels of smaller caliber. These emboli cause infarction with hemorrhage secondary to occlusion of the vessel. Other examples of emboli include gas bubbles from deep-sea decompression, fat from bone fractures, or amniotic fluid in obstetric complications. *(Rubin and Farber, pp 265–268)*

250. **The answer is C (2,4).** Acute grief often causes waves of somatic distress and hallucinations and illusions of the deceased. A substantial portion of bereaved individuals develop depressive syndrome. Antidepressant therapy usually is not indicated in uncomplicated grief reaction, which usually subsides in time with completion of the grief work. *(Lindemann)*

251. **The answer is D (4).** The ventral posterior lateral nucleus of the thalamus receives input from the primary sensory tracts originating in noncranial structures of the body. It projects, in turn, to the primary sensory cortex of the cerebrum. The sensory input from the face is relayed in the ventral posterior medial nucleus. *(Heimer, pp 175–176, 331–335)*

252. The answer is B (1,3). Postextrasystolic potentiation is a well-known phenomenon in which premature ventricular systole is followed by (1) a subnormal premature contraction, (2) a compensating pause, (3) a supernormal contraction, and (4) persistence for several beats of the potentiated response. Inadequate filling of the ventricle just before the premature beat contributes to (1). Exaggerated filling during (2) contributes to the postextrasystolic potentiation of (3). In addition to Frank-Starling mechanisms, the movement of intracellular Ca^{2+} during contraction and relaxation appears to underlie this phenomenon. The premature beat occurs when Ca^+ is relatively unavailable for contraction. The postextrasystolic beat occurs after a compensatory pause, and there is an abundance of Ca^{2+} available for contraction. *(Berne and Levy pp 177–178)*

253. The answer is E (all). The most versatile carrier of one-carbon groups in mammals is tetrahydrofolate. Methyl ($-CH_3$), methylene ($-CH_2-$), formyl ($-CHO$), formimino ($-CHNH$), and methenyl ($-CH=$) groups can all be carried by tetrahydrofolate. In amino acid, purine, and pyrimidine biosynthesis, it serves as a donor. In degradative reactions, it serves as an acceptor. Although tetrahydrofolate does carry methyl groups in certain reactions, the major donor of methyl groups is S-adenosylmethionine. CO_2 is not carried by tetrahydrofolate. Biotin is the carrier of CO_2. Humans obtain tetrahydrofolate from their diet or from bacteria of the intestinal tract. *(Stryer, pp 580–583)*

254. The answer is A (1,2,3). Phagocytic cells, such as macrophages and neutrophils, have receptors for C3b. B lymphocytes also react with C3b. However, T lymphocytes appear to lack a membrane receptor for this molecule. It is the presence of the C3b receptor on phagocytic cells that is responsible for the opsonization of bacteria and other foreign materials by antibody and complement. The antibody reacts with an antigen on the bacterial surface, and the complement cascade is activated. During this activation, C3b is deposited onto the surface of the organism, and it interacts with the receptor in the phagocyte membrane to bring the two cells together, thus facilitating the phagocytic process. *(Joklik et al, pp 206–207,229,268,280–282,287,351,373)*

255. The answer is D (4). The changes in the nucleus seen in various forms of cell injury include pyknosis, which is a condensation and destruction of the nuclear protein, karyolysis, which is a lysis or disruption of the nuclear material, and karyorrhexis, which has a similar disruptive and irreversible effect. Swelling of the rough endoplasmic reticulum usually occurs in earlier forms of cell injury and is not related to nuclear changes and in some respects, therefore, is reversible. This is typically seen in so-called cloudy swelling and similar cytoplasmic changes recognizable in cell injury. *(Rubin and Farber, pp 14–20)*

256. The answer is E (all). Although a depressed mood is common among patients with the depressive syndrome, there may be apathy and anhedonia as well. Anorexia is common, but overeating also may occur. *(Leigh and Reiser, pp 99–141)*

257. The answer is E (all). The hypothalamus, which comprises the floor and walls of the third ventricle of the brain, is the site of control for the autonomic nervous system and many of the endocrine axes. It receives input from many areas, and one of the major routes is the rather diffuse medial forebrain bundle. Efferent fibers pass via the bundle and other tracts to brain stem nuclear areas as well as the spinal cord. *(Heimer, pp 293–307)*

258. The answer is C (2,4). The tympanic reflex may be set in motion by strong acoustic stimuli. The reflex consists of the contraction of the muscles of the middle ear, including the tensor tympani. This produces an inward movement of the maleus and an outward movement of the foot plate of the stapes, with the result that conduction of sound waves through the ossicles is attenuated. It is believed that the tympanic reflex protects the cochlea from sustained loud sounds. *(Ganong, p 146)*

259. The answer is E (all). All cells, except liver, phosphorylate glucose to glucose 6-phosphate with a hexokinase. In the liver, a glucokinase catalyzes the phosphorylation of glucose. In contrast to hexokinases, liver glucokinase has a very high K_m and, thus, a low affinity for glucose. This is necessary to allow free glucose to perfuse from the liver back out into the blood when blood sugar levels are low. Glucose 6-phosphate, derived from gluconeogenesis or from glycogenolysis, is dephosphorylated in the liver by glucose 6-phosphatase, so that it can cross the liver plasma membrane as free glucose. The other enzymes listed in the question, pyruvate carboxylase and fructose 1,6-diphosphatase, are enzymes of gluconeogenesis, a process that occurs only in the liver and kidneys. *(Stryer, pp 361, 438–440, 454–455, 637–639)*

260. The answer is E (all). IgM is composed of a μ heavy chains and either κ or λ light chains. The pentamer is held together by one J (joining) chain. The immune system of an animal would react to all of these different components of the molecule and would produce a wide variety of antibodies specific to the different determinant groups of the molecule. Some of the antibodies would be to linear portions of the polypeptide chains, whereas others could be specific to a tripeptide complex that results from the folding of the peptide and is composed of two amino acids of one peptide chain and one amino acid of another. These particular determinant groups would be lost on dissociation of the peptides or through mild proteolysis. *(Joklik et al, p 187)*

261. The answer is A (1,2,3). Three types of reactions may be seen in the skin following the sting of a bee, wasp, or hornet. Two of the responses, the acute necrotic and subacute inflammatory types, are histologically nonspecific. The chronic lymphoid response to these stings and to tick bites is referred to as persistent arthropod sting. It may have a pseudolymphomatous appearance. It is, therefore, considered to be one of the pseudolymphomatous dermatoses. Affected persons show a dense lymphoid and histiocytic infiltrate in the dermis that also may extend into the subcutaneous adipose tissue. Eosinophils and plasma cells may be identified, as may multinucleated cells, hyperchromatic nuclei, and lymphoid follicles with germinal centers. The presence of such follicles is one feature that suggests a benign, reactive process in these skin lesions. A necrotizing granulomatous response is not described in association with these stings.*(Lever and Schaumburg-Lever, pp 219–220, 753)*

262. The answer is E (all) Obsessive neurosis is conceptualized to be a result of the separation of affect from ideas through the defense mechanisms of undoing and isolation. Affected patients are thought to regress to the anal sadistic level, with rigid and punitive superego activity. *(Kaplan et al, pp 631–728)*

263. The answer is D (4). Complete unilateral deafness is almost always a result of damage to the auditory nerve or organ of Corti of that side. The fibers originating in the spiral ganglion reach both the dorsal and ventral cochlear nuclei. Hence, destruction of one nucleus would diminish the ability to process information from the ear of the affected side. The majority of the fibers from the cochlear nuclei pass to the thalamus in the contralateral side of the brain stem. *(Heimer, pp 261–275)*

264. The answer is B (1,3). The figure that accompanies the question represents a typical ventricular function curve. A shift up and to the left, such as occurred from A to B, is indicative of increased contractility of the heart. All other things being held constant, a number of conditions will produce this increase in contractility, including norepinephrine infusion and sympathetic stimulation. Both of these effects presumably work via stimulation of

myocardial β receptors. Lowering the temperature of the heart and blocking the movement of calcium might be expected to have much the opposite effect and thus reduce cardiac contractility. *(Berne and Levy, pp 161,169–173)*

265. The answer is A (1,2,3). Regions of the chromosome that are being actively transcribed are referred to as transcriptionally active chromatin. The DNA in these domains is especially sensitive to digestion by the enzyme DNase I. It is assumed that this reflects some altered conformation of the chromatin in these regions. The high mobility group nonhistone proteins HMG 14 and HMG 17 often are found associated with active chromatin. The C-5 position of cytosine in a majority of the CpG dinucleotides in the genomes of mammalian DNA is methylated. It has been found that transcriptionally active chromatin has a lower degree of methylation than bulk chromatin. Histone levels have not been correlated with gene activity. *(Stryer, pp 842–844)*

266. The answer is A (1,2,3). The hypervariable regions of the antibody molecule are responsible for the serologic specificity of the molecule. They occur in the *N*-terminal region of both heavy and light polypeptide chains of the molecule and hence are in the Fab region of the molecule. Fc fragment is composed of the C-terminal half of the heavy chains. It is the product of papain digestion of the antibody molecule and is the portion of the molecule to which most of the carbohydrate is attached. Here resides the portion of the immunoglobulin molecule that controls its ability to cross the placenta, bind to mast cells, activate complement, and participate in the several different activities characteristic of the various immunoglobulin classes. *(Joklik et al, pp 186–187)*

267. The answer is C (2,4). Drug-induced vasculitis may be caused by a variety of drugs, the most common of which are phenylbutazone, chlorothiazide, the sulfonamides, and ampicillin. Two forms of drug-induced vasculitis may be identified. The less common form, the leukocytoclastic type, is characterized by an infiltrate with a predominance of neutrophils around and within the walls of the dermal blood vessels. The vessel walls often show fibrinoid necrosis. Most cases of drug-induced vasculitis are of the lymphocytic type. The form is characterized by a mononuclear and eosinophilic infiltrate in and around the small dermal vessels. Generally, fibroid necrosis is not evident. Two clinical patterns of the lymphocytic type can be recognized. In one pattern, the vasculitis tends to produce a maculopapular eruption over the extremities and is limited to involvement of the skin. In the second pattern, all skin surfaces may be involved by purpuric lesions. Additionally, various organs (heart, liver, and kidneys) may be involved, and death may result. An underlying panniculitis is not associated with drug-induced vasculitis. (*Lever and Schaumburg-Lever, pp 168, 259*)

268. **The answer is B (1,3).** Captopril inhibits angiotensin-converting enzyme (peptidyl dipeptidase), which is identical to kininase II. The immediate effect of this inhibition is to decrease conversion of angiotensin I to angiotensin II and to inhibit degradation of bradykinin. Both of these effects contribute to the vasodilatation caused by captopril. Captopril indirectly decreases aldosterone production. (*Gilman et al, p 649*)

269. **The answer is A (1,2,3).** Psychologic defense mechanisms are exaggerated under stressful conditions, such as hospitalization. They are adaptive in certain illness states, as the effectiveness of defense mechanisms seems to be inversely correlated with autonomic arousal. Defense mechanisms are mobilized unconsciously (automatically). (*Leigh and Reiser, pp 77–98*)

270. **The answer is C (2,4).** The organ of Corti, the neural transducer for sound, is located in the cochlear duct. It is activated by pressure changes within the perilymph that originates at the oval window, pass through the scala vestibuli, the heicotrema, and scala tympani, and end at the round window. The cochlear duct containing the organ of Corti is filled with endolymph. The organ of Corti is attached to the basilar membrane, which is the floor of the cochlear duct. The tectorial membrane is attached to the limbus of the spiral lamina. (*Heimer, pp 261–270*)

271. **The answer is B (1,3).** CCK is released by endocrine cells of the small intestine in response to the presence of fat and protein digestion products. In addition to stimulating secretion of pancreatic enzymes, CCK will competitively block the action of gastrin on gastric parietal cells. By itself, CCK has only a small effect on the secretion of pancreatic juice. However, it markedly enhances the stimulatory action of secretin. (*Davenport, 1978, pp 39–41*)

272. **The answer is D (4).** Prokaryotic DNA and eukaryotic DNA are replicated in a semiconservative manner. However, many differences exist between the two types. Bacterial DNA is circular, whereas eukaryotic nuclear DNA is linear and unbranched. Eukaryotic nuclear DNA is arranged in chromosomes composed of molecules at least 100 times as large as bacterial DNA. In addition, chromosomes are composed of histone–DNA complexes, a structural arrangement not found in bacteria. (*Stryer, pp 79–84*)

273. **The answer is A (1,2,3).** Rickettsiae, like other bacteria, have cell walls, nuclear material, and ribosomes. They divide by binary fission and are susceptible to antibacterial antibiotics. They are obligate intracellular parasites, not facultative, but this characteristic has nothing to do with being bacteria-like. (*Joklik et al, pp 593–595*)

274. **The answer is A (1,2,3).** The development of the fetal lungs essentially takes place in two stages. The trachea, bronchi, and bronchioles develop during the first half of gestational life. At about 7 mo gestation, the alveoli begin to develop. At first, they have thick walls with abundant inter- and intralobular connective tissue. The blood vessels, necessary for the exchange of gases, are located deep within this connective tissue and thus are removed from the air spaces. A cuboidal epithelium that is not an effective oxygen exchanger lines the alveolar spaces. As maturation takes place, the cuboidal lining thins out, there is loss of the connective tissue substance, and the alveolar spaces enlarge. All this brings the vascular network into proximity with the alveolar air spaces. At term, alveoli are still small, septa are still thick, and connective tissue is still prominent—as compared to the adult lung. The underdeveloped lungs in the low-weight, immature or premature infant, therefore, may contribute to the most common causes of death in such infants—respiratory distress and hypoxia, often complicated by infection. Current medical intervention, however, often is successful in salvaging many of these infants. (*Robbins et al, pp 476–486*)

275. **The correct answer is C (2,4).** Digoxin is the prototypic cardiac glycoside that is used to treat congestive heart failure and, to a lesser extent, atrial fibrillation and flutter. The beneficial effects of digoxin are all explained on the basis of increased contractile force of the myocardium or positive inotropy. The mechanisms underlying the positive inotropy are unclear but involve, in part, inhibition of membrane bound Na^+,K^+-ATPase activity and increase in slow inward current during the action potential of the heart. The electrophysiologic effects of digoxin contribute to a minor extent to its use as an antiarrhythmic drug and principally to its untoward cardiovascular effects. The mechanisms underlying these electrophysiologic effects are both direct (increased abnormal automaticity) and indirect (vagal—increased refractory period of atrioventricular node and decreased conduction velocity—and sympathetic—increased abnormal automaticity). Digoxin is extremely toxic and has a low therapeutic index. Loading doses of digoxin frequently are required, since the half-time of elimination is relatively long compared to the desired time to reach therapeutic effect. The term "digitizing" has arisen from the need for this form of multiple dosage therapy. *(Gilman et al, pp 716–743)*

276. The answer is E (all). Patients perceive their symptoms to be less serious when they are common, familiar, and predictable. They are perceived to be more serious if the degree of threat or personal loss is believed to be great, as occurs when a patient coughs up blood, for example. *(Leigh and Reiser, pp 3–15)*

277. The answer is A (1,2,3). Layer V of the cerebral cortex, the internal pyramidal layer, contains medium and large pyramidal cells as well as the giant pyramidal cells of Betz. This layer gives rise to many corticifugal fibers. Layers II and III, the external granular and external pyramidal layers, contain small- and medium-sized pyramidal cells that project to subcortical structures and to areas in the ipsilateral and contralateral cortex. Layer I, the molecular layer, is a fiber layer. *(Heimer, pp 338–339)*

278. The answer is E (all). Retinols, or A vitamins, are essential components in the synthesis of rhodopsin, the visual pigment of rods, as well as in the synthesis of the photosensitive pigments of cones. An early sign of a deficiency in vitamin A is the inability to see at night (nyctalopia). This effect may be reversed by the administration of vitamin A. However, a long-lasting deficiency may lead to the degeneration of both types of photoreceptor cells and then to the degeneration of neurons in the retina. *(Ganong, p 135)*

279. The answer is A (1,2,3). An unesterified hydroxyl group is left on the C-1' atom of the glycerol backbone of phospholipids by the action of phospholipase A_1, which releases a free fatty acid, on the C-2' atom by the action of phospholipase A_2, which also releases a free fatty acid, and on the C-3' atom by the action of phospholipase C, which releases choline phosphate. Phospholipase D cleaves off the choline group, leaving phosphatidic acid. *(Stryer, p 552)*

280. The answer is E (all). The cell wall of virtually all bacteria contains peptidoglycan, which consists of a backbone of *N*-acetylmuramic acid and *N*-acetylglucosamine in a β-1,4 linkage, a tetrapeptide, and a peptide bridge from the terminal COOH of one tetrapeptide to a reactive group (usually a free NH_2 group) of a neighboring tetrapeptide. Lysozyme hydrolyzes the glucosidic linkage between the two substituted sugar components and destroys the cell wall, thus making the cell susceptible to osmotic pressure changes. *(Joklik et al, pp 21, 64–65)*

281. The answer is E (all). Many chemicals are now recognized as inducing cancer in humans. These include industrial chemicals, such as vinyl chloride, asbestos, nickel, chromium compounds, 4-aminobiphenyl, benzidine, and 2-naphthylamine; drugs, such as diethylstilbestrol and phenacetin; chemical mixtures, such as cigarette tars, soots, and oils; chemical additives, such as saccharin; and natural compounds, such as betel nuts and aflatoxins. Vinyl chloride is a compound used in the production of polyvinylchloride in the plastic industry. It is highly carcinogenic in animals and also causes rare cases of hemangiosarcoma of the liver in workers with high exposure levels. Aflatoxin B is a mold formed by strains of *Aspergillus flavus,* which grows on peanuts and nuts. It is a highly potent carcinogen in animals, causing hepatocellular carcinoma, and it has been implicated in human cases of hepatoma in regions where there are high aflatoxin levels in the diet. Betel nuts are chewed in many countries and are thought to cause a markedly increased rate of carcinoma of the mucous membranes in the oral cavities of individuals who chew large amounts of these nuts combined with other substances. 2-Naphthylamine is an aromatic amine that is used in the aniline dye and rubber industries. It is absorbed through the skin and lungs and is excreted in the urine. This compound has been correlated with the development of cancers of the bladder. *(Kissane, pp 546–548)*

282. The answer is C (2,4). Digoxin is a cardiac glycoside with a narrow margin of safety that is not metabolized to a great extent by the liver but is excreted virtually in unchanged form in the kidney. Accordingly, decreased renal perfusion will increase circulating levels of digoxin, whereas little change will be associated with altered hepatic function. Inappropriate ingestion of too large a dose of any drug can potentially increase its circulating levels. Similarly, circulating levels of any drug are inversely related to its volume of distribution, and thus a decrease in volume of distribution of digoxin caused unexplainedly by quinidine is a common means by which digoxin levels have been reported to increase. *(Gilman et al, pp 741–743)*

283. The answer is A (1,2,3). Increased stress level, anxiety concerning symptoms, and upper socioeconomic class have been shown to increase the likelihood of a person's seeking medical help for an illness. An unpleasant experience with a physician, on the other hand, is likely to interfere with the tendency to seek future help from a physician. *(Leigh and Reiser, pp 3–15; Mechanic)*

284. The answer is D (4). The pharyngeal pouches are diverticulae of the cranial foregut (primitive pharynx). None of them normally communicate with the cervical sinus, which is formed from the externally situated pharyngeal (branchial) clefts. As outpouchings of the primitive pharynx, the pouches by definition would be located internal (posterior) to the buccopharyngeal membrane. The third pharyngeal pouch gives rise to the inferior parathyroid glands and thymus bilaterally. The first pouch contributes to the formation of the eustachian tube and middle ear cavity. *(Moore, pp 179–197)*

285. The answer is C (2,4). The endolymph, which bathes the apical surfaces of the hair cells in the cochlea, is unusual in that it has a high concentration of potassium ions. The endocochlear potential is the steady potential difference of about 80 mV that can be recorded between the endolymph and the surrounding, low-potassium perilymph. Ion pumps in the stria vascularis are responsible for generating and maintaining this potential difference. Deformation of the basilar membrane cannot produce such a steady potential difference. The generator potential of the hair cells is the change in cell membrane potential that leads to activation of the afferent nerve fibers in response to acoustic stimuli. *(Ganong, pp 139–140)*

286. The answer is A (1,2,3). The immediate source of carbons for fatty acid synthesis is acetyl-CoA, which is converted to malonyl-CoA in the first step of fatty acid synthesis. Thus, any precursor of acteyl-CoA can be a source of carbon atoms for fatty acids. Glucose and other carbohydrates that are converted to glycolytic intermediates, as well as ketogenic amino acids derived from protein degradation, can contribute carbon atoms to acetyl-CoA. Citrate is the major carrier of mitochondrial acetyl-CoA carbons to the cytosol for fatty acid synthesis, since acetyl-CoA itself cannot move across the inner mitochondrial membrane. Once citrate has diffused into the cytosol, it is cleaved into acetyl-CoA and oxaloacetate by the citrate cleavage enzyme (citrate lyase). Steroids, all of which are derived from cholesterol in humans, cannot be degraded. Bile excretion is the main route of disposal of the cholesterol nucleus. Thus, although acetyl-CoA is a precursor of cholesterol, once incorporated, the carbon atoms of cholesterol are unavailable for biosynthesis of other compounds. *(Stryer, pp 480–481)*

287. The answer is A (1,2,3). The rabies virus is a rhabdovirus containing single-stranded RNA. The *G* gene of the rabies virus genome is responsible for the synthesis of a glycoprotein that constitutes the spikes on the rabies virus surface and is responsible for the attachment of the rabies virus on the host cells. Susceptible cells, such as the cells of the CNS, have receptors on which the glycoprotein spikes can attach and thus allow the rabies virus to enter the nerve cell and multiply. Salivary glands are tissues with dense innervation. Therefore, large amounts of rabies virus may be found in the salivary glands, from which the virus is excreted in the saliva of such infected carnivorous animals as dogs, cats, bats, foxes, and other animals. *(Joklik et al, pp 848–849)*

288. The answer is B (1,3). There are three major patterns of rejection of a tissue transplant: hyperacute, acute, and chronic rejection. With the kidney as the example, hyperacute rejection occurs within minutes after the transplantation. Acute rejection manifests itself as sudden deterioration of renal function within days or months to years following transplantation. Two histologic types of acute renal rejection are recognized and may overlap in any given patient. Acute cellular rejection demonstrates an interstitial mononuclear cell infiltrate and edema with mild interstitial hemorrhage. Focal tubular necrosis due to mononuclear cell infiltration may occur. In the absence of an arteritis, this type of rejection responds to immunosuppressive therapy. Acute humoral rejection or rejection vasculitis produces a necrotizing arteritis with endothelial necrosis, neutrophilic infiltration, deposition of immunoglobulin, complement, and fibrin, and thrombosis. This leads to severe glomerular and cortical damage that fails to respond to immunosuppressive therapy. Chronic rejection is a progressive dysfunction of the kidney with gradual increase in serum creatinine levels during a 4- to 6-mo period. *(Robbins et al, pp 171–176)*

289. The answer is D (4). A basic principle of pharmacology is that the effect of a drug is directly proportional to the concentration of drug–receptor complex. Quantitative measures of dose–response relationships are complex but can be described by (1) potency or the location of a dose–response curve along the dose axis and (2) maximal efficacy as reflected in the plateau of a dose–response curve. Although potency has useful information regarding how much of a dose of drug X is required to produce a certain effect, the ultimate use of a drug is better manifest in its efficacy. Accordingly, low potency is a disadvantage only if effective dose is so large that it is awkward to administer. The affinity of drugs for receptors is an intrinsic property of this interaction and may be unrelated to the drug's ability to bring about a response. Frequently many steps downstream from drug–receptor complex, including intracellular signalling and biochemical and physiologic coupling, contribute to the ultimate response. Antagonists are drugs that bind to receptors but bring about no response, in contrast to partial agonists that also bind to receptors but bring about less than complete responses. *(Gilman et al, pp 44–46)*

290. The answer is E (all). The basic element of informed consent include the following: a reasonable explanation of the procedures and their purposes, a description of potential risks, a description of potential benefits, a discussion of potential alternatives, inviting questions and providing answers to them, and advising patients that they are free to withdraw the consent at any time without adversely affecting their relationship with the physician or institution. *(Balis, pp 352–357)*

291. The answer is B (1,3). The major efferent pathways from the cerebellum exit by way of the superior cerebellar peduncle or the brachium conjunctivum. Fibers exiting from the cerebellum and passing to the reticular formation and vestibular nuclei do so by way of the inferior cerebellar peduncle, or restiform body. The major number of fibers in the inferior cerebellar peduncle are afferent to the cerebellum and are derived from the dorsal spinocerebellar tracts and vestibulocerebellar system. The middle cerebellar peduncle, or brachium pontis, consists of fibers entering the cerebellum from the pontine nuclei. *(Heimer, pp 211–224)*

292. The answer is D (4). A number of physiologic adjustments occur during exercise, including increased sympathetic nervous stimulation, adrenal medullary secretion of epinephrine, vasodilatation of contracting muscle, and contraction of muscles around blood vessels. It is the combined effect on the heart and peripheral vascular beds that underlies a large increase in cardiac output without much change in filling pressure. Venoconstriction will decrease venous capacitance and effectively increase circulating blood volume. Sympathetic stimulation of the heart increases its contractility and rate and thus further aids in increasing output with little change in right atrial pressure. Increased cardiac function by itself would lead to only a modest increase in cardiac output if venous return were not increased. During exercise, extreme dilatation in the skeletal muscle vasculature along with decreased venous capacitance leads to a large decrease in peripheral vascular resistance. *(Guyton, pp 276–277)*

293. The answer is C (2,4). Bile salts are derivatives of cholesterol that contain both polar and nonpolar portions. This property allows them to solubilize dietary lipids, which, in turn, aids in the intestinal absorption of lipids and facilitates their digestion by pancreatic lipase. *(Stryer, p 559)*

294. The answer is B (1,3). The varicella-herpes zoster virus has a tropism for nerve cells, and readily establishes a latent infection in nerve tissue. Exacerbation of the infection results in shingles, which is characterized by myalgia, fever, malaise, and skin lesions that consist of groups of small vesicles on inflammatory bases. These lesions occur in cutaneous areas supplied by certain nerve trunks. Varicella-zoster is a DNA virus that multiplies in the nucleus of the cell. Cytomegalic cells are characteristic of cytomegalovirus, another member of the Herpesviridae. *(Joklik et al, pp 794–796)*

295. The answer is A (1,2,3). The lesion shown in the question is multiple emboli in the lung, occluding arteries. Pulmonary emboli are a frequent complication of bedrest and are seen in debilitated elderly people. They originate in deep leg veins from thrombi that are dislodged and sent into the peripheral circulation via the inferior vena cava, where they obstruct the pulmonary arterial circulation. They may cause pulmonary hemorrhage or infarction, depending on the amount of collateral blood supply. If they are large and obstruct major blood vessels, they may cause sudden death by interrupting cardiac output. If the emboli are multiple, over time they may lead to chronic pulmonary damage and fibrosis, with pulmonary hypertension and right-sided heart failure. *(Rubin and Farber, pp 265–268)*

296. The answer is B (1,3). Aminoglycoside antibiotics may cause a rise in serum creatinine levels because of slow accumulation in renal tissue. Studies on humans and animals suggest that tobramycin is slightly less nephrotoxic than gentamicin, but the clinical significance of this small difference is unclear. Ototoxicity manifests itself as auditory or vestibular dysfunction. Aminoglycosides are not hepatotoxic. However, they are weak bases and do not contain a sodium ion, which might pose a problem for patients with congestive heart failure. *(Gilman et al, pp 1157–1160)*

297. The answer is C (2,4). Anxiety increases sympathetic tone. Anxiety is associated with increased performance up to a point. Anxiety may be a classically conditioned response. Although an anxiety-provoking situation may be repressed (unconscious), anxiety itself as an affect is not unconscious. It may be attenuated, however, as in signal anxiety, which occurs in the face of psychologic conflict, ushering in defense mechanisms. *(Leigh and Reiser, pp 41–76)*

298. The answer is E (all). Each branchial arch contains, at some time during development, an aortic arch artery, a cartilaginous plate or rod, a cranial nerve or major branch of a cranial nerve, and mesenchyme to form muscle tissue and other connective tissue. Neural crest tissue in the head region contributes to the undifferentiated mesenchyme in the branchial arches and also forms the sensory neurons related to cranial nerves III through XII. *(Moore, pp 179–197)*

299. The answer is B (1,3). The Henderson-Hasselbalch equation enables one to predict the ratio of ionized and un-ionized species of a compound for a given pH. Renal clearance of a substance can be augmented by increasing the concentration of ionized species (nonreabsorbable) in the kidneys and increasing urine flow. A weak acid ($pK = 7.2$) will have a significant increase in ionized species when pH is raised. Thus, bicarbonate infusion to alkalinize the urine is useful. Osmotic diuresis with mannitol will increase urine flow and subsequently phenobarbital clearance. Lowering the ventilatory rate will increase H^+ secretion and lower urine pH. Vasopressin will reduce urine flow. *(Guyton, pp 439–441)*

300. The answer is A (1,2,3). Insulin and glucagon are antagonistic in the maintenance of blood glucose levels and glucose use by tissues. Calcitonin and parathyroid hormone are antagonistic in the maintenance of calcium levels and metabolism of calcium. Histamine and serotonin are antagonistic in the maintenance of vasomotor tone. Epinephrine and norepinephrine are not antagonistic. The adrenal hormone epinephrine and its neurotransmitter counterpart, norepinephrine, both stimulate similar hormone receptors that lead to the production of cyclic AMP in muscle and adipocytes. These catecholamines stimulate lipolysis and glycogenolysis. *(Stryer, pp 591–592,636–637)*

301. The answer is E (all). One early clue to human immunodeficiency virus (HIV) infection (AIDS) is a decrease of the CD-4+ helper T cells, since the HIV multiplies in and destroys these cells. This situation frequently leads to such opportunistic infections as *P. carinii* pneumonia, cytomegalovirus pneumonia, retinitis, encephalitis, *Candida albicans* esophagitis, and *Toxoplasma gondii* encephalitis. Malignancies, such as Kaposi's sarcoma or non-Hodgkin's B cell lymphomas and sarcomas of the rectum or tongue, constitute the hallmarks of AIDS. *(Joklik et al, pp 865–866)*

302. The answer is B (1,3). The process described as apoptosis is one that for many years was largely overlooked but has now become well recognized as a major form of individual cell deletion in which the nuclear material shrinks within the cell cytoplasm and the cytoplasm shrinks around it, forming small dense bodies. Such bodies are often phagocytosed and removed without disruption of the cell as classically seen in other forms of necrosis. It is clear that this type of cell deletion may occur in people in the normal aging process and in certain types of so-called atrophic processes in the body, including such structures as the endometrium. It is, therefore, a normal regulatory and aging process and distinctly different from the other forms of cell death and necrosis. *(Rubin and Farber, p 15; Lewis and Rowden, pp 103–109)*

303. The answer is E (all). Cholestyramine, a bile acid sequestrant, reduces plasma cholesterol levels by decreasing concentrations of low-density lipoproteins. Orally administered drugs may be bound by cholestryamine as well, including chlorothiazide, penylbutazone, phenobarbital, oral anticoagulants, thyroxine, and digitalis glycosides. This problem may be avoided to a large extent by administering other drugs at least 1 hr before or 4 hr after cholestyramine. Steatorrhea may be another side effect, impairing absorption of fat-soluble vitamins. If this condition develops, vitamin supplementation is recommended. *(Gilman et al, pp 840–841)*

304. The answer is A (1,2,3). Relative risk of developing a certain disease is defined as the rate of disease in the exposed group divided by the rate of disease in the nonexposed group, in this example $2.27/0.07 = 32$. The attributable risk is the rate of disease in the exposed group that can be attributed to exposure—that is, the rate of disease in the exposed group less the rate in the unexposed group ($2.27 - 0.07 = 2.20$). Since 2.20 deaths per 1,000 among heavy smokers (out of 2.27 lung cancer deaths per 1,000) can be attributed to smoking, 2.20/2.27, or 97 percent, of the total risk of death from lung cancer is accounted for by heavy smoking. The population attributable risk depends on the lung cancer death rate observed for the total population, which was not stated in the problem. *(MacMahon and Pugh, pp 232–234)*

305. The answer is B (1,3). DNA polymerase III holoenzyme is a multisubunit enzyme that is responsible for the replication of most of the DNA comprising the *E. coli* chromosome. All known DNA polymerases can catalyze the synthesis of DNA only in the 5' to 3' direction. In addition, most DNA polymerases have the ability to cleave the terminal nucleotide from the growing DNA strand if it is improperly base paired with the template. This activity is referred to as "proofreading" and is catalyzed by a 3' to 5' exonuclease. *(Stryer, pp 668–669, 673)*

306. The answer is E (all). The proximal renal tubules consist of highly metabolic active epithelial cells with extensive brush borders to facilitate much of the resorptive and secretory processes of the kidneys. More than 65 percent of water filtered in the glomerulus is absorbed at this site. Glucose, proteins, and amino acids are virtually completely reabsorbed from the filtrate, and a significant fraction of Na^+, Cl^-, and HCO_3^- and K^+ also is reabsorbed. *(Mountcastle, pp 1167,1176–1179)*

307. The answer is C (2,4). Dicumarol and warfarin are antagonists of vitamin K. Under normal conditions, a vitamin K-dependent γ-carboxylation of certain glutamate residues of prothrombin occurs after translation. In the presence of either warfarin or dicumarol, abnormal prothrombin with unchanged glutamate residues is produced. The abnormal prothrombin is unable to bind calcium and participate in the clotting process. Vitamin K is normally produced by intestinal bacteria. *(Stryer, pp 251–252)*

308. The answer is C (2,4). There are numerous antigenic types of *H. influenzae* and *S. pyogenes*. However, these are genetically stable and do not change during a particular infectious episode. Such is not the case with *T. gambiense* and *B. recurrentis*, both of which readily change their antigenic expression within the host, thus permitting exacerbations or relapses in the disease process. *(Hoeprich, pp 1149,1245–1246)*

309. The answer is E (all). Honeycomb lung, or diffuse interstitial fibrosis, is a general term for pulmonary fibrosis, which is secondary to many environmental and occupational hazards. It is characterized by diffuse obliteration of the alveolar septa with fibrosis and thickening, bronchiolar dilatation, cyst formation, and squamous metaplasia. Alveolar capillary block leads to dyspnea, tachycardia, cyanosis, and right heart failure. The causes are numerous, including environmental factors, such as silica, *T. polyspora* (farmer's lung), talc, synthetic fibers, beryllium, asbestos, coal dust (anthrocosis), nitrogen dioxide (silo-filler's disease), and flax (byssinosis); connective tissue diseases, such as rheumatoid arthritis, systemic lupus erythematosus, scleroderma, and sarcoidosis; drugs, such as bulsulfan and bleomycin; oxygen; and idiopathic etiologies. *(Kissane, pp 880–882,907–915)*

310. The answer is E (all). Benzoyl peroxide is bactericidal to anaerobic and microaerophilic bacteria, since it slowly releases oxygen. Ethanol is most effective against staphylococci at concentrations of between 40 and 60 percent. However, 70 percent ethanol has a faster action, whereas concentrations above 80 percent have lower efficacy. Iodine is still widely used because of its efficacy, economics, and low toxicity to tissues. Elemental iodine is a potent, rapidly acting agent that is lethal to microflora, microzoa, and viruses. Local toxicity is low when compared with its germicidal potency. However, some individuals may demonstrate hypersensitivity to iodine. A 2 percent tincture of iodine solution is used in preoperative scrubbing, whereas a 0.5 to 1.0 percent solution is suitable for wounds and abrasions. Phenol and its derivatives may be bacteriostatic, bactericidal, and fungicidal. Their germicidal activity is a consequence of denaturing proteins. *(Gilman et al, pp 968–970)*

311. The answer is E (all). Delinquency and psychiatric disorders often are accompanied by reading difficulties. The significance of the association is not definitely established. Organic brain dysfunction and specific temperament features are among the factors that may predispose the child to a multiple of such conditions. *(Rutter et al)*

BIBLIOGRAPHY

Anatomy

Carpenter MB, and Sutin J. *Human Neuroanatomy*. 8th ed. Baltimore, Md: Williams and Wilkins, 1983.

Gardner E, Gray DS, O'Rahilly R. *Anatomy: A Regional Study of Human Structure*. 5th ed. Philadelphia: WB Saunders, 1986.

Heimer L. *The Human Brain and Spinal Cord*. New York: Springer-Verlag, New York, Inc., 1983.

Moore K. *The Developing Human*. 3rd ed. Philadelphia: WB Saunders, 1982.

Woodburne, RT. *Essentials of Human Anatomy*. 8th ed. New York: Oxford University Press, 1988.

Physiology

Berne RM, Levy, MN. *Cardiovascular Physiology*. 4th ed. St. Louis: CV Mosby Co., 1981.

Davenport, HW. *A Digest of Digestion*. 2nd ed. Chicago: Year Book Medical Publishers, Inc., 1978.

Ganong WF. *Review of Medical Physiology*. 14th ed. Los Altos, Calif: Lange Medical Publications, 1989.

Guyton AC. *Textbook of Medical Physiology*. 7th ed. Philadelphia: WB Saunders Co, 1986.

Mountcastle VB. *Medical Physiology*. 14th ed. St. Louis: CV Mosby Co, 1980.

Petersen OH, Maruyama Y. Calcium-activated potassium channels and their role in secretion. *Nature*. February 1984; 693–696.

Biochemistry

Lehninger AL. *Biochemistry*. 2nd ed. New York: Worth Publishers, Inc, 1977.

Stryer L. *Biochemistry*. 3rd ed. San Francisco: WH Freeman and Co, 1988.

Microbiology

Jawetz E, Melnick JL, Adelberg EA, et al. *Review of Medical Microbiology*. 17th ed. Norwalk, Conn.: Appleton & Lange; 1987.

Joklik WK, Willett HP, Amos DB, Wilfert CM. *Zinsser Microbiology*. 19th ed. Norwalk, Conn.: Appleton & Lange; 1988.

Roitt IM, Brostoff J, Male DK. *Immunology*. St. Louis, Mo.: C.V. Mosby Company; 1985.

Pathology

Hutt MSR, Burkitt DP. *The Geography of Non-Infectious Disease*. Oxford: Oxford University Press, 1986.

Kissane JM. *Anderson's Pathology*. 8th ed. St. Louis: CV Mosby Co, 1985.

Lever W, and Schaumburg-Lever G. *Histopathology of the Skin* 6th ed. Philadelphia: JB Lippincott Co, 1983.

Lewis MG, Rowden G. *Histopathology: A Step-by-Step Approach*. Boston: Little, Brown and Co, 1984.

Robbins, SL, Cotran RS, Kumar V. *Pathologic Basis of Disease*. 3rd ed. Philadelphia: WB Saunders Co, 1984.

Rubin E, Farber JL. *Pathology*. Philadelphia: JB Lippincott Co, 1988.

Pharmacology

Craig CR, Stitzel RE, eds. *Modern Pharmacology*. 2nd ed. Boston: Little, Brown and Co, 1986.

Gilman AG, Goodman LS, Rall TW, Murad F. *The Pharmacological Basis of Therapeutics*. 7th ed. New York: Macmillan Inc, 1985.

Katcher BS, Young LY, Koda-Kimble MA. *Applied Therapeutics: The Clinical Use of Drugs*. 3rd ed. San Francisco: Applied Therapeutics, Inc, 1983.

Lewis JH, Zimmerman HJ, Ishak KG, Mullick FG. Enflurance hepatotoxicity: A clinicopathologic study of 24 cases. *Ann Intern Med*. June 1983; 984–992.

Lindeman RD, Papper S. Therapy of fluid and electrolyte disorders. *Ann Intern Med*. January 1975; 64–70

Wyngaarden JB, Smith LH. *Cecil Textbook of Medicine*. 16th ed. Philadelphia: WB Saunders Co, 1982.

Behavioral Sciences

American Psychiatric Association. *Diagnostic and Statistical Manual of Mental Disorders*. 3rd ed. rev. (*DSM-III-R*). Washington, DC: American Psychiatric Association, 1987.

Balis GU, ed. *The Behavioral and Social Sciences and the Practice of Medicine*. Vol. II. *The Psychiatric Foundations of Medicine*. Stoneham, Mass.: Butterworth Publishers, Inc, 1978.

Erikson EH. *Identity and the Life Cycle*. Vol. I. *Psychological Issues*. New York: International Universities Press, 1959.

Hine FR, Carson RC, Maddox GL, Thompson RJ, Williams RB. *Introduction to Behavioral Science in Medicine*. New York: Springer-Verlag New York, Inc, 1983.

Kaplan HI, Sadock, BJ, eds. *Comprehensive Textbook of Psychiatry*. 4th ed. Baltimore: Williams & Wilkins Co, 1985.

Leigh H, Reiser MF. *The Patient. Biological, Psychological, and Social Dimensions of Medical Practice*. 2nd ed. New York: Plenum Publishing Corp, 1985.

Lennenberg EH. *Biological Foundation of Language*. New York: John Wiley & Sons, Inc, 1967.

Lindemann E. Symptomatology and management of acute grief. *Am J Psychiatry* May 1944; 141–148.

MacMahon B, Pugh T. *Epidemiology, Principles and Methods*. Boston: Little, Brown & Co, 1970.

Mechanic D. Social psychologic factors affecting the presentation of bodily complaints. *N Engl J Med*. May 5, 1972; 1132–1139.

Rutter M, Tizard J, Whitmore K. *Education, Health, and Behavior*. London: Longman Group, Ltd, 1970.

Simons, RC, ed. *Understanding Human Behavior in Health and Illness*. 3rd ed. Baltimore: Williams & Wilkins Co, 1985.

Practice Test Subspeciality List

ANATOMY

1. Peripheral circulation
4. Musculoskeletal
7. Embryology
   Respiratory System
11. Cardiovascular system
15. Peripheral nervous system
20. Endocrine system
25. Lymphatic system
32. Heart and great vessels
39. Peripheral nervous system
46. Peripheral nervous system
53. Urinary system
60. Peripheral circulation
67. Digestive system
74. Digestive system
81. GU system
88. Female genital system
95. Peripheral nervous system
102. Genital system
109. Respiratory system
116. Nervous system
123. Nervous system
130. Nervous system
137. Nervous system
162. Autonomic nervous system
163. Autonomic nervous system
164. Autonomic nervous system
165. Autonomic nervous system
195. Peripheral nervous system
196. Peripheral nervous system
197. Peripheral nervous system
216. Embryology Nervous system
217. Embryology Nervous system
218. Embryology Nervous system
245. Embryology Nervous system
251. Embryology Nervous system
257. Embryology Nervous system
263. Embryology Nervous system
270. Embryology Nervous system
277. Embryology Nervous system
284. Embryology Pharynx; branchial arches
291. Nervous system

298. Embryology Pharynx; branchial arches

PHYSIOLOGY

10. Cardiovascular regulation
12. Cardiovascular regulation
16. Cardiovascular regulation
21. Cardiac electrophysiology
26. Cardiac electrophysiology
33. Endocrinology
40. Gastrointestinal
47. Endocrinology
54. Endocrinology
61. Endocrinology
68. Endocrinology
75. Endocrinology
82. Endocrinology
89. Endocrinology
96. Endocrinology
103. Nervous System
110. Circulation in specific organs
117. Circulation in specific organs
124. Circulation in specific organs
131. Hemodynamics
138. Cardiac cycle
144. Endocrinology
145. Endocrinology
146. Endocrinology
147. Endocrinology
166. Cardiac electrophysiology
167. Cardiac electrophysiology
168. Cardiac electrophysiology
198. Cardiac electrophysiology
199. Cardiac electrophysiology
219. Nervous System
220. Nervous System
221. Nervous System
246. Excretory function
252. Cardiovascular regulation
258. Special senses
264. Cardiac cycle
271. Gastrointestinal

278. Special senses
285. Special senses
292. Hemodynamics
299. Excretory function
306. Excretory function

BIOCHEMISTRY

2. Lipids
5. Vitamins
8. pH
13. Nutrition
17. Amino acids
22. Amino acids
27. Amino acids
34. Protein
41. Protein
48. Protein
55. Blood
62. Blood
69. Blood
76. Small molecule metabolism
83. Small molecule metabolism
90. Carbohydrate metabolism
97. Carbohydrate metabolism
104. Enzymes
111. Molecular biology
118. Molecular biology
125. Enzymes
132. Lipids
139. Integration of metabolism
148. Enzymes
149. Enzymes
150. Enzymes
169. Molecular biology
170. Molecular biology
171. Molecular biology
200. Carbohydrates
201. Carbohydrates
202. Carbohydrates
222. Molecular biology
223. Molecular biology
224. Molecular biology
233. Small molecule metabolism
235. Amino acids
237. Protein
241. Integration of metabolism
247. Small molecule metabolism
253. Small molecule metabolism
259. Carbohydrate metabolism
265. Molecular biology
272. Molecular biology
279. Lipids
286. Lipids
293. Lipids
300. Hormones
305. Molecular Biology
307. Blood

MICROBIOLOGY

28. Immune response
35. Immune response
42. Physiology
49. Pathogenic bacteriology
56. Virology
63. Virology
70. Virology
77. Immune deficiency disease
84. Physiology
91. Antigen-antibody reaction Serology
98. Antigen-antibody reaction Serology
105. Immunology Transplantation
112. Immunology Transplantation
119. Immune response
126. Immune response
133. Mycology
140. Pathogenic bacteriology
151. Virology
152. Virology
153. Virology
172. Pathogenic bacteriology
173. Pathogenic bacteriology
174. Physiology
203. Antigens
204. Immune response
225. Exotoxins
226. Exotoxins
231. Pathogenic bacteriology
232. Virology
234. Virology
236. Virology
238. Virology
242. Virology
248. Virology
254. Cellular immunology
260. Antibody structure
266. Antibody structure
273. Physiology
280. Physiology
287. Virology
294. Virology
301. Virology
308. Pathogenic bacteriology

PATHOLOGY

3. Endocrine system
6. Respiratory system
9. Respiratory system
14. Miscellaneous
18. Cardiovascular system
23. Kidney and urinary system
29. Circulatory system
36. Processes of neoplasia
43. Endocrine system
50. Blood and lymphatic system

57. Kidney and urinary system
64. Genetic syndromes and metabolic diseases
71. Cardiovascular system
78. Inflammation
85. Genetic syndromes and metabolic diseases
92. Miscellaneous
99. Genital system
106. Processes of neoplasia
113. Circulatory system
120. Processes of neoplasia
127. Inflammation
134. Circulatory system
141. Inflammation
175. Genetic syndromes and metabolic diseases
176. Genetic syndromes and metabolic diseases
177. Genetic syndromes and metabolic diseases
178. Genetic syndromes and metabolic diseases
205. Central Nervous system
206. Central Nervous system
227. Blood and lymphatic system
228. Blood and lymphatic system
239. Processes of neoplasia
243. Processes of neoplasia
249. Circulatory system
255. Cell injury
261. Nongenetic syndromes
267. Nongenetic syndromes
274. Abnormal growth
281. Processes of neoplasia
288. Immunopathology
295. Respiratory system
302. Cell injury and response
309. Respiratory system

PHARMACOLOGY

30. Central and peripheral nervous systems
37. Endocrine system
44. Poisoning and therapy of intoxication
51. Central and peripheral nervous systems
58. Antibiotics
65. General principles
72. Endocrine system
79. Blood and blood-forming organs
86. Cardiovascular and respiratory systems
93. Cardiovascular and respiratory systems
100. Autonomic nervous system
107. CNS drugs/Gas anesthetics
114. CNS drugs/Gas anesthetics
121. Kidneys, fluid, electrolytes
128. Central and peripheral nervous systems analgesics
135. Central and peripheral nervous systems psychotherapeutic agents
142. Hormone-like drugs/Oral hypoglycemics
154. Cardiovascular and respiratory systems/Antihypertensive agents
155. Cardiovascular and respiratory systems/Antihypertensive agents

156. Cardiovascular and respiratory systems/Antihypertensive agents
157. Cardiovascular and respiratory systems/Antihypertensive agents
179. Autonomic nervous system
180. Autonomic nervous system
181. Autonomic nervous system
182. Autonomic nervous system
183. Autonomic nervous system
184. Autonomic nervous system
190. Antimicrobial agents
191. Antimicrobial agents
192. Antimicrobial agents
193. Antimicrobial agents
194. Antimicrobial agents
207. Cardiovascular Antihypertensive agents
208. Cardiovascular Antihypertensive agents
229. Immunosuppression
230. Immunosuppression
268. Cardiovascular and respiratory systems
275. Cardiovascular and respiratory systems Congestive heart failure
282. General principles
289. General principles
296. Antibiotics
303. Cardiovascular and respiratory systems Drugs affecting cholesterol and lipid metabolism
310. Chemotherapeutic agents

BEHAVIORAL SCIENCES

19. Individual dynamics
24. Medical sociology
31. Learning theory
38. Brain/behavior
45. Anxiety/psychopharmacology
52. Aggression
59. Individual dynamics
66. Individual dynamics
73. Suicide/epidemiology
80. Pain/neurophysiology
87. Psychopharmacology
94. Suicide/epidemiology
101. Sleep and dreaming
108. Doctor-patient relationship
115. Medical sociology
122. Grief/depression
129. Patient management/individual dynamics
136. Human sexuality
143. Epidemiology
158. Child psychology
159. Child psychology
160. Child psychology
161. Child psychology
185. Child psychology
186. Child psychology
187. Child psychology
188. Child psychology

189. Child psychology
209. Learning theory
210. Learning theory
211. Learning theory
212. Learning theory
213. Learning theory
214. Learning theory
215. Learning theory
240. Suicide/sociology/depression
244. Depression

250. Depression/grief/emotions
256. Depression/emotions
262. Individual dynamics
269. Individual dynamics
276. Medical sociology
283. Medical sociology
290. Law and medical ethics
297. Anxiety/learning theory
304. Epidemiology
311. Child psychology

NAME _____
Last   First   Middle

ADDRESS _____
Street

_____
City   State   Zip

DIRECTIONS Mark your social security number from top to bottom in the appropriate boxes on the right. Refer to the section "HOW TO TAKE THE PRACTICE TEST" in the introduction to the book for more information. PLEASE USE NO.2 PENCIL ONLY.

MAKE ERASURES COMPLETE

SOC SEC NUMBER

	0 1 2 3 4 5 6 7 8 9
	0 1 2 3 4 5 6 7 8 9
	0 1 2 3 4 5 6 7 8 9
	0 1 2 3 4 5 6 7 8 9
	0 1 2 3 4 5 6 7 8 9
	0 1 2 3 4 5 6 7 8 9
	0 1 2 3 4 5 6 7 8 9
	0 1 2 3 4 5 6 7 8 9
	0 1 2 3 4 5 6 7 8 9

PAGE 1 2
TYPE 1 2 3

1 A B C D E   2 A B C D E   3 A B C D E   4 A B C D E   5 A B C D E   6 A B C D E   7 A B C D E   8 A B C D E

9 A B C D E   10 A B C D E   11 A B C D E   12 A B C D E   13 A B C D E   14 A B C D E   15 A B C D E   16 A B C D E

17 A B C D E   18 A B C D E   19 A B C D E   20 A B C D E   21 A B C D E   22 A B C D E   23 A B C D E   24 A B C D E

25 A B C D E   26 A B C D E   27 A B C D E   28 A B C D E   29 A B C D E   30 A B C D E   31 A B C D E   32 A B C D E

33 A B C D E   34 A B C D E   35 A B C D E   36 A B C D E   37 A B C D E   38 A B C D E   39 A B C D E   40 A B C D E

41 A B C D E   42 A B C D E   43 A B C D E   44 A B C D E   45 A B C D E   46 A B C D E   47 A B C D E   48 A B C D E

49 A B C D E   50 A B C D E   51 A B C D E   52 A B C D E   53 A B C D E   54 A B C D E   55 A B C D E   56 A B C D E

57 A B C D E   58 A B C D E   59 A B C D E   60 A B C D E   61 A B C D E   62 A B C D E   63 A B C D E   64 A B C D E

65 A B C D E   66 A B C D E   67 A B C D E   68 A B C D E   69 A B C D E   70 A B C D E   71 A B C D E   72 A B C D E

73 A B C D E   74 A B C D E   75 A B C D E   76 A B C D E   77 A B C D E   78 A B C D E   79 A B C D E   80 A B C D E

81 A B C D E   82 A B C D E   83 A B C D E   84 A B C D E   85 A B C D E   86 A B C D E   87 A B C D E   88 A B C D E

89 A B C D E   90 A B C D E   91 A B C D E   92 A B C D E   93 A B C D E   94 A B C D E   95 A B C D E   96 A B C D E

97 A B C D E   98 A B C D E   99 A B C D E   100 A B C D E   101 A B C D E   102 A B C D E   103 A B C D E   104 A B C D E

105 A B C D E   106 A B C D E   107 A B C D E   108 A B C D E   109 A B C D E   110 A B C D E   111 A B C D E   112 A B C D E

113 A B C D E   114 A B C D E   115 A B C D E   116 A B C D E   117 A B C D E   118 A B C D E   119 A B C D E   120 A B C D E

121 A B C D E   122 A B C D E   123 A B C D E   124 A B C D E   125 A B C D E   126 A B C D E   127 A B C D E   128 A B C D E

129 A B C D E   130 A B C D E   131 A B C D E   132 A B C D E   133 A B C D E   134 A B C D E   135 A B C D E   136 A B C D E

137 A B C D E   138 A B C D E   139 A B C D E   140 A B C D E   141 A B C D E   142 A B C D E   143 A B C D E   144 A B C D E

145 A B C D E   146 A B C D E   147 A B C D E   148 A B C D E   149 A B C D E   150 A B C D E   151 A B C D E   152 A B C D E

153 A B C D E   154 A B C D E   155 A B C D E   156 A B C D E   157 A B C D E   158 A B C D E   159 A B C D E   160 A B C D E

S O C | S E C | N U M B E R

	0	1	2	3	4	5	6	7	8	9
	0	1	2	3	4	5	6	7	8	9
	0	1	2	3	4	5	6	7	8	9
	0	1	2	3	4	5	6	7	8	9
	0	1	2	3	4	5	6	7	8	9
	0	1	2	3	4	5	6	7	8	9
	0	1	2	3	4	5	6	7	8	9
	0	1	2	3	4	5	6	7	8	9
	0	1	2	3	4	5	6	7	8	9

PAGE 1 2
TYPE 1 2 3

161 A B C D E 162 A B C D E 163 A B C D E 164 A B C D E 165 A B C D E 166 A B C D E 167 A B C D E 168 A B C D E

169 A B C D E 170 A B C D E 171 A B C D E 172 A B C D E 173 A B C D E 174 A B C D E 175 A B C D E 176 A B C D E

177 A B C D E 178 A B C D E 179 A B C D E 180 A B C D E 181 A B C D E 182 A B C D E 183 A B C D E 184 A B C D E

185 A B C D E 186 A B C D E 187 A B C D E 188 A B C D E 189 A B C D E 190 A B C D E 191 A B C D E 192 A B C D E

193 A B C D E 194 A B C D E 195 A B C D E 196 A B C D E 197 A B C D E 198 A B C D E 199 A B C D E 200 A B C D E

201 A B C D E 202 A B C D E 203 A B C D E 204 A B C D E 205 A B C D E 206 A B C D E 207 A B C D E 208 A B C D E

209 A B C D E 210 A B C D E 211 A B C D E 212 A B C D E 213 A B C D E 214 A B C D E 215 A B C D E 216 A B C D E

217 A B C D E 218 A B C D E 219 A B C D E 220 A B C D E 221 A B C D E 222 A B C D E 223 A B C D E 224 A B C D E

225 A B C D E 226 A B C D E 227 A B C D E 228 A B C D E 229 A B C D E 230 A B C D E 231 A B C D E 232 A B C D E

233 A B C D E 234 A B C D E 235 A B C D E 236 A B C D E 237 A B C D E 238 A B C D E 239 A B C D E 240 A B C D E

241 A B C D E 242 A B C D E 243 A B C D E 244 A B C D E 245 A B C D E 246 A B C D E 247 A B C D E 248 A B C D E

249 A B C D E 250 A B C D E 251 A B C D E 252 A B C D E 253 A B C D E 254 A B C D E 255 A B C D E 256 A B C D E

257 A B C D E 258 A B C D E 259 A B C D E 260 A B C D E 261 A B C D E 262 A B C D E 263 A B C D E 264 A B C D E

265 A B C D E 266 A B C D E 267 A B C D E 268 A B C D E 269 A B C D E 270 A B C D E 271 A B C D E 272 A B C D E

273 A B C D E 274 A B C D E 275 A B C D E 276 A B C D E 277 A B C D E 278 A B C D E 279 A B C D E 280 A B C D E

281 A B C D E 282 A B C D E 283 A B C D E 284 A B C D E 285 A B C D E 286 A B C D E 287 A B C D E 288 A B C D E

289 A B C D E 290 A B C D E 291 A B C D E 292 A B C D E 293 A B C D E 294 A B C D E 295 A B C D E 296 A B C D E

297 A B C D E 298 A B C D E 299 A B C D E 300 A B C D E 301 A B C D E 302 A B C D E 303 A B C D E 304 A B C D E

305 A B C D E 306 A B C D E 307 A B C D E 308 A B C D E 309 A B C D E 310 A B C D E 311 A B C D E 312 A B C D E

313 A B C D E 314 A B C D E 315 A B C D E 316 A B C D E 317 A B C D E 318 A B C D E 319 A B C D E 320 A B C D E